Critical Care Skills

Critical Care Skills

Editors

Kemba D. DeGroot, R.N., B.A., C.C.R.N.

Marilyn B. Damato, R.N., B.S.N., C.N.R.N.

The Methodist Hospital
Texas Medical Center
Houston, Texas

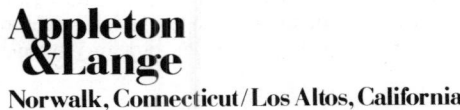

Appleton &Lange

Norwalk, Connecticut / Los Altos, California

87 88 89 90 91 / 10 9 8 7 6 5 4 3 2 1

Prentice-Hall of Australia, Pty. Ltd., Sydney
Prentice-Hall Canada, Inc.
Prentice-Hall Hispanoamericana, S.A., Mexico
Prentice-Hall of India Private Limited, New Delhi
Prentice-Hall International (UK) Limited, London
Prentice-Hall of Japan, Inc., Tokyo
Prentice-Hall of Southeast Asia (Pte.) Ltd., Singapore
Whitehall Books Ltd., Wellington, New Zealand
Editora Prentice-Hall do Brasil Ltda., Rio de Janeiro

Library of Congress Cataloging-in-Publication Data

Critical care skills.

   Includes bibliographies and index.
   1. Intensive care nursing. I. DeGroot, Kemba Dianne.
II. Damato, Marilyn B. III. Methodist Hospital
(Houston, Tex.) [DNLM: 1. Critical Care—methods—
nurses' instruction. WY 154 C9345]
RT120.I5C78   1986   610.73'61   86-10934
ISBN 0-8385-1240-2

Design: M. Chandler Martylewski

PRINTED IN THE UNITED STATES OF AMERICA

To our peers and our colleagues,
to our patients and their families . . .
for all they have shared,
for all we have learned.

Contributors

THE METHODIST HOSPITAL, TEXAS MEDICAL CENTER, HOUSTON, TEXAS

Adrianne Ward Cosby, R.N., M.S.N.
Assistant Manager, Nursing Service

Marilyn B. Damato, R.N., B.S.N., C.N.R.N.
Neurosurgical Nurse Specialist; Clinical Practitioner-Teacher, Level II, Department of Central Education

Kemba D. DeGroot, R.N., B.A., C.C.R.N.
Cardiovascular Nurse Specialist; Head Nurse Manager, Alkek 7, Surgical Nursing Service

Carol W. La Croix, R.N., B.S.N.
Head Nurse Manager, General Clinical Research Center, Medical Nursing Service

Imelda Clare Otte, R.N.
Emergency Ambulatory Nurse Practitioner, Surgical Nursing Service

Ann Lorene Quinn, R.N., B.S.N.
Neurosurgical Nurse Specialist; Head Nurse Manager, Neurosurgical Intensive Care and Intermediate Care, Surgical Nursing Service

Dian Gayle Teinert, R.N., M.S.
Coordinator, Department of Central Education

Theresa Ann Zimmerman, R.N., B.S., C.C.R.N.
Cardiovascular Nurse Specialist; Clinical Practitioner-Teacher, Level II, Department of Central Education

Contents

Foreword

*The critical care nurse shall be competent and current in critical care nursing.**

Competent critical care nursing practice requires that the nurse master both an expansive knowledge base and an extensive repertoire of clinical skills. The attainment and maintenance of competency poses a formidable challenge to the critical care nurse because of the continual and rapid evolution of this area of nursing practice. Without timely and thorough updating, the knowledge soon becomes obsolete and incomplete, and clinical skills become outdated. Without purposeful integration of this knowledge base into a nursing practice perspective, much of its relevance for the daily provision of critical care nursing is lost.

A number of texts are available to assist the nurse in acquiring the cognitive basis for critical care nursing. Few resources exist for the equally important consideration of clinical skills. This book addresses those skills the nurse needs to gain proficiency in bedside critical care nursing practice.

Nurse educators who prepare new critical care staff recognize that a major concern for orientees is acquiring competency in clinical and technical skills. Following orientation, critical care inservice and continuing education programs focus heavily on the maintenance and augmentation of these assessment and procedural skills. In order for critical care patients to receive safe and optimal nursing care, the nurses who provide this care must be able to daily and/or periodically demonstrate that they can apply their knowledge and skills in an effective manner.

Critical Care Skills is a carefully selected compendium of the clinical skills requisite for critical care nursing practice. The editors devote attention to the assessment techniques and procedures most relevant for the bedside nurse. Rather than merely presenting a fragmented litany of technical procedures, DeGroot and Damato incorporate nursing diagnosis as a pivotal thread in the fabric of critical care nursing. Their coverage includes an admixture of physical and clinical assessment skills, technical skills, and related information useful for planning, implementing, and evaluating nursing care of the critically ill patient. Their work represents a welcome addition to the critical care nursing literature.

JoAnn Grif Alspach, R.N., M.S.N., C.C.R.N.
Consultant, Critical Care Nursing Education
Editor, *Critical Care Nurse* Journal

---

*American Association of Critical-Care Nurses. *Standards for nursing care of the critically ill* (Standard VIII). Reston, VA: Reston Publishing, 1981, p. 41.

Preface

Caring for critically ill patients in a highly technical setting demands the application of multi-level nursing skills:

- Skill as a clinical practitioner, operating in a sophisticated technical environment
- Skill as an independent diagnostician, using scientific information to identify and treat the patient's response to illness
- Skill as an interdependent health care team member, practicing within the context of team relationships

Because of recent legislative changes, acutely ill patients move quickly through the ICU setting. Skills once practiced only during the intensive care phase of hospitalization must now be mastered with increasing frequency by practitioners in non-ICU settings. Developing these skills to ever higher levels in any setting is an on-going challenge; one that must be continually anticipated and utilized for the benefit of the patient, the health care institution, and the nursing profession.

Critical Care Skills is intended to help the clinician practice cognitive processes and clinical skills which promote independent nursing interventions. It is designed as a bedside tool, with a format that encourages immediate use in critical care nursing situations.

Chapters 1 through 7 focus on assessment skills and technical procedures related to a specific body system. The assessment sections examine the data bases obtained from the patient's biopsychosocial history, physical examinations, and laboratory results. By studying the listed parameters, findings, and possible etiologies, the practitioner can quickly generate an index of suspicion or list of possible nursing diagnoses. In the technical procedures section of each chapter, a specific nursing diagnosis* serves as the focus. Detailed nursing interventions, criteria for outcome, and documentation guidelines are outlines for each procedure. Chapter 8, *Psychosocial Factors,* details common conditions caused by the psychological and spiritual impact of illness. The information in every chapter is supplemented by photographs, tables, drawings, graphs, a glossary, and a bibliography. In addition, Chapter 8 contains an Appendix on religious attitudes and requirements which may influence patient behavior.

In this book, we have attempted to provide a practical, up-to-date reference for learners, practitioners, and educators, as well as those involved with formulation of policies and procedures. We welcome the opportunity to present a body of knowledge that has come from critical care research and look forward to expanding and applying this knowledge toward a constant professional goal: patient wellness.

Kemba D. DeGroot, R.N.

Marilyn B. Damato, R.N.

---

*Nursing diagnoses are taken from Kim, M. J., McFarland, G. K., & McLane, A. M. (Eds.). *Pocket guide to nursing diagnoses*. St. Louis: Mosby, 1984, with permission.

Acknowledgments

No project of this complexity would ever reach fruition without the support and assistance of many individuals, "up front" and "behind the scenes." We, as editors, are indebted to each and every one of you.

First and foremost, we wish to thank the Administration of The Methodist Hospital. Without their initial support for our efforts, this project could never have begun. To Peggy Woods and to LaDonna Doud, for their availability, guidance, and encouragement throughout the project, we are especially grateful.

The willingness of the contributing authors to share their knowledge and skills as well as their time and energies only served to reinforce our pride in our profession. All their efforts are most gratefully acknowledged.

Several nursing experts were selected by the publisher to review the manuscript. We wish to thank them all for their direction. The reviews of Joann Grif Alspach and Martha A. O. Curley, in particular, challenged each of us as clinicians and as writers.

We particularly want to thank Bob DeGroot, M.Ed., Licensed Professional Counselor, and Associate School Psychologist. He generously gave his time and expertise during multiple consultations regarding content for Chapter 8, Psychosocial Factors. His support for the project has been unwavering.

A special acknowledgment goes to JoAnn McBride and her staff in the Word Processing Service of The Methodist Hospital. Without their expert assistance, we would still be penciling in corrections and additions.

The staff of the Department of Medical Photography and Television at The Methodist Hospital enabled us to provide the photographs for each chapter. The on-site photographs were taken by Peter Traylor, Medical Photographer. Shirley Hudson and Gloria Flucas assisted with processing and scheduling.

The long hours of posing under hot lights by our models Bob DeGroot and Kevin Dominque deserve special thanks. One picture *is* worth a thousand words.

To Rick Weimer, for his support and belief in this project, we are truly indebted.

To Nancy Greenberg, Production Editor, Appleton & Lange, for her endless patience, attention to detail, and gentle guidance, we would like to express our sincere gratitude.

Kemba D. DeGroot, R.N.
Marilyn B. Damato, R.N.

Critical Care Skills

1

CARDIOVASCULAR SYSTEM

Theresa Ann Zimmerman

Assessment of the Pertinent Cardiovascular History

RATIONALE

Assimilation of the pertinent information obtained from the cardiovascular history alerts the critical care nurse to the potential development of related disorders. This data collection is also essential for the development of an individualized, comprehensive nursing care plan.

PARAMETERS	FINDINGS	IMPLICATIONS FOR NURSING CARE
1. Family history	1. Diabetes mellitus Marfan's syndrome Cardiovascular disease, such as hypertension, cerebrovascular accident, myocardial infarction	1. Predisposes patient to development of diabetes with potential for cardiovascular disease Transmitted as a hereditary, autosomal dominant trait Poses a predisposition to the development of cardiovascular disease in the patient.
2. Past health history	2. Hypertension Myocardial infarction Recent weight gain Diabetes mellitus Rheumatic fever Heart murmur Cardiovascular surgical procedures Infective endocarditis Permanent pacemaker Marfan's syndrome	2. Predisposes the patient to the development of cardiovascular disease or cerebrovascular accident Predisposes the patient to congestive heart failure or myocardial infarction May be an indication of congestive heart failure and associated fluid retention Predisposes the patient to the development of cardiovascular disease Predisposes the patient to the development of cardiac valve dysfunction Indication of cardiac dysfunction, such as valve dysfunction, ventricular or atrial septal defect May indicate disease progression Predisposition to emboli and cardiac valve dysfunction Potential for decreased cardiac output or pacemaker malfunction Potential for development of aortic dissection
3. Patient profile	3. Smoking Low-sodium diet Current medications	3. Predisposes patient to cardiovascular disease Noncompliance may predispose patient to or cause exacerbation of congestive heart failure or hypertension Knowledge of current medications will alert nurse to possible drug incompatibilities or toxicities as well as to specific disease entities requiring pharmacological control
4. Present problem	4. Chest pain Edema Dysrhythmias Claudication Dyspnea, orthopnea, paroxysmal nocturnal dyspnea, dyspnea on exertion Peripheral cyanosis	4. May indicate myocardial ischemia, impending myocardial infarction, pericarditis, or valve dysfunction Should alert nurse to possible presence of congestive heart failure or decreased cardiac output May indicate decrease in coronary artery perfusion, electrolyte abnormalities, or drug toxicity; also may predispose patient to decrease in cardiac output Indication of partial arterial occlusion Indicates fluid retention or congestive heart failure May indicate decreased cardiac output
5. Review of systems	5. A. Cardiovascular system	5. A. Activity intolerance, potential Cardiac output, alteration in: decreased Fluid volume, alteration in: excess

		Skin integrity, impairment of: potential
		Tissue perfusion, alteration in: cardiopulmonary
	B. Pulmonary system	**B.** Breathing pattern, ineffective
		Gas exchange, impaired
	C. Renal system	**C.** Fluid volume, alteration in: excess

Assessment of the Cardiovascular System by Inspection and Palpation

RATIONALE

Inspection and palpation of the cardiovascular system are performed as part of a cardiovascular assessment in order to alert the nurse to the possibility of any underlying abnormal conditions of the heart and circulation.

PARAMETERS	FINDINGS	POSSIBLE ETIOLOGIES	DOCUMENTATION
Inspection 1. Precordium 2. Neck veins 3. Epigastric area **Palpation (Fig. 1–3)**	For inspection of the precordium, the patient should be supine, with the head of the bed elevated approximately 30 degrees. Stand at the patient's right side and use tangential lighting (light rays coming from the side of the patient). This will enhance the visibility of precordial movements. The apical impulse is the only pulsation that should normally be visible over the precordium. 1. **A.** Left ventricular heave or lift characterized by an increase in the size and amplitude of the impulse **B.** Sustained apical impulse **C.** Rapid, diffuse, forceful apical impulse **D.** Right ventricular heave or lift **E.** Paradoxical movement of left anterior chest 2. Distended jugular veins (Figs. 1–1 and 1–2). External jugular veins in the neck are normally visible and frequently distended when the patient is lying flat. When the head of the bed is raised 30 degrees, the veins should collapse. Persistent venous distention with the head of the bed elevated 45 to 90 degrees is an indication of increased volume in the venous system which may be caused by fluid retention or obstruction in the superior vena cava 3. Forceful pulsations Palpation of the precordium should be performed with the the patient supine and the trunk elevated approximately 30 degrees.	1. **A.** Left ventricular hypertrophy **B.** Aortic stenosis **C.** Aortic insufficiency **D.** Right ventricular hypertrophy **E.** Left ventricular aneurysm 2. Right heart failure Tricuspid insufficiency or stenosis Hypervolemia Cardiac tamponade Superior vena cava obstruction Pulmonary hypertension Congestive heart failure 3. Abdominal aortic aneurysm	• Location and characteristics of impulses • Time the impulses occur in relation to the cardiac cycle • Phase of cardiac cycle during which thrills occur • Degree of neck vein distention • Rate of arterial pulses • Quality and characteristics of arterial pulses • Bilateral equality of arterial pulses

1. Apical impulse (point of maximal impulse)	1. **A.** Forceful, lateral displacement **B.** Sustained **C.** Diffuse (greater than 3 cm area) **D.** Systolic thrill (palpable vibration associated with turbulent flow) **E.** Diastolic thrill	1. **A.** Aortic insufficiency Left ventricular hypertrophy **B.** Aortic stenosis Left ventricular hypertrophy **C.** Left ventricular hypertrophy **D.** Mitral insufficiency **E.** Mitral stenosis
2. Right ventricular area	2. **A.** Heave or lift **B.** Diastolic thrill **C.** Systolic thrill	2. **A.** Right ventricular hypertrophy May also be present in hyperdynamic states such as hyperthyroidism or fever **B.** Tricuspid stenosis Mitral stenosis **C.** Severe tricuspid regurgitation Ventricular septal defect
3. Aortic area	3. **A.** Accentuated impulse **B.** Systolic thrill	3. **A.** Systemic hypertension **B.** Aortic stenosis
4. Pulmonic area	4. **A.** Accentuated impulse **B.** Forceful and sustained impulse **C.** Systolic thrill	4. **A.** Pulmonary hypertension **B.** Mitral stenosis **C.** Pulmonic stenosis
5. Epigastric area	5. Strong impulse	5. Abdominal aortic aneurysm Right ventricular hypertrophy
6. Bilateral peripheral arterial pulses: Carotid, brachial, radial, femoral, popliteal, dorsalis pedis, posterior tibial (Figs. 1–4 to 1–10) Extreme caution must be taken when palpating the carotid artery because of the risk of baroreceptor stimulation, which can cause severe bradycardia. *Do not palpate both carotid arteries simultaneously.*	6. **A.** Pulsus magnus (bounding pulse) **B.** Pulsus parvus (weak pulse) **C.** Bigeminal pulse (pulse beats occur in pairs) **D.** Peripheral pulse deficit (number of pulse beats counted at a peripheral artery is less than those counted in the same period of time at the apex of the heart) **E.** Pulsus paradoxus (decrease in pulse amplitude greater than 10 mm Hg during normal inspiration) **F.** Pulsus bisferiens (two impulses palpated during systole) **G.** Pulsus alternans (every other beat weaker than preceding beat)	6. **A.** Hypertension Aortic insufficiency Patent ductus arteriosus Anemia Anxiety Hyperthyroidism Arteriosclerosis **B.** Left ventricular failure Severe aortic stenosis **C.** Bigeminal premature ectopic beats **D.** Premature extrasystoles Atrial fibrillation **E.** Cardiac tamponade Positive pressure ventilation **F.** Aortic insufficiency Idiopathic hypertrophic subaortic stenosis **G.** Left ventricular failure

POSSIBLE NURSING DIAGNOSES

- Cardiac output, alteration in: decreased
- Tissue perfusion, alteration in: cardiopulmonary

SPECIAL NOTE

Grading

The strength of arterial pulses may be rated using the following scale:

0	Absent
1+	Thready, weak, easily obliterated with pressure
2+	May be difficult to palpate but stronger than 1+
3+	Normal
4+	Bounding

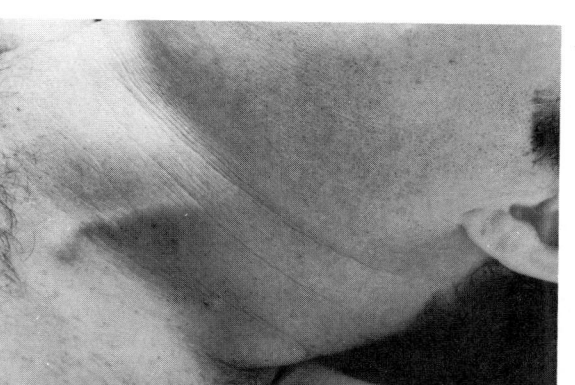

Figure 1–1. Noninvasive CVP measurement.

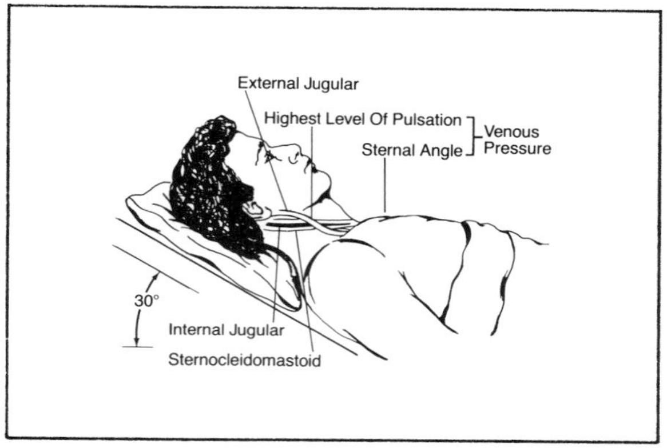

Figure 1–2. Noninvasive CVP monitoring. Central venous pressure may be estimated noninvasively by: (1) Adjusting the height of the head of the bed until the internal jugular vein can be detected; (2) Identifying the highest point of internal jugular pulsations; and (3) Measuring the vertical distance between the highest point of pulsation and the sternal angle.

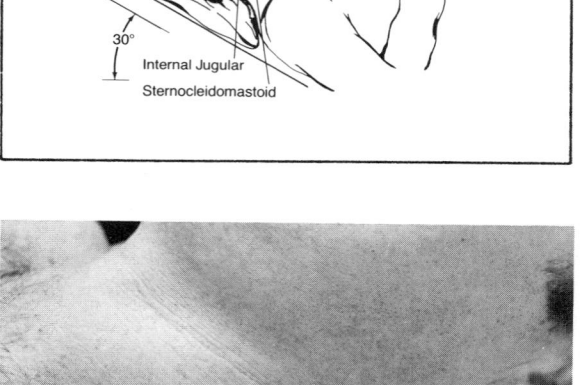

Figure 1–3. Palpation areas. Normal location of cardiac impulses: apical area—point of maximal impulse (fifth intercostal space, midclavicular line), right ventricular area (lower left sternal border, third to fifth intercostal space), aortic area (second intercostal space to right of sternum), and pulmonic area (second intercostal space to left of sternum).

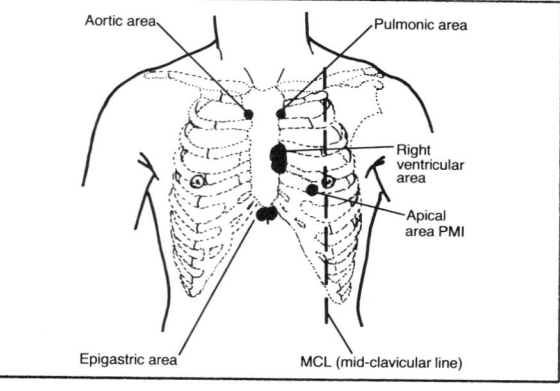

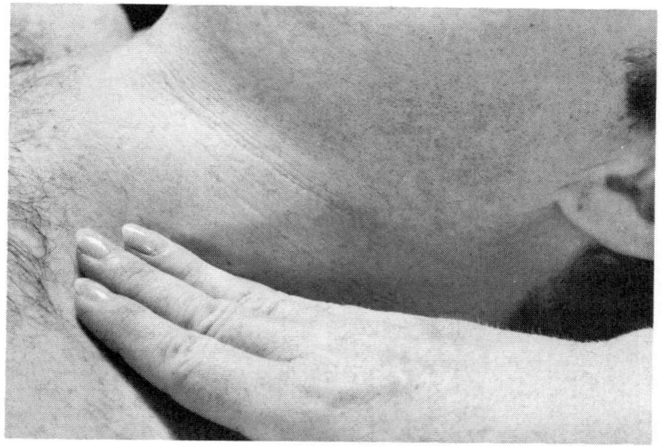

Figure 1–4. Palpating carotid pulse.

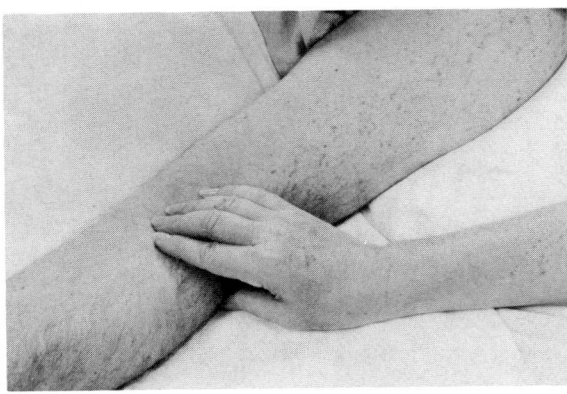

Figure 1–5. Palpating brachial pulse.

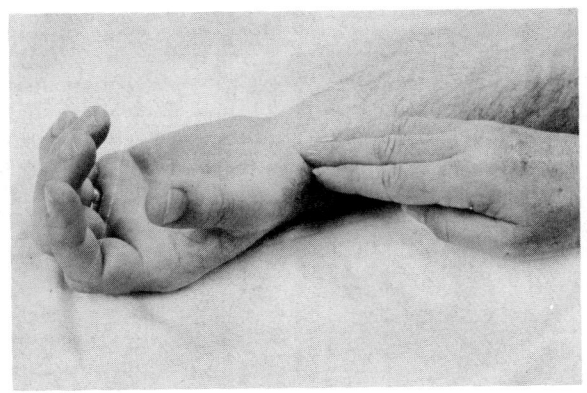

Figure 1–6. Palpating radial pulse.

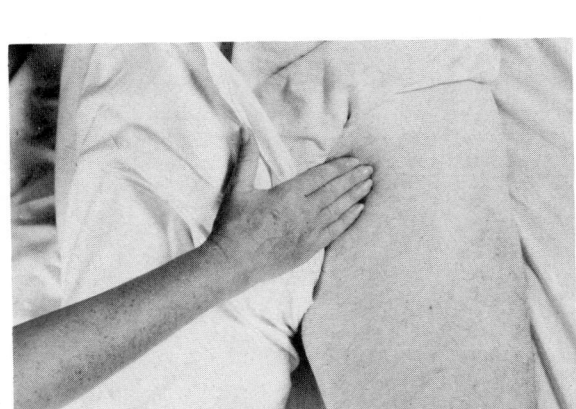

Figure 1–7. Palpating femoral pulse.

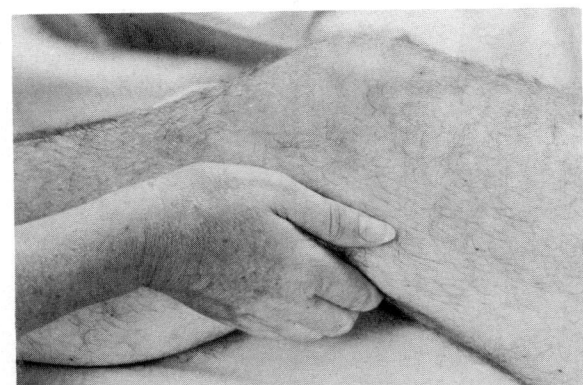

Figure 1–8. Palpating popliteal pulse.

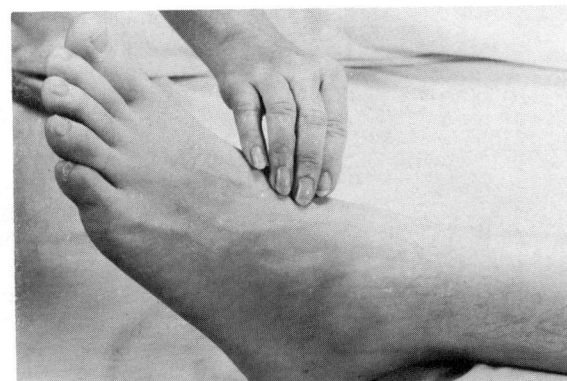

Figure 1–9. Palpating dorsalis pedis pulse.

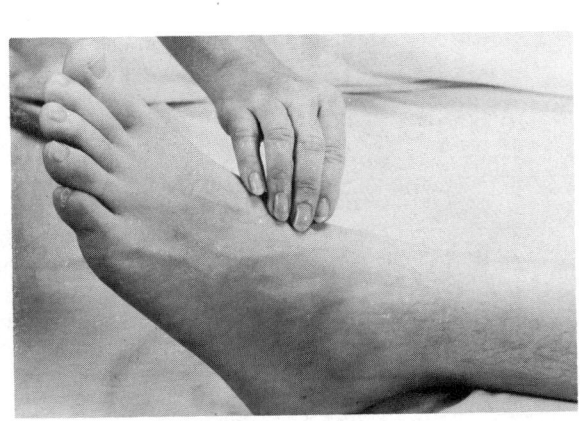

Figure 1–10. Palpating posterior tibial pulse.

Assessment of Cardiac Auscultatory Findings

RATIONALE

Cardiac auscultation is an invaluable skill for the critical care nurse to develop. Early changes in the heart sounds, which may indicate a change in the patient's condition or a need for therapeutic intervention, can be detected by the skilled practitioner.

PARAMETERS	FINDINGS	POSSIBLE ETIOLOGIES	DOCUMENTATION
1. Valve closure sounds (Figs. 1–11 to 1–15)	1. **A.** First heart sound (S_1). S_1 is heard best with the diaphragm of the stethoscope, at the apex of the heart **B.** Second heart sound (S_2). S_2 is heard best with the diaphragm of the stethoscope, at the base of the heart (Fig. 1–16) **a.** Split S_2 (physiologic) **b.** Fixed splitting **c.** Wide splitting **d.** Paradoxical splitting	1. **A.** S_1 is a normal heart sound caused by closure of the mitral and tricuspid valves; it occurs with carotid pulse or immediately following the QRS of the ECG tracing. **B.** S_2 is a normal heart sound caused by closure of the aortic and pulmonary valves. **a.** Two components of S_2: aortic (A_2) and pulmonic (P_2). Both of these components are sometimes heard because the aortic valve normally closes first and there is a slight delay in pulmonary valve closure, especially during inspiration when venous return to the right ventricle is augmented. This is normal physiological splitting **b.** Fixed splitting refers to the auscultation of both components of S_2 during both inspiration and expiration; it is usually associated with an atrial septal defect, which will slow pulmonary valve closure because of volume overload in the right ventricle **c.** Wide splitting is caused by a delay in pulmonary valve closure often related to right bundle branch block, pulmonary stenosis, right ventricular failure, and pulmonary hypertension **d.** Paradoxical splitting results when the pulmonary valve closes at the correct time but aortic valve closure is delayed due to impedance to left ventricular emptying, as seen with aortic stenosis, left bundle branch block, left ventricular failure, and systemic hypertension. Because A_2 is the louder of the two components of S_2, the second component heard	• Pitch of sound, i.e., high or low pitch • Intensity • Location where sound is best heard • Radiation of sound • Timing, i.e., systolic or diastolic • Duration, e.g., holosystolic (heard throughout systole) • Quality, e.g., blowing, musical • Effect of respiratory cycle on sound

2. Ventricular filling sounds (gallops)	**2. A.** Third heart sound (S_3). If an S_3 is present, it will be heard just after S_2. The rhythm it creates may sound like the word "Kentucky" (Fig. 1–17). An S_3 is a soft, low-pitched sound best heard using the bell of the stethoscope, at the apex of the heart **B.** Fourth heart sound (S_4). If an S_4 is present, it will be heard before S_1. The rhythm it creates may sound like the word "Tennessee" (Fig. 1–18). An S_4 is a low-pitched sound best heard using the bell of the stethoscope, at the apex of the heart. An S_4 originating from the right ventricle will usually be louder on inspiration. One originating from the left ventricle is usually louder on exhalation **C.** Summation gallop	in the paradoxically split S_2 will be the loudest **2. A.** S_3, or ventricular gallop, may occur when there is decreased ventricular compliance resulting in abrupt cessation to ventricular filling. Its presence is the hallmark of heart failure. **B.** S_4, or atrial gallop, is related to atrial contraction against a high ventricular pressure. Caused by atrial contraction, it is never present in the patient with atrial fibrillation or atrial flutter. An S_4 is often heard in acute myocardial infarction, congestive heart failure, aortic stenosis, hypertension, and hyperdynamic states. **C.** Summation gallop results when both an S_3 and an S_4 are present with a tachycardia. The two sounds merge together as one loud sound usually heard in middiastole. It is frequently present in advanced heart failure
3. Murmurs	**3. A.** Systolic murmur **B.** Diastolic murmur Murmurs are sometimes graded using the following intensity scale: Grade I — Very faint murmur Grade II — Faint murmur but easily audible Grade III — Moderate intensity Grade IV — Loud murmur associated with a thrill Grade V — Loud murmur, may be heard with stethoscope just slightly off chest Grade VI — Can be heard without stethoscope Because there are varying grading scales used in assessing murmur intensity, the	**3. A.** Systolic murmurs (heard between S_1 and S_2) **a.** Aortic stenosis **b.** Pulmonary stenosis **c.** Mitral insufficiency **d.** Tricuspid insufficiency **e.** Ventricular septal defect **B.** Diastolic murmurs (heard between S_2 and the next S_1) **a.** Mitral stenosis **b.** Tricuspid stenosis **c.** Aortic insufficiency **d.** Pulmonary insufficiency

(continued)

PARAMETERS	FINDINGS	POSSIBLE ETIOLOGIES	DOCUMENTATION
4. Extracardiac sounds	scale used should be recorded, e.g., when using the above scale, a grade II murmur would be documented as "II/VI" 4. Pericardial friction rub	4. A pericardial friction rub has a grating, scratchy, high-pitched sound resulting from inflammation of the pericardial sac. It is often heard during ventricular systole in the patient with pericarditis, acute myocardial infarction, and in the postoperative cardiac surgery patient	

POSSIBLE NURSING DIAGNOSES

- Activity intolerance, potential
- Cardiac output, alteration in: decreased
- Fluid volume, alteration in: excess
- Tissue perfusion, alteration in: cardiopulmonary

SPECIAL NOTE

Characteristics

The following are some of the characteristics of heart murmurs:

Condition	Location	Timing*	Quality*	Pitch
Aortic stenosis	Second right intercostal space (ICS)	Midsystole	Harsh, crescendo–decrescendo	Medium
Aortic insufficiency	Second right ICS—lower left sternal border	Holosystolic	Blowing, decrescendo	High
Mitral stenosis	Apex	Middiastolic or presystolic	Rumbling	Low
Mitral insufficiency	Apex	Holosystolic	Blowing	High
Pulmonary stenosis	Second left ICS	Midsystole	Harsh, crescendo–decrescendo	Medium to high
Pulmonary insufficiency	Second left ICS	Early diastole	Blowing, decrescendo	High
Tricuspid stenosis	Fourth ICS—left sternal border	Middiastole	Rumbling, decrescendo	Low
Tricuspid insufficiency	Lower left sternal border	Holosystolic	Harsh	High
Ventricular septal defect	Lower left sternal border	Holosystolic	Harsh	High

*See Figure 1–19 for an illustration of timing and quality.

Figure 1–11. Auscultation areas. Sounds are projected in the direction of flow, therefore the following areas are auscultated for the various valvular components of heart sounds: aortic (second intercostal space to the right of the sternum), pulmonic (second intercostal space to the left of the sternum), tricuspid (fourth to fifth intercostal space, left lower sternal border), and mitral (fifth intercostal space, midclavicular line, to the left of the sternum). *(Adapted from Neel, C. J., & Wallerstein, M. B. A pocket guide for medical-surgical nursing. Bowie, Md.: Brady, 1985, p. 123, with permission.)*

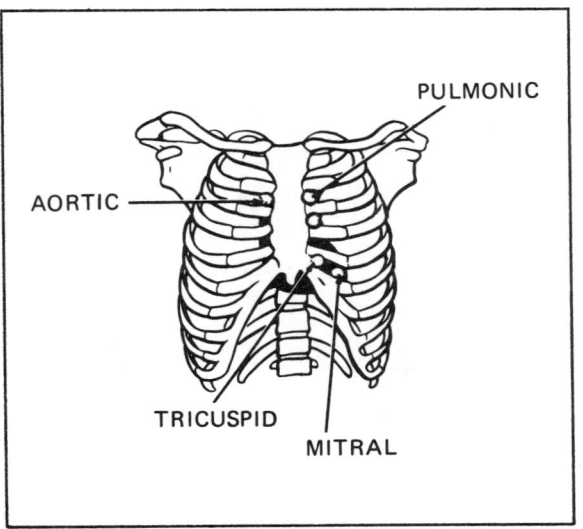

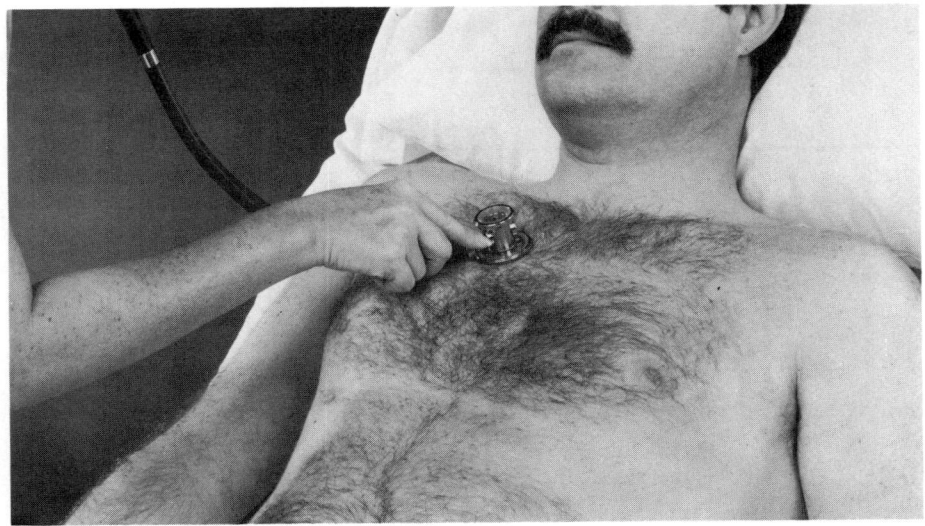

Figure 1–12. Auscultating aortic area.

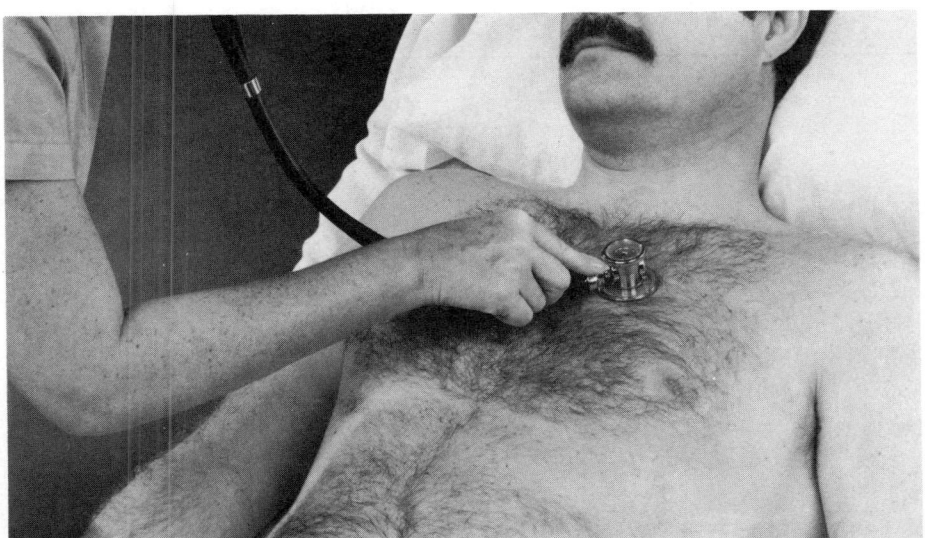

Figure 1–13. Auscultating pulmonic area.

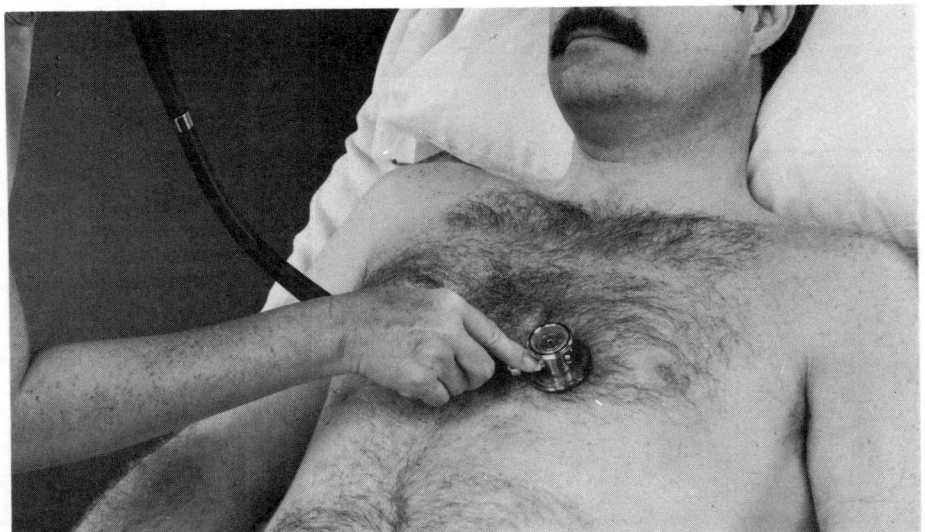

Figure 1–14. Auscultating tricuspid area.

(continued)

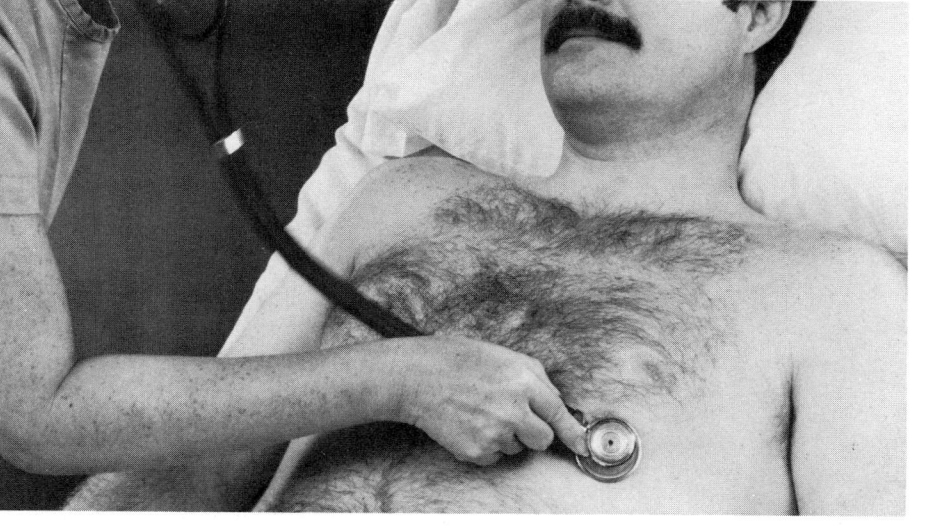

Figure 1–15. Auscultating mitral area.

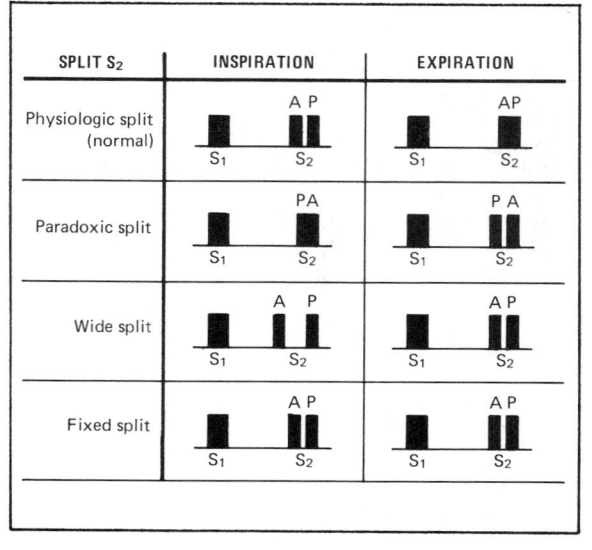

Figure 1–16. Split S_2.

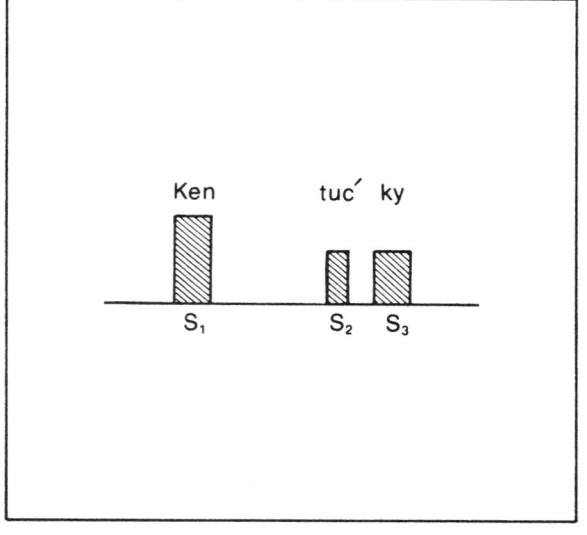

Figure 1–17. S_3. *(From Borg, N., Nikas, D. L., Stark, J., & Williams, S. M. (Eds.). Core curriculum for critical care nursing (2nd ed.). Philadelphia: Saunders, 1981, p. 101, with permission.)*

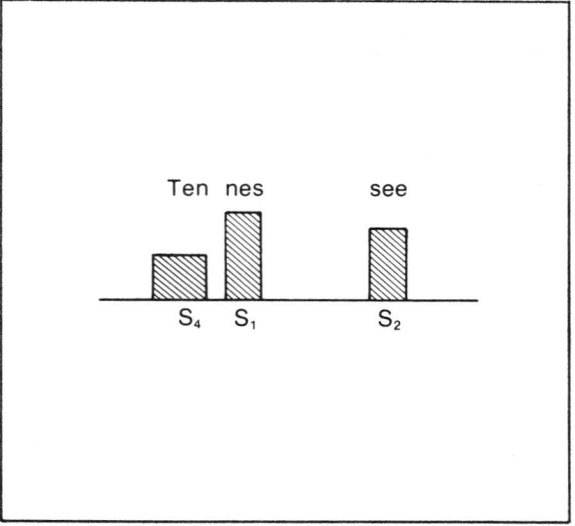

Figure 1–18. S_4. *(From Borg, N., Nikas, D. L., Stark, J., & Williams, S. M. (Eds.). Core curriculum for critical care nursing (2nd ed.). Philadelphia: Saunders, 1981, p. 102, with permission.)*

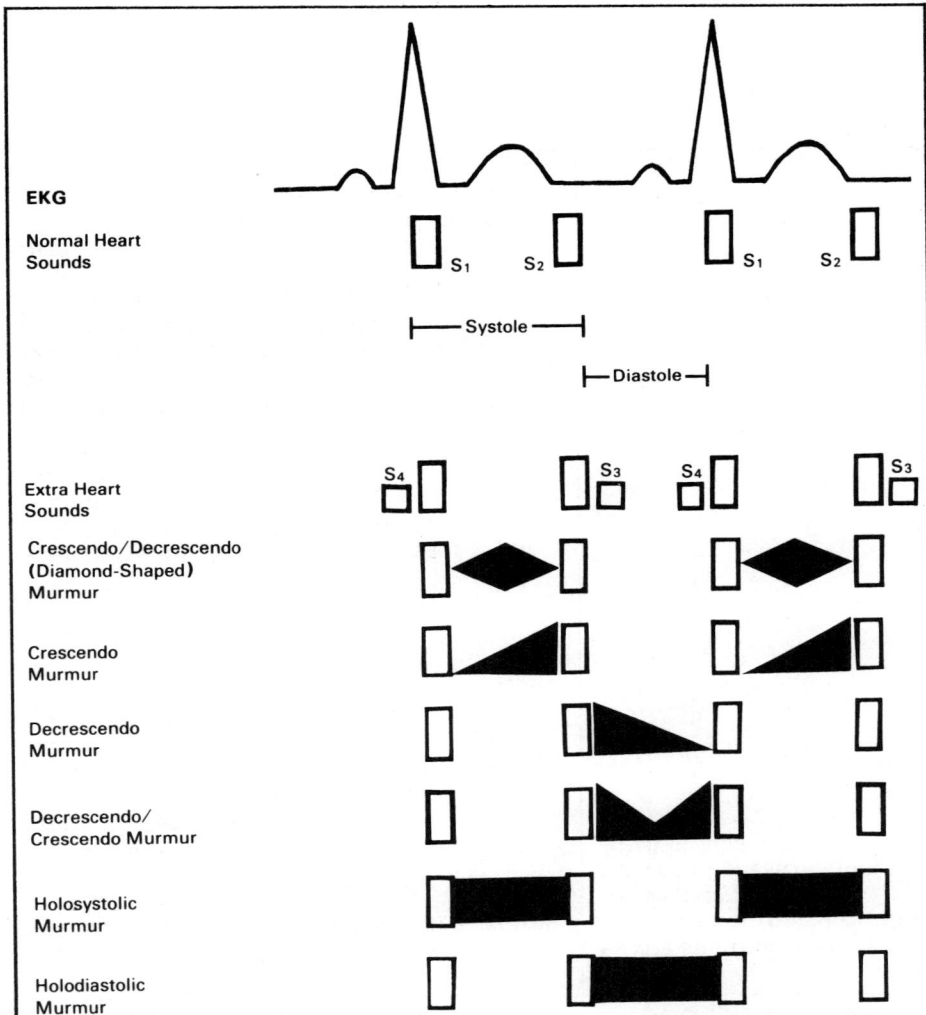

Figure 1–19. Timing and quality of heart sounds. Crescendo murmurs start out soft and become progressively louder. Decrescendo murmurs start out loud and become progressively softer. Crescendo/decrescendo murmurs start out soft, progressively increase in loudness, and then become softer again. Decrescendo/crescendo murmurs start out loud, progressively decrease in loudness, and then become loud again. Holosystolic murmurs are heard throughout systole. Holodiastolic murmurs are heard throughout diastole. *(Adapted from Partridge, S. A. Cardiac auscultation.* Dimensions of critical care nursing, *1982, 1(3), 158, with permission.)*

Assessment of Serum Enzymes

RATIONALE

Cardiac enzymes are those enzymes that are found in greater quantity in the cardiac tissue when compared to other body tissues. Because enzymes are released from damaged tissues, an elevated level is a useful tool in the diagnosis of various disease states. No one enzyme is specific for one disease state due to the overlap of these enzymes in various cells of the body. This section is limited to cardiac etiologies of enzyme abnormalities.

PARAMETERS	FINDINGS	POSSIBLE ETIOLOGIES	DOCUMENTATION
1. Creatine kinase (CK)	1. CK elevated above normal: Male, 5–55 mU/ml; female, 5–35 mU/ml	1. Acute myocardial infarction: Increase seen in 3–6 hours, peaks in first 24 hours, and returns to normal in 3–4 days Myocarditis Postcardioversion Prolonged tachycardia	• Date and time blood sample was drawn and results of laboratory test • Name of physician notified of laboratory results
2. Creatine kinase-MB (myocardial band): An isoenzyme of CK located only in heart muscle and therefore considered the most reliable enzyme to be evaluated in the diagnosis of myocardial infarction	2. CK-MB detected (normal CK-MB 0%)	2. Acute myocardial infarction: Detected in 4–6 hours, peaks in 12–18 hours, and returns to normal in 2–5 days Following cardiac surgery	
3. Serum glutamic oxalo-acetic transaminase (SGOT)	3. SGOT elevated above normal, 8–33 U/ml	3. Acute myocardial infarction: Increase seen in 6–12 hours, peaks in 24–48 hours, and returns to normal in 4–7 days Myocarditis Postcardioversion Pericarditis Dissecting aortic aneurysm	
4. Lactic dehydrogenase (LDH)	4. LDH elevated above normal, 75–200 IU/L	4. Acute myocardial infarction: Increase seen in 12–24 hours, peaks in 48–72 hours, and returns to normal within 8–14 days Bacterial pericarditis Following cardiac surgery Hemolysis from prosthetic heart valves	
5. Hydroxybutyric dehydrogenase (HBD)	5. HBD elevated above normal, 135–275 IU/L	5. Acute myocardial infarction: Increase seen within 12 hours, peaks in 48–72 hours, and returns to normal within 11–16 days	

POSSIBLE NURSING DIAGNOSES

• Cardiac output, alteration in: decreased
• Tissue perfusion, alteration in: cardiopulmonary

Interpretation

The normal laboratory values stated may vary depending on the laboratory methods used. They are also sometimes reported in quantitative values other than those listed. Before attempting to interpret a laboratory result, ascertain the normal values used by the particular laboratory in which the test was performed

CK-MB

CK-MB may be present in the serum following an infarction even in the absence of an elevated CK. Because CK-MB may be released during cardiac surgery, its elevation cannot be used as an indication of a myocardial infarction during the immediate postoperative period

Assessment of Arterial Waveforms

RATIONALE

The effects of heart rate and rhythm on cardiac output can often be ascertained by observation of the arterial pulse waveform. More importantly, careful examination can provide valuable information regarding the patient's hemodynamic and physiological status. The knowledgeable critical care nurse, familiar with waveforms characteristic of selected abnormal conditions, can integrate these findings with other assessment parameters.

PARAMETERS	FINDINGS	POSSIBLE ETIOLOGIES	DOCUMENTATION
1. Normal tracing (Fig. 1–20)	1. Rapid upstroke; dicrotic notch, signifying closure of the aortic valve and the onset of diastole, is present; smooth, round contour; pulse pressure (difference between systolic and diastolic pressure) between 30 and 40 mm Hg	1. Normal	• Characteristics of the arterial waveform including any alteration noted during the respiratory cycle • Systolic and diastolic pulse and their comparison to the blood pressure taken by cuff. Normally the systolic pressure obtained via an arterial catheter is 5–20 mm Hg higher than that obtained via an indirect method
2. Dampened tracing (Fig. 1–21)	2. Flattened, rounded appearance, slow upstroke, narrow pulse pressure, and difficult to discern dicrotic notch	2. Clot on tip of catheter or catheter tip against the arterial wall	
3. Pulsus alternans (Fig. 1–22)	3. Pulse waveform pattern is regular, but the size and intensity of the pulses vary	3. Left ventricular failure	
4. Bigeminal pulse (Fig. 1–23)	4. Pulse waveform pattern is irregular. Every other pulse is premature and smaller in size than the normal pulse due to shorter diastolic filling time	4. Ventricular bigeminy	
5. Pulsus paradoxus (Fig. 1–24)	5. Diminished amplitude of pulse waveform during spontaneous inspiration greater than normal diminution of less than 10 mm Hg	5. Cardiac tamponade Severe lung disease Patient on positive pressure mechanical ventilator	
6. Pulsus bisferiens (Fig. 1–25)	6. Double systolic impulse	6. Combined aortic stenosis and insufficiency Aortic insufficiency alone Idiopathic hypertrophic subaortic stenosis	

POSSIBLE NURSING DIAGNOSES

• Cardiac output, alteration in: decreased
• Fluid volume, deficit: actual

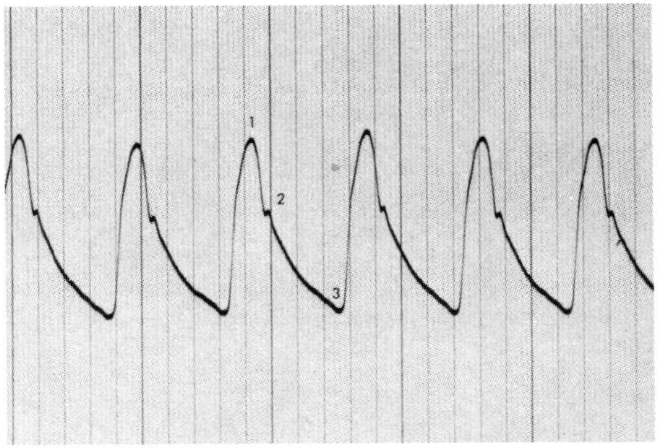

Figure 1–20. Normal waveform: peak systole (1), dicrotic notch (2), and end diastole (3). *Daily, E. K., & Schroeder, J. S. Hemodynamic waveforms: Exercises in identification and analysis. St. Louis, Mo.: Mosby, 1983, p. 100, with permission.)*

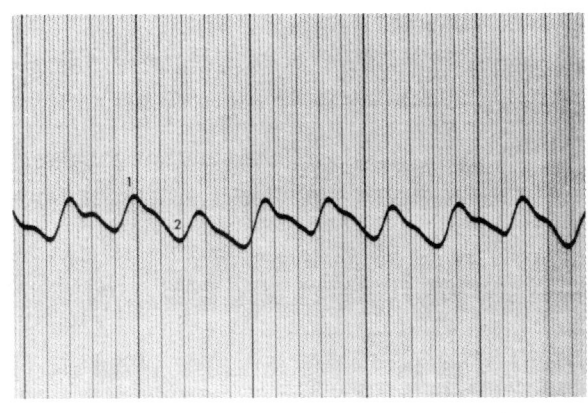

Figure 1–21. Dampened waveform. *(From Daily, E. K., & Schroeder, J. S. Hemodynamic waveforms: Exercises in identification and analysis. St. Louis, Mo.: Mosby, 1983, p. 107, with permission.)*

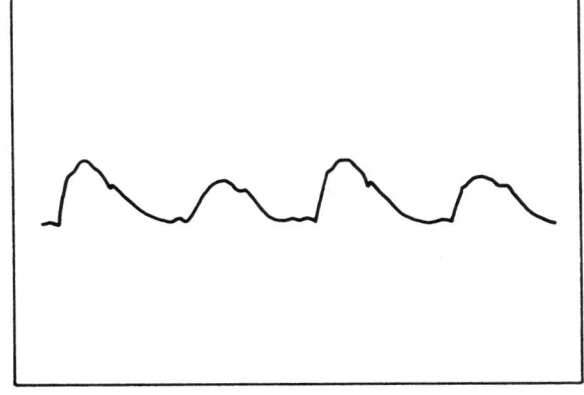

Figure 1–22. Pulsus alternans. *(From Andreoli, K. G., Fowkes, V. K., Zipes, D. P., & Wallace, A. G. (Eds.). Comprehensive cardiac care (5th ed.). St. Louis, Mo.: Mosby, 1983, p. 42, with permission.)*

Figure 1–23. Bigeminal pulse. *(From Andreoli, K. G., Fowkes, V. K., Zipes, D. P., & Wallace A. G. (Eds.). Comprehensive cardiac care (5th ed.). St. Louis, Mo.: Mosby, 1983, p. 42, with permission.)*

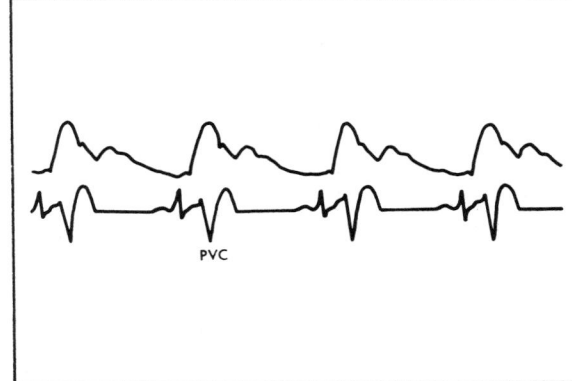

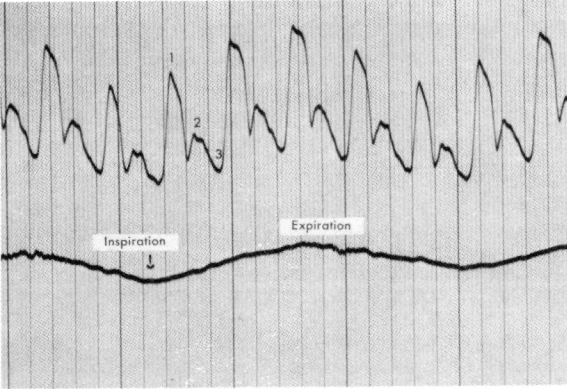

Figure 1–24. Pulsus paradoxus. *(From Daily, E. K., & Schroeder, J. S. Hemodynamic waveforms: Exercises in identification and analysis. St. Louis, Mo.: Mosby, 1983, p. 113, with permission.)*

Figure 1–25. Pulsus bisferiens. *(From Fowler, N. O. Examination of the heart. Part two: Inspection and palpation of venous and arterial pulses. Dallas, Tex.: American Heart Association, 1972, p. 27, with permission of the American Heart Association, Inc.)*

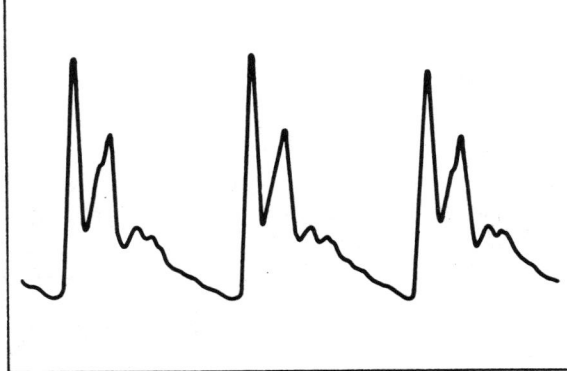

Assessment of Cardiac Function with the Pulmonary Artery Catheter

RATIONALE

Pulmonary artery catheters are inserted to assess the hemodynamic status of critically ill patients. The measurements obtained provide valuable information regarding left ventricular function as well as the response of the patient to fluid therapy or medications (Figs. 1–26 and 1–27).

Left ventricular end diastolic pressure (LVEDP) provides the most accurate estimate of the left ventricular function. It is an indication of the myocardial fiber stretch during diastole. In the absence of pulmonary vascular obstruction, the LVEDP can be obtained with the pulmonary artery catheter.

When the mitral valve is open at the end of diastole, the pressure among the left atrium, left ventricle, pulmonary veins, pulmonary capillaries, and pulmonary artery equilibrates. The pulmonary artery diastolic and pulmonary capillary wedge pressure measurements obtained are therefore equal to LVEDP and left atrial pressure.

PARAMETERS	FINDINGS	POSSIBLE ETIOLOGIES	DOCUMENTATION
1. Right atrial pressure (Figs. 1–28 and 1–29)	1. A. Right atrial (RA) pressure elevated above normal of 2–6 mm Hg B. Right atrial pressure below normal range	1. A. Cardiac tamponade Right ventricular failure Pulmonary embolism Pulmonary hypertension Hypervolemia Atrial septal defect Tricuspid stenosis or insufficiency B. Hypovolemia Peripheral vasodilatation	• RA pressure as catheter is being inserted and on subsequent measurements obtained from proximal port of catheter • RV pressure as catheter is being inserted • PAP and PCWP obtained during catheter insertion and on subsequent measurements • Amount of air needed to wedge catheter balloon • Cardiac output and cardiac index calculations, if obtained • Results of mixed venous oxygen saturation measurements, if obtained • Systemic vascular resistance, if obtained
2. Right ventricular pressure (Figs. 1–30 and 1–31)	2. A. Right ventricular (RV) pressure elevated above normal systolic range of 20–30 mm Hg and diastolic range of 0–5 mm Hg B. Right ventricular pressure below normal range	2. A. Ventricular septal defect Right ventricular failure Pulmonary embolism Pulmonary hypertension Pulmonary valvular stenosis Constrictive pericarditis Atrial septal defect B. Hypovolemia Peripheral vasodilatation	
3. Pulmonary artery pressure (Figs. 1–32 and 1–33)	3. Pulmonary artery pressure (PAP) elevated above normal systolic range of 20–30 mm Hg and diastolic range of 8–10 mm Hg	3. Chronic obstructive pulmonary disease Pulmonary edema Pulmonary embolism Hypervolemia Pulmonary hypertension Mitral stenosis Left ventricular failure Atrial septal defect Ventricular septal defect	

		Adult respiratory distress syndrome Pneumothorax Positive pressure mechanical ventilation Positive end expiratory pressure (PEEP) Continuous positive airway pressure (CPAP)
4. Pulmonary capillary wedge pressure (Figs. 1–34 and 1–35)	**4. A.** Pulmonary capillary wedge pressure (PCWP) elevated above normal systolic range of 5–12 mm Hg **B.** Pulmonary capillary wedge pressure below normal range	**4. A.** Hypervolemia Pulmonary edema Left ventricular dysfunction Mitral stenosis or insufficiency Elevated systemic vascular resistance **B.** Hypovolemia
5. Cardiac output/cardiac index (calculated by dividing the cardiac output by the patient's body surface area, which can be obtained from height–weight tables)	**5. A.** Cardiac output elevated above normal range of 4–8 L/min; cardiac index elevated above normal range of 2.5–4.0 L/min/m² **B.** Cardiac output below normal range; cardiac index below normal range	**5. A.** Anemia Sympathetic stimulation of myocardium Fever Arteriovenous fistula Hyperthyroidism Hypoxia (causes vasodilatation and decrease in systemic vascular resistance) **B.** Myocardial infarction Left ventricular aneurysm Cardiac tamponade Elevated systemic vascular resistance Hypovolemia Left ventricular failure
6. Mixed venous oxygen saturation	**6. A.** Mixed venous oxygen saturation elevated above normal of 75% **B.** Mixed venous oxygen saturation below 65%	**6. A.** Increased oxygen delivery, e.g., increased FIo_2 Decreased oxygen demand, e.g., hypothermia **B.** Decreased oxygen delivery, e.g., anemia, hypoxemia, decreased cardiac output, carbon monoxide poisoning Increased oxygen demand, e.g., hyperthermia
7. Systemic vascular resistance: $$\frac{\text{Mean arterial pressure} - \text{CVP}}{\text{Cardiac output}} \times 80$$	**7. A.** Systemic vascular resistance elevated above normal range of 900–1600 dynes/sec/cm^{-5} **B.** Systemic vascular resistance below normal range	**7. A.** Vasoconstriction **B.** Vasodilatation

POSSIBLE NURSING DIAGNOSES

- Cardiac output, alteration in: decreased
- Fluid volume, alteration in: excess
- Fluid volume, deficit, actual
- Gas exchange, impaired
- Tissue perfusion, alteration in: cardiopulmonary

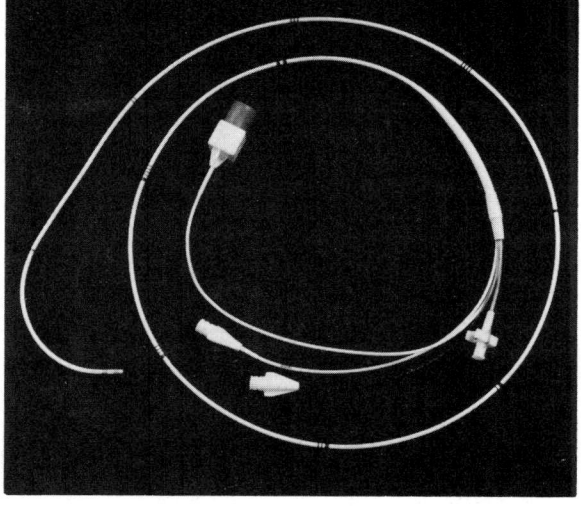

Figure 1–26. Pulmonary artery catheter.

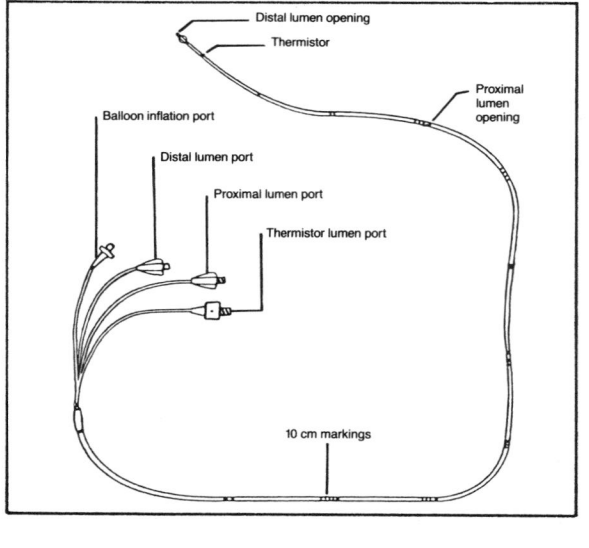

Figure 1–27. PA catheter. When the pulmonary artery catheter is properly positioned, the opening of the proximal port is located in the right atrium allowing for central venous pressure readings to be obtained. It is the distal port which is attached to a transducer system allowing for monitor display of the pulmonary artery wedge pressures. Mixed venous blood samples may be obtained from the distal port. *(From Bustin, D.* Hemodynamic monitoring for critical care. *Norwalk, Conn.: Appleton-Century-Crofts, 1986, p. 12, with permission.)*

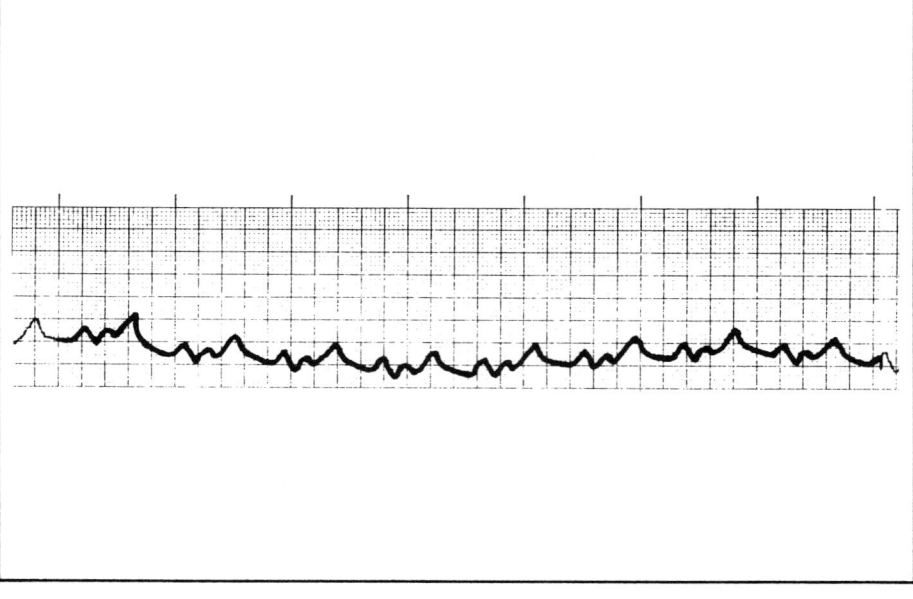

Figure 1–28. PA catheter waveform, right atrium.

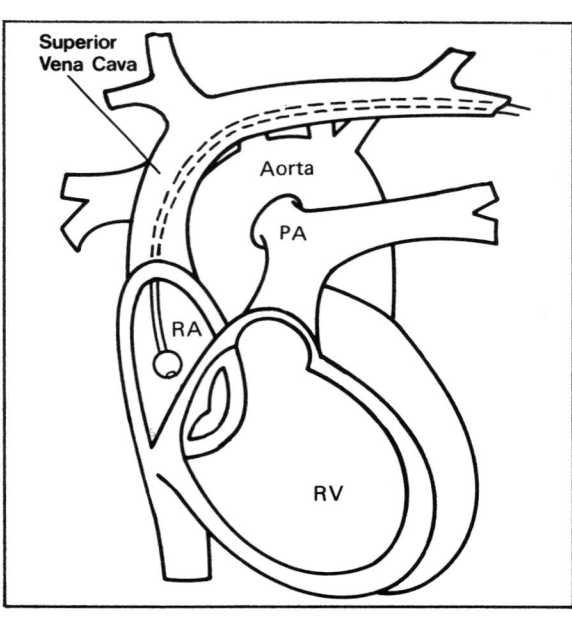

Figure 1–29. PA catheter placement, right atrium.

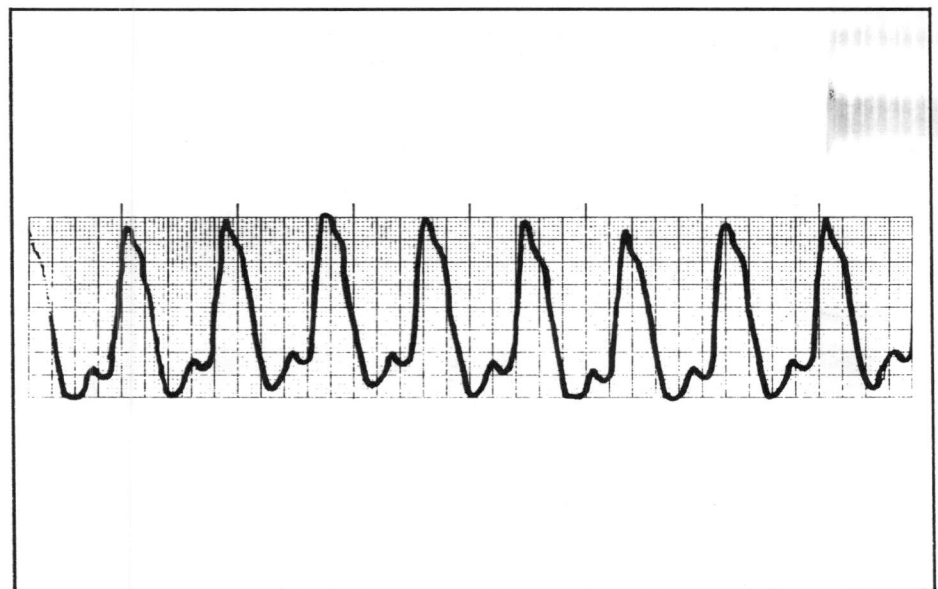

Figure 1–30. PA catheter waveform, right ventricle.

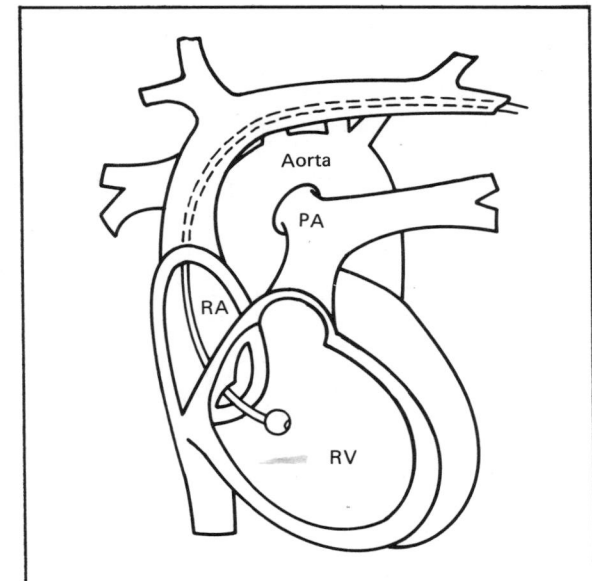

Figure 1–31. PA catheter placement, right ventricle.

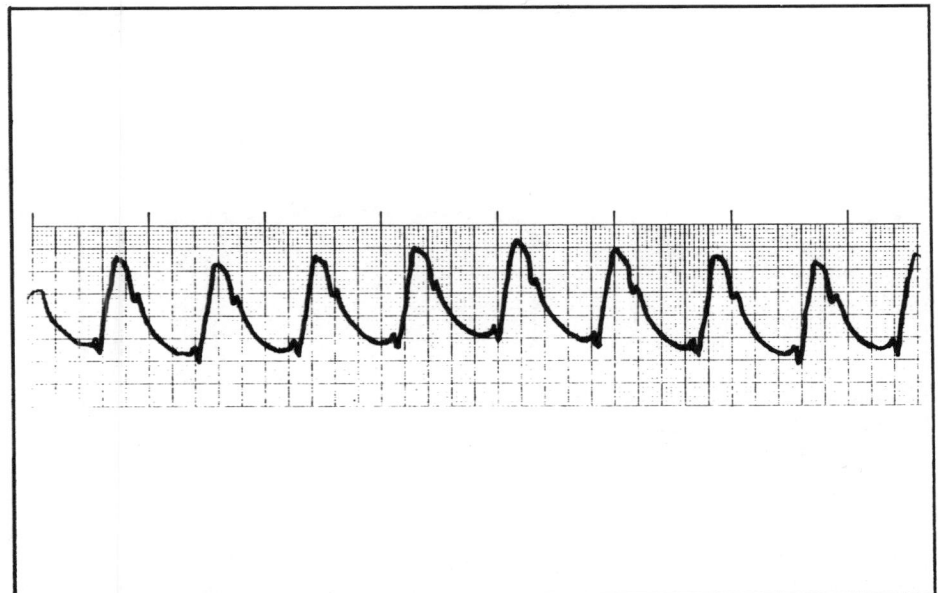

Figure 1–32. PA catheter waveform, pulmonary artery.

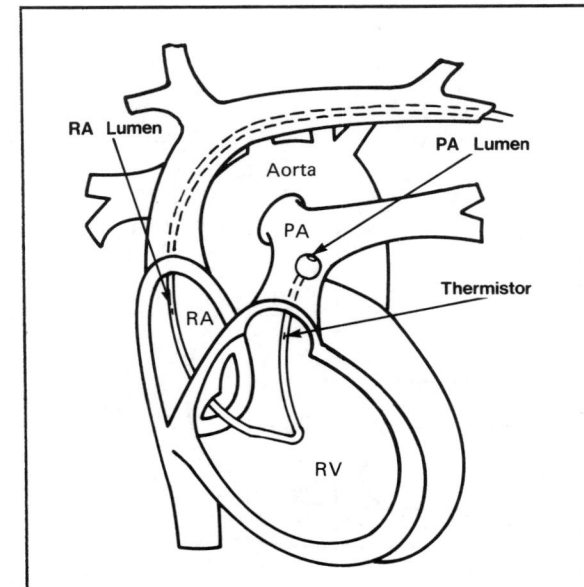

Figure 1–33. PA catheter placement, pulmonary artery.

(continued)

CARDIOVASCULAR SYSTEM: ASSESSMENT OF CARDIAC FUNCTION WITH THE PULMONARY ARTERY CATHETER **21**

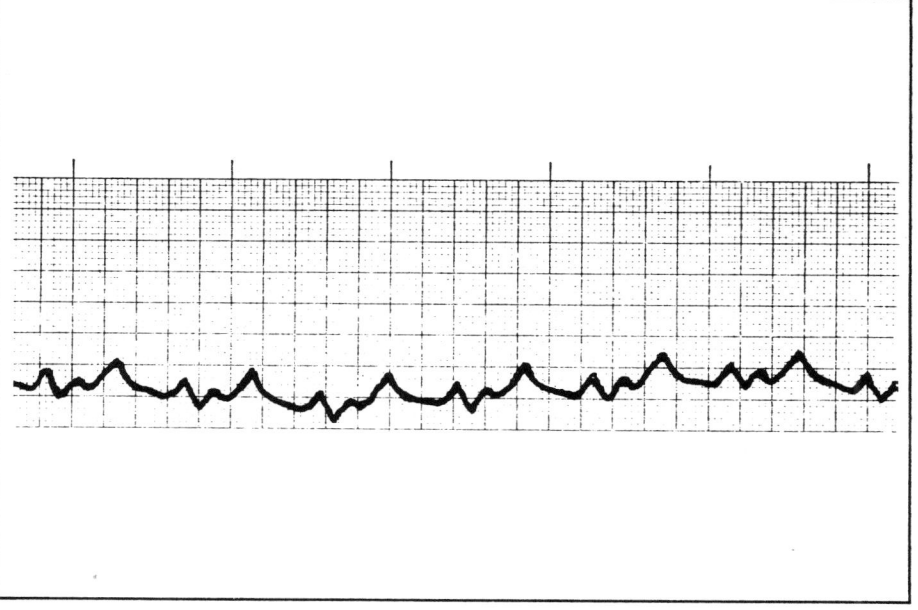

Figure 1–34. PA catheter waveform, pulmonary capillary wedge.

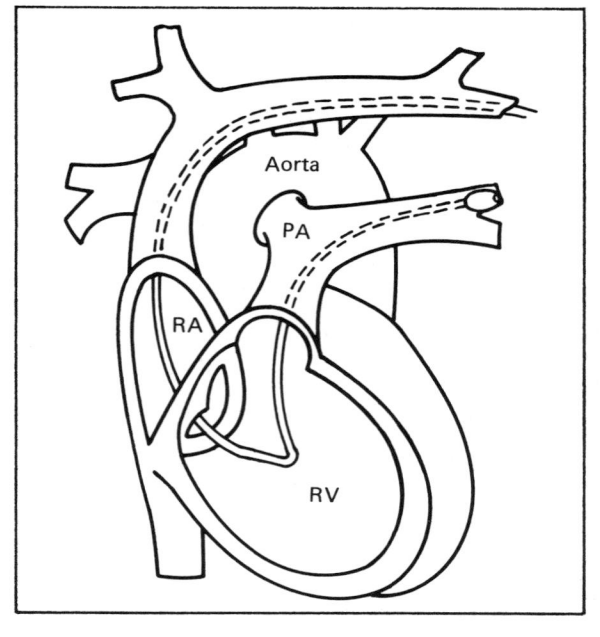

Figure 1–35. PA catheter placement, pulmonary capillary wedge.

Care of the Patient with an Intra-arterial Catheter

NURSING DIAGNOSIS	RATIONALE	DEFINING CHARACTERISTICS	EXPECTED OUTCOME

Injury, potential for	Intra-arterial catheters are frequently inserted in the critical care patient to provide direct, continuous blood pressure monitoring. Techniques employed in equipment assembly, catheter insertion, and frequent manipulations involved in catheter use may result in multiple complications for the patient. Because of the risk involved, the nurse must assess the patient astutely for signs and symptoms indicative of developing complications. Meticulous technique regarding care of the catheter and related equipment is imperative.
	1. Hemorrhage
	
	2. Air embolism
	
	3. Thrombosis
	
	4. Hematoma
	
	5. Infection
	
	6. Arterial spasm
		Potential sources of injury to the patient with an intra-arterial catheter and their defining characteristics include:
		
		1. Bleeding from disconnected tubing
		   Insertion site dressing saturated with blood
		2. Elevation of heart rate
		   Decrease in blood pressure
		   Elevated central venous pressure (CVP)
		   Elevated pulmonary artery pressure (PAP)
		   Decrease in systemic vascular resistance
		   Dampened waveform
		3. Dampened waveform
		   Weak or absent pulses below insertion site
		   Decreased warmth and sensation distal to insertion site
		   Pain distal to insertion site
		   Pallor or cyanosis distal to insertion site
		4. Ecchymosis at insertion site
		   Swelling at insertion site
		5. Elevated temperature
		   Elevation of heart rate
		   Purulent drainage at insertion site
		   Redness, edema, and warmth at insertion site
		6. Intermittent decrease in pulse below insertion site
		   Intermittent pallor or cyanosis below insertion site
		   Pain around and distal to insertion site
			No injury will result from use of an indwelling intra-arterial catheter

NURSING INTERVENTIONS

Preinsertion

Perform Allen's test prior to insertion of radial arterial catheter (Figs. 1–36, 1–37, and 1–38).

During Insertion

1. Verify security of all tubing connections at time of insertion, then at beginning of each shift and following any manipulation
2. Maintain aseptic technique during catheter insertion

After Insertion

1. Set monitor alarm limit at 20 mm Hg greater than patient's systolic pressure and 10 mm Hg less than patient diastolic pressure
2. Keep insertion site exposed, if possible
3. Check pressure tubing for air bubbles at beginning of shift and following tubing change
4. Assess pulses, color, sensation, and temperature distal to insertion site q2–4h
5. Assess for swelling or ecchymosis at insertion site q2–4h
6. Check patient's temperature, pulse, blood pressure, and respiratory rate at least q1–2h
7. Change insertion site dressing q24h and assess site for any drainage or signs of inflammation
8. Question patient to ascertain any sensation of pain distal to insertion site
9. Apply direct pressure over insertion site for 5–10 minutes following removal of catheter from brachial, radial, axillary, and dorsalis pedis arteries. Apply pressure for 10–15 minutes following removal of femoral arterial catheter

OUTCOME CRITERIA

1. There will be no bleeding from insertion site
2. Vital signs, CVP, and PAP will remain within patient's normal limits
3. Strong pulses and normal color, temperature, and sensation distal to insertion site
4. There will be no swelling or ecchymosis around insertion site while catheter is in place
5. Insertion site will be free of purulent drainage, and there will be no signs of inflammation
6. Patient will have no complaints of pain around or distal to insertion site

DOCUMENTATION

- Time, size of catheter, insertion site, and by whom the catheter was inserted
- Patient's blood pressure by cuff and alarm limits set on monitor every shift
- Presence or absence of bleeding from insertion site at the beginning of shift and with any change
- Pulse quality, color, temperature, and sensation distal to insertion site q2–4h
- Presence or absence of swelling or ecchymosis at insertion site q2–4h
- Patient's temperature, pulse, blood pressure, and respiratory rate at least q1–2h
- Time of dressing change and presence or absence of inflammation or purulent drainage noted at insertion site
- Any complaints of pain distal to insertion site
- Name of physician removing catheter and the length of time pressure was applied
- Presence or absence of swelling or ecchymosis immediately following catheter removal, 1 hour postremoval, and q2h for 24 hours

(continued)

SPECIAL NOTE

Placement

Intra-arterial catheters for pressure monitoring may be inserted via the radial, brachial, femoral, axillary, and dorsalis pedis arteries. If a catheter is inserted via the radial or brachial arteries, it is important that the extremity be supported on an armboard splint to prevent catheter dislodgement through inadvertent flexion.

Femoral Insertion

Femoral lines are frequently inserted during an emergency because the femoral artery is often the easiest to palpate during periods of decreased blood pressure. One disadvantage to femoral arterial catheterization, however, is the potential for massive occult bleeding from a damaged artery. A second disadvantage is related to the large diameter of the artery, frequently causing difficulty in attaining hemostasis following catheter removal.

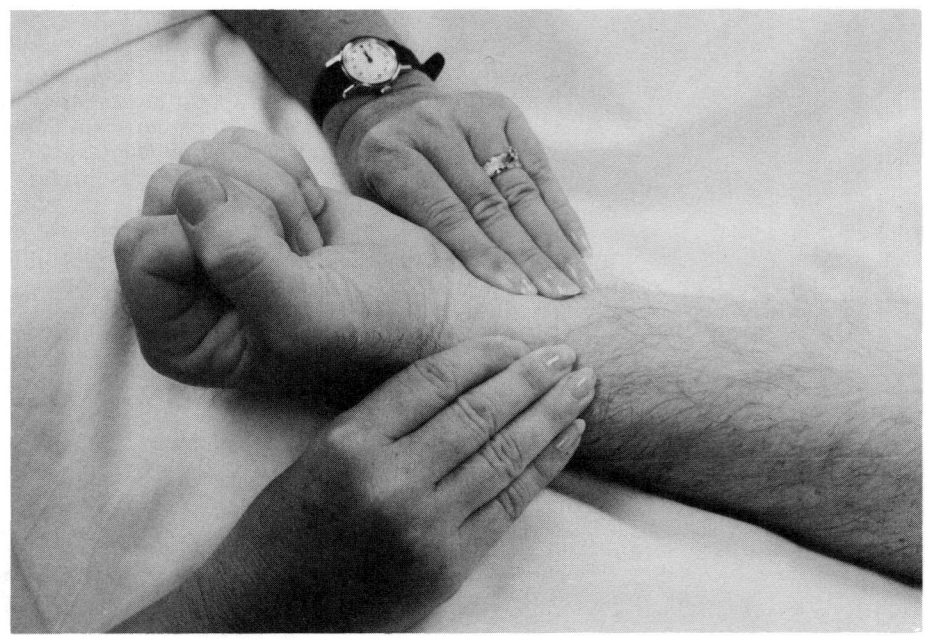

Figure 1–36. Allen test should always be performed prior to the insertion of a radial arterial line in order to assess blood flow to the hand via the ulnar artery. To perform the Allen test (step 1): Compress the patient's ulnar and radial arteries simultaneously for approximately one minute while the patient is clenching and unclenching his fist.

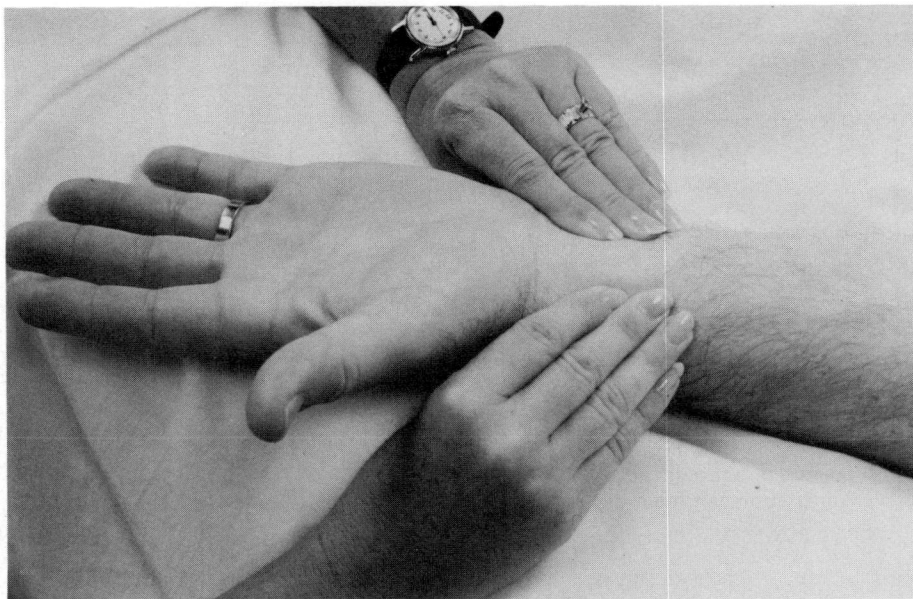

Figure 1–37. Allen's test (step 2): Have the patient unclench his hand; release the pressure on the ulnar artery.

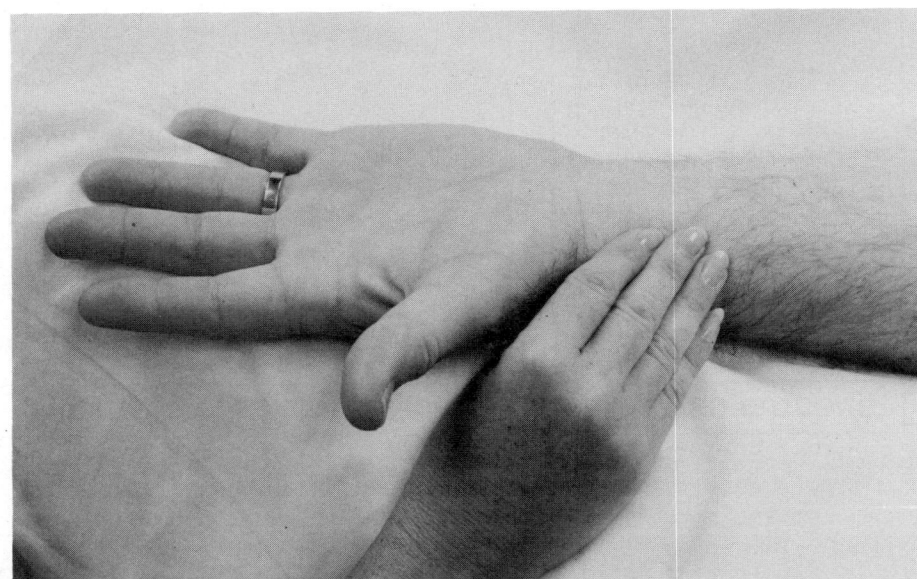

Figure 1–38. Allen's test (step 3): If the palm turns pink in 5 seconds or less, ulnar arterial blood flow to the hand is considered adequate.

Care of the Patient with a Pulmonary Artery Catheter

NURSING DIAGNOSES	RATIONALE	DEFINING CHARACTERISTICS	EXPECTED OUTCOME
1. Cardiac output, alteration in: decreased	1. Cardiac output may be decreased by many factors including myocardial infarction, left ventricular aneurysm, dysrhythmias, hypovolemia, cardiac tamponade, and increased systemic vascular resistance	1. Decrease in systolic blood pressure below patient's normal level Decrease in urine output Cool, clammy skin Pallor, possible cyanosis Mental confusion	1. Cardiac output is maintained within optimal range
2. Gas exchange, impaired	2. Gas exchange may be impaired by alveolar hypoventilation, inadequate FIo_2, and ventilation–perfusion abnormalities	2. Abnormal arterial blood gas results Dyspnea, shortness of breath Altered mental status	2. Gas exchange is maintained at an optimal level
3. Fluid volume, alteration in: excess	3. Fluid volume excess may occur from the administration of excessive fluid to the patient or an inadequate cardiac output	3. Edema Rales Jugular vein distention Dyspnea, tachypnea Increase in blood pressure above patient's normal range	3. Fluid volume excess is reduced
4. Fluid volume, deficit, actual	4. Fluid volume may be deficient because of inadequate fluid intake or excessive fluid loss	4. Poor skin turgor Decrease in urine output Weak, rapid pulse Decrease in blood pressure below patient's normal range	4. Fluid volume status is maintained within optimal range
5. Injury, potential for	5. Injury to the patient may occur from pulmonary artery infarction, pulmonary embolism, pulmonary artery perforation, pneumothorax (following insertion via subclavian vein), or infection. Dysrhythmias may result from irritation of the right ventricular wall during insertion or from migration of the distal tip back into the right ventricle	5. Hemoptysis Tachycardia Tachypnea Substernal pain Pallor Hypotension Dyspnea Absent or diminished breath sounds on one side Decreased chest expansion on one side Premature ventricular complexes or ventricular tachycardia Elevated temperature Inflammation or purulent drainage at insertion site	5. No complications related to pulmonary artery catheter will occur

NURSING INTERVENTIONS

Preinsertion

1. Obtain baseline heart rate, blood pressure, temperature, and respiratory rate
2. Explain procedure to patient
3. Assemble monitoring equipment using aseptic technique and ascertain the absence of air bubbles in the pressure tubing
4. Attach transducer system to cardiac monitor
5. Flush proximal and distal ports of catheter immediately before insertion
6. Inflate balloon and check for patency (Fig. 1–39)

During Insertion

1. Assist physician with catheter insertion, maintaining aseptic technique
2. Monitor pressure waveforms as catheter is being inserted
3. Closely monitor ECG for the development of dysrhythmias as catheter is passing through the right ventricle

After Insertion

1. Obtain order for chest x-ray to assess catheter position and verify absence of pneumothorax
2. Apply sterile dressing to insertion site and change dressing q24h using aseptic technique
3. Assess bilateral breath sounds and chest expansion for the development of pneumothorax immediately following insertion and q2h
4. Check vital signs at least q1–2h
5. Maintain patency of proximal port by continuous infusion of ordered intravenous solution
6. Maintain patency of distal port by continuous infusion of heparinized flush solution
7. Obtain pulmonary capillary wedge pressure (PCWP) and CVP q1–2h or more frequently if ordered
8. Before measuring the pulmonary artery and pulmonary capillary wedge pressures, ensure that the equipment is properly calibrated and that the transducer is level with the patient's right atrium. It is not necessary to lay the patient flat for pressure readings; however, the patient should be in the same position for each reading, if possible. All readings are taken at the end of patient exhalation
9. After obtaining the pulmonary artery pressure, slowly inject air (amount not to exceed balloon capacity as indicated on catheter, usually 1.5 cc) into the balloon port while simultaneously observing the monitor for a wedge tracing. Stop injecting air as soon as this tracing is displayed. After obtaining the wedge pressure, allow the balloon to deflate passively by removing the syringe; avoid manual deflation by aspiration, which may cause a tear in the balloon (Fig. 1–40). A pulmonary artery pressure tracing should then be observed on the monitor
10. Continuously monitor pressure tracing for signs of dampening waveform (Fig. 1–41)
11. Monitor patient continuously for the development of hemoptysis (which may indicate pulmonary artery perforation) or chest pain (which may indicate pulmonary artery infarction, pulmonary embolism, or pneumothorax) following catheter insertion
12. If the monitor displays a right ventricular pressure tracing after catheter insertion, it is an indication that the catheter tip has moved back into the right ventricle. Inflation of the balloon for a few seconds may cause the tip to float back into the pulmonary artery. If the tip remains in the RV after this attempt, the catheter must be removed by the physician because of the risk of ventricular irritability
13. If the monitor displays a PCW tracing when the balloon is not inflated, it indicates distal migration of the catheter tip into a narrow branch of the pulmonary artery. While the tip is in this position there is an impedance to blood flow to that area, which can cause pulmonary infarction. Notify the physician immediately to withdraw the catheter tip back to the main pulmonary artery
14. The cardiac output can be measured via the thermodilution technique in the patient with a pulmonary artery catheter equipped with a thermistor. The thermistor port is attached to a cardiac output computer,

(continued)

which has the capability of calculating the cardiac output based on changes in the blood temperature in the pulmonary artery. Using this technique, a specified amount of sterile fluid (usually 10ml) is rapidly injected (4 seconds or less) into the proximal port of the catheter, where it then mixes with the blood in that area. The lowered temperature of that blood as it passes the thermistor in the pulmonary artery is measured by the computer, and from this the computer calculates the cardiac output from a temperature concentration curve. The temperature of the fluid being injected may be room temperature or iced. In general, at least three consecutive measurements are obtained and averaged to calculate the cardiac output

OUTCOME CRITERIA

1. Maintenance or return of optimal cardiac output
2. Maintenance or return of optimal arterial blood gases
3. Alleviation of fluid volume excess as evidenced by pulmonary capillary wedge pressure and central venous pressure within patient's normal range
4. Restoration of adequate fluid volume
5. No complications from pulmonary artery catheterization

DOCUMENTATION

- Temperature, heart rate, blood pressure, and respiratory rate prior to catheter insertion
- Proximal and distal ports were flushed
- Balloon patency checked prior to insertion
- Time catheter was inserted, name of physician inserting catheter, catheter size, and insertion site
- RA, RV, PA, and PCWP pressures as catheter is being inserted
- Presence or absence of PVCs or ventricular tachycardia noted during catheter insertion
- Time chest x-ray was obtained
- Time of dressing change and presence or absence of inflammation or purulent drainage
- Presence of bilateral breath sounds and chest expansion
- Type of solution infusing into proximal port and patency of port
- Continuous infusion into distal port
- PAP, PCWP, and CVP with each reading
- Amount of air used to inflate balloon and presence or absence of slight resistance during inflation
- Presence or absence of signs of dampening

SPECIAL NOTE

Flow-directed Placement

Pulmonary artery catheters are frequently inserted via the subclavian vein. Other common insertion sites include the internal jugular vein, the femoral vein, and the antecubital vein. After the catheter has been advanced through the superior vena cava into the right atrium, the balloon should be inflated. With the balloon inflated, the catheter tip will float into the right ventricle and then out to the pulmonary artery. When the balloon has reached a very narrow branch of the pulmonary artery it will become wedged in the vessel, displaying the pulmonary capillary wedge pressure (PCWP) waveform on the monitor. The balloon is then deflated, and the catheter tip should float back from this narrow branch, again displaying the pulmonary artery pressure waveform.

Waveforms

The right atrial, right ventricular, pulmonary artery, and pulmonary capillary wedge each have a characteristic pressure waveform. To determine the position of the catheter tip, it is imperative that the distal port of the catheter be attached to a transducer system before insertion and that the pressure waveform be displayed on the monitor oscilloscope.

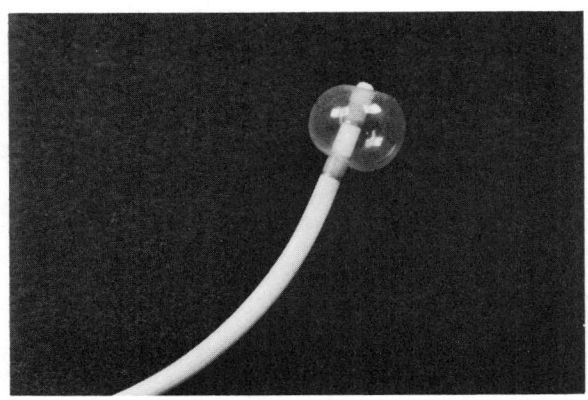

Figure 1–39. Balloon inflated (close-up of tip).

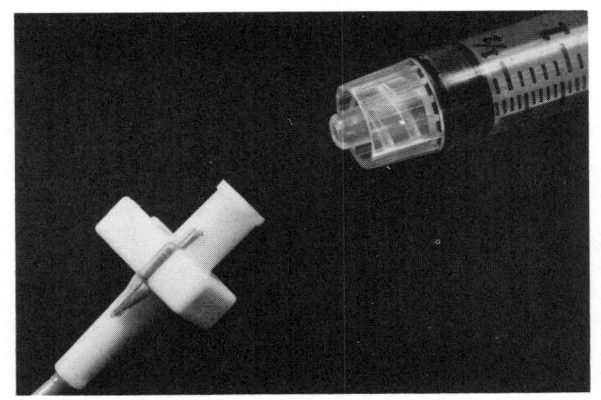

Figure 1–40. Removal of syringe to deflate balloon following PCWP.

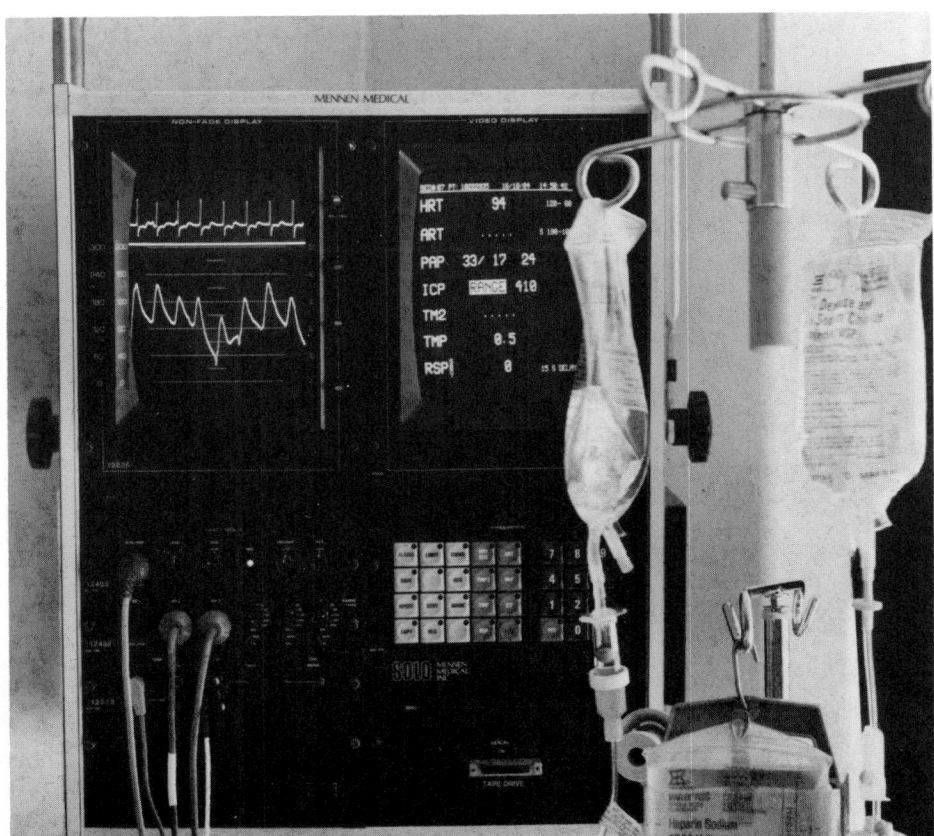

Figure 1–41. Monitor.

Care of the Patient Requiring Electrical Defibrillation or Cardioversion

NURSING DIAGNOSES	RATIONALE	DEFINING CHARACTERISTICS	EXPECTED OUTCOME
	Electrical defibrillation is the delivery of a nonsynchronized direct electrical current to the myocardium in an attempt to terminate ventricular fibrillation. Cardioversion is electrical current, synchronized with the patient's R wave, delivered in an attempt to terminate ventricular tachycardia or supraventricular tachydysrhythmias that compromise cardiac output.		
1. Cardiac output, alteration in: decreased	1. Cardiac output will be absent or minimal in the patient during ventricular fibrillation. A decreased or absent cardiac output may also occur following attempted cardioversion if the patient is converted to a more lethal rhythm, e.g., supraventricular rhythm or ventricular tachycardia to ventricular fibrillation	1. Deterioration of cardiac rhythm Severe hypotension or absence of blood pressure Absence of palpable pulse Loss of consciousness (if not already present) Cardiac arrest	1. Hemodynamically stable rhythm and adequate cardiac output will be restored
2. Skin integrity, impairment of: potential	2. Skin integrity may be impaired through skin burns if excessive gel paste or saline is used on paddles and electrical bridging between paddles occurs	2. Painful burns on patient's skin in area where paddles were applied or in area between paddles	2. No burns will occur

NURSING INTERVENTIONS

Preprocedure

1. Explain procedure to patient (if patient is alert)
2. Determine serum potassium level prior to elective cardioversion, if possible. Hypokalemia enhances electrical instability, which may cause postconversion dysrhythmias
3. Clean skin, if moist, prior to procedure. High salt content present in perspiration may lead to skin burns
4. Avoid excessive gel paste or saline on paddles to avoid electrical bridging between paddles resulting in skin burns
5. Ensure synchronous mode setting for cardioversion to prevent electrical charge from occurring during vulnerable period of cardiac cycle, which may cause more lethal rhythm
6. Ensure proper energy selection*:
   A. Adult defibrillation
      200–300 joules for first two attempts
      360 joules for subsequent attempts

---

*American Heart Association standards.

B. Internal defibrillation (open-chest; internal paddles applied directly to heart) 5–40 joules
C. Emergency cardioversion
Patient with pulse: 20–100 joules
Unconscious patient: 200 joules
7. Obtain baseline ECG strip
8. Ensure proper grounding of equipment

During Procedure

1. Ensure proper paddle placement
   A. Standard: One paddle to the right of the sternum at the second intercostal space; second paddle on the left side to the left of the nipple, in the midclavicular line (Fig. 1–42)
   B. Anterior–posterior: One paddle over the precordium and the second paddle posteriorly, below the left scapula (Fig. 1–43)
   C. Patient with permanent pacemaker: Avoid placing paddles over pulse generator, since it may cause damage to generator (Fig. 1–44)
2. Ensure the use of firm paddle pressure (25–30 pounds per paddle)
3. Continuously run ECG strip
4. Ensure that operator is standing on a dry floor
5. Verify that all personnel are clear of bed before discharging paddles
6. If cardioversion is being performed, ensure that synchronizer switch is activated and that discharge buttons are held until the machine delivers the current
7. If initial attempt at defibrillation or emergency cardioversion is unsuccessful, repeat the countershock as soon as possible. If second countershock is unsuccessful, continue CPR and provide additional advanced cardiac life support measures, e.g., medications, oxygen

After Procedure

1. Check monitor and obtain ECG strip
2. Check for palpable pulse
3. Institute CPR if needed
4. Ensure patency of airway
5. Obtain 12-lead ECG as ordered

OUTCOME CRITERIA

1. Patient's rhythm is restored to one that is hemodynamically stable
2. Patient's skin is intact and free of burns

DOCUMENTATION

- Serum potassium level, if obtained prior to procedure
- Application of gel paste or saline to paddles
- Establishment of synchronous mode setting prior to cardioversion
- Amount of energy selection used for each countershock delivered
- Attachment of rhythm strip obtained before and after procedure to nurse's notes
- Name of physician performing procedure, paddle placement, time of procedure, and number of attempts
- Time CPR was instituted, if applicable
- Patency of airway
- Time and results of 12-lead ECG

(continued)

SPECIAL NOTE

Precautions

The potential for injury to the patient and medical staff is heightened when safety precautions are not observed. The critical care nurse plays a vital role in ensuring that all safety precautions are followed and injury is avoided.

1. Ensure that all electrical equipment is grounded
2. Ensure that operator is standing on a dry floor
3. Verify that all personnel are clear of the bed prior to discharging the paddles

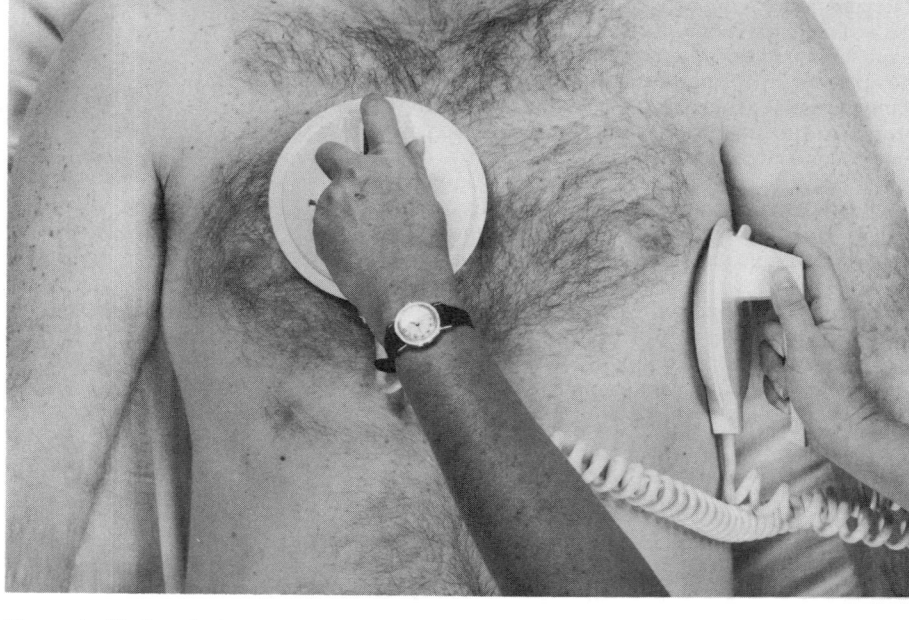

Figure 1–42. Standard paddle placement.

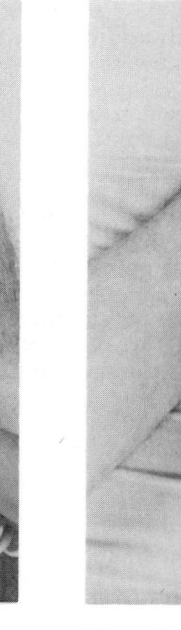

Figure 1–43. AP paddle placement.

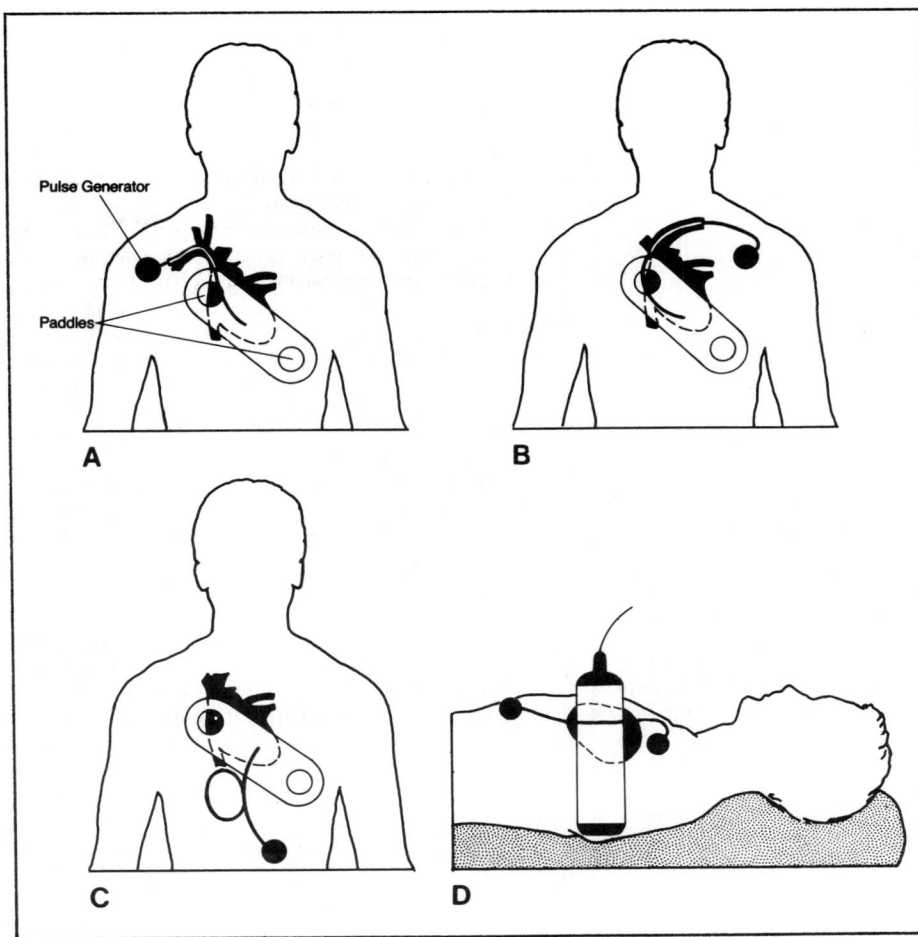

Figure 1–44. Paddle placement with pacemaker. **A.** Anterior–anterior placement when pulse generator in upper right chest. **B.** Anterior–anterior placement when pulse generator in upper left chest. **C.** Anterior–anterior placement when pulse generator in lower left abdomen. **D.** Anterior–posterior placement when pulse generator in either upper chest or lower abdomen. *(Adapted from Springrose, S. Recommended defibrillation procedures for pacemaker patients. CPI Tech Issues, 1980, 6, 2, with permission of Cardiac Pacemakers, Inc.)*

Care of the Patient Requiring Temporary Cardiac Pacing

NURSING DIAGNOSES	RATIONALE	DEFINING CHARACTERISTICS	EXPECTED OUTCOME
	Temporary pacemaker insertion can be a lifesaving procedure for the patient with a hemodynamically unstable rhythm. This hemodynamic instability may be caused by an inability of the heart to initiate or conduct its own impulse at a sufficient rate or by a refractory tachydysrhythmia. Displacement of the pacemaker catheter or malfunction of the pacemaker generator may cause serious complications and injury to the patient. The critical care nurse must closely assess the patient and the ECG to detect early pacemaker malfunction.		
1. Cardiac output, alterations in: decreased	1. Cardiac output may be decreased in the patient requiring cardiac pacing from dysrhythmias, such as sinus arrest, sick sinus syndrome, symptomatic sinus bradycardia, second- and third-degree heart block, persistent ventricular tachycardia, and some supraventricular tachy-dysrhythmias	1. Decrease in blood pressure Changes in mental status, e.g., restlessness, confusion Cool, clammy skin	1. Cardiac output is restored to within normal limits
2. Injury, potential for	2. Injury to the patient related to cardiac pacing may be caused by pacemaker failure or malfunction, right ventricular or interventricular septal perforation from the catheter lead, and microshock	2. Pacemaker failure or malfunction • Failure to sense patient's spontaneous beats: Pacer spikes occur at regular intervals regardless of patient's rhythm (Fig. 1–45) • Failure to capture: Pacer spikes visible but ventricles do not respond (Fig. 1–46) • Absence of generator discharge: Complete or intermittent absence of pacer spikes, and rate of patient's own rhythm is slower than preset rate of pulse generator (Fig. 1–47) Right ventricular or interventricular septal perforation may be characterized by signs and symptoms of cardiac tamponade, possible loss of capture, hiccoughs if the electrode is pacing the diaphragm, and change in pacing waveform configuration Microshock to the patient may occur if electric safety precautions are not taken; may result in ventricular fibrillation	2. No complications related to cardiac pacing occur

NURSING INTERVENTIONS

Preinsertion

1. Explain procedure to patient, if possible
2. Shave area around insertion site
3. Change generator batteries if needed
4. Ascertain proper grounding of all surrounding equipment
5. Attach patient to ECG monitor

During Insertion

1. Assist physician with insertion, maintaining aseptic technique
2. Monitor ECG for dysrhythmias as pacemaker lead is being inserted

After Insertion

1. Apply sterile dressing to insertion site and change dressing q24h using aseptic technique
2. Obtain baseline 12-lead ECG
3. Obtain chest x-ray to check for lead placement
4. Check patient temperature, blood pressure, and respiratory rate q1–2h
5. Monitor heart rate continuously
6. Secure all pacemaker system connections
7. Attach ECG rhythm strip to nurses notes q4–8h
8. Restrict range of motion in extremity in which catheter is inserted
9. Monitor for alteration of QRS configuration initiated by pacemaker
10. Wear latex rubber gloves when handling metal portion of pacemaker electrodes to prevent microshock hazard to patient
11. Set heart rate low alarm limit on monitor just below generator rate
12. Assess generator settings every shift (Fig. 1–48)
13. Check and record pacing threshold q8h. This is the lowest energy level needed to capture the ventricle and can be determined by decreasing the generator energy output (MA) until capture ceases; the MA is then increased until capture is regained

OUTCOME CRITERIA

1. Adequate cardiac output will be restored and maintained
2. Complications related to catheter placement or cardiac pacing will be avoided

DOCUMENTATION

- Time of insertion, name of physician inserting catheter, site of insertion, type of catheter used, and reason for catheter insertion
- Time 12-lead ECG was obtained
- Time chest x-ray was performed
- Vital signs
- Attachment of ECG rhythm strip to nurse's notes, existing rhythm, and pacemaker functioning
- Heart rate alarm limits set on monitor
- Rate, MA, and sensitivity settings every shift
- Threshold potential every shift
- Any noted change in QRS configuration initiated by pacemaker
- Maintenance of restricted range of motion in area of catheter insertion
- Time of dressing change and condition of insertion site

(continued)

SPECIAL NOTE

Methods of Pacing

1. Transthoracic pacing: Pacing wire is inserted into the heart through a needle in the anterior chest; this method is only used in emergency situations
2. Epicardial pacing: Electrodes are placed on the surface of the heart; this is used most commonly following open-heart surgery
3. Endocardial pacing: Pacing catheter is inserted transvenously, then threaded through the vena cava, the right atrium, and then into the right ventricle (Fig. 1–49).

ICHD Codes

Pacemaker functions are described using the three-letter code developed by the Inter-Society Commission for Heart Diseases Resources (ICHD):

First Letter	Second Letter	Third Letter	Description
Chamber Paced	*Chamber Sensed*	*Mode of Response*	
V	D	D	Ventricular pacing, no sensing
A	D	D	Atrial pacing, no sensing
V	V	I	Demand ventricular pacing; ventricular pacing and sensing, inhibited mode
V	V	T	Ventricular pacing and sensing, triggered mode
A	A	I	Demand atrial pacing; inhibited mode
V	A	T	Ventricular pacing, atrial sensing
D	V	I	Dual chamber pacing, ventricular sensing; inhibited mode

Abbreviations: A = Atrium; D = Dual chamber; I = Inhibited; T = Triggered; V = Ventricle.
(Adapted from Parsonnet V., et al.: Implantable cardiac pacemakers status report and resource guideline. Circulation, 1974, 50(4), A21–35.)

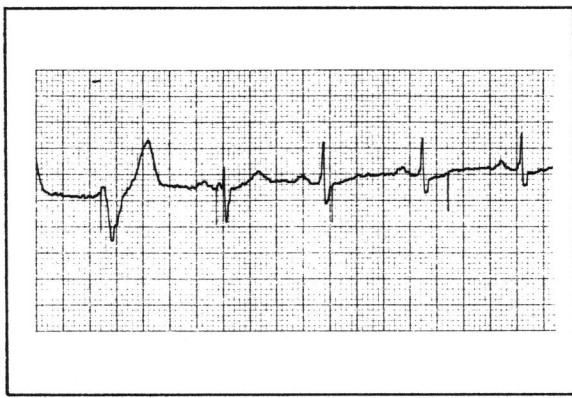

Figure 1–45. Failure to sense.

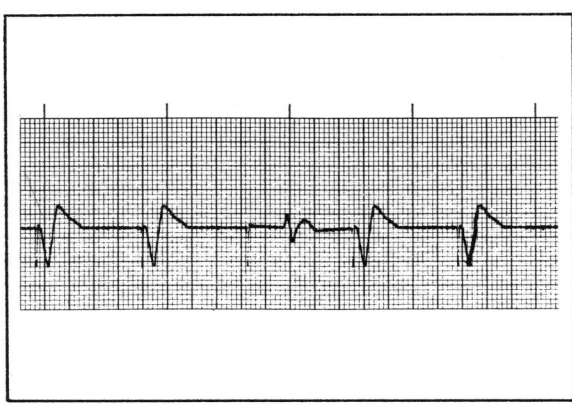

Figure 1–46. Failure to capture.

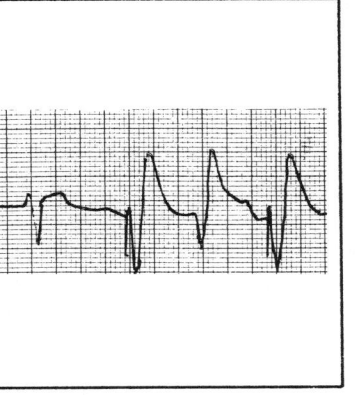

Figure 1–47. Failure to pace. *(From Seidel, J. C. (Ed.). Electrocardiography: A modular approach. St. Louis, Mo.: Mosby, 1986, p. 176, with permission.)*

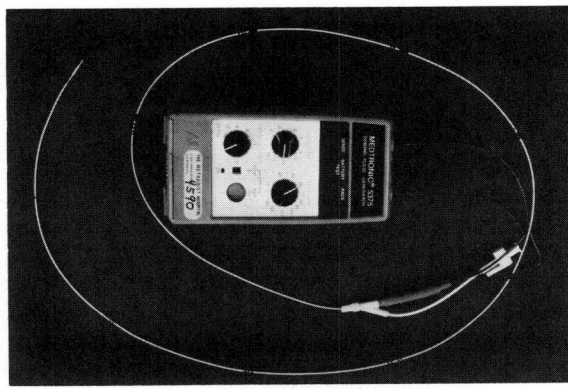

Figure 1–48. Close-up of temporary pacer and lead.

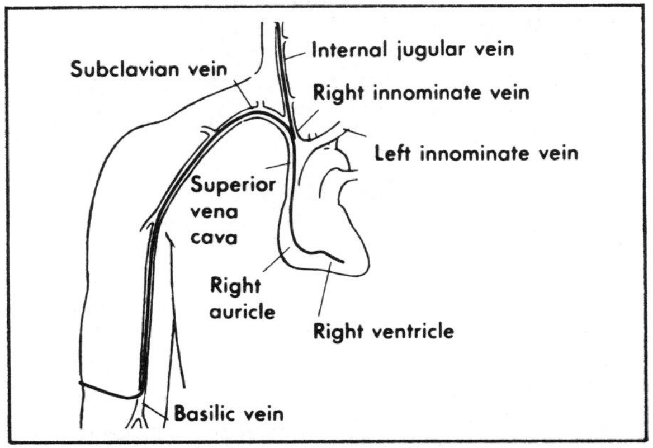

Figure 1–49. Transvenous pacing catheter in place. *(From Andreoli, K. G., Fowkes, V. H., Zipes, D. P., & Wallace, A. G. Comprehensive cardiac care (4th ed.). St. Louis, Mo.: Mosby, 1979, p. 260, with permission.)*

Subclavian vein

Internal jugular vein

Right innominate vein

Left innominate vein

Superior vena cava

Right auricle

Right ventricle

Basilic vein

Care of the Patient Requiring Circulatory Assist by Intra-aortic Balloon Counterpulsation

NURSING DIAGNOSES	RATIONALE	DEFINING CHARACTERISTICS	EXPECTED OUTCOME
	Intra-aortic balloon counterpulsation (IABP) assists the left ventricle by decreasing afterload and augmenting diastolic pressure. This pressure augmentation leads to an increase in coronary artery blood flow and improves the perfusion of other vital organs (Figs. 1–50 and 1–51). Some of the indications for use of the intra-aortic balloon include: • Hemodynamic instability following an acute myocardial infarction • Unstable angina refractory to medication • Inability to wean from cardiopulmonary bypass • Circulatory support for the preoperative and postoperative cardiac surgery patient		
1. Cardiac output, alteration in: decreased	1. Cardiac output may be decreased as a result of many factors, including myocardial infarction, left ventricular aneurysm, and increased systemic vascular resistance. Hemodynamic instability may also occur from improper balloon timing	1. Cardiac output below normal range of 4–8 L/min Decrease in systolic blood pressure below patient's normal level Decrease in urine output Cool, clammy skin Pallor Mental confusion Tachycardia	1. Cardiac output is restored to or maintained within normal limits
2. Injury, potential for	2. Although the intra-aortic balloon pump can be a life-sustaining treatment modality, it may also cause serious complications. These include hemorrhage or hematoma at the insertion site, aortic rupture, aortic dissection, hemolysis, infection and thrombus formation	2. Hemorrhage or hematoma at insertion site Aortic rupture characterized by weak, rapid pulse, pallor, profound hypotension Aortic dissection manifested by back pain, hypotension, decrease in renal function, unequal pulses and blood pressure in right and left extremities, and decreased quality of peripheral pulses Hemolysis characterized by abnormal coagulation studies and bleeding from invasive monitoring or intravenous insertion sites Infection manifested by an elevated temperature, inflammation or purulent drainage at the insertion site, with elevation of the white blood cell count	2. No complications related to intra-aortic balloon pumping will occur

		Thrombus formation causing weak or absent pulses in the affected extremity, pain, blanching or mottling, and a cool–cold extremity Immobility potentially leading to atelectasis and decubitus ulcer formation	
3. Tissue perfusion, alteration in: peripheral	**3.** Decreased tissue perfusion may be the result of leg ischemia distal to the balloon insertion site or ischemia to the left arm due to occlusion of the left subclavian artery	**3.** Ischemia of the leg distal to the insertion site or of the left arm as characterized by diminished distal pulses, pain, loss of sensation, and blanching or mottling	**3.** Adequate tissue perfusion is maintained

NURSING INTERVENTIONS

Every 15–30 Minutes

Check blood pressure, heart rate, and respiratory rate

Every Hour

1. Measure urine output
2. Check temperature
3. Check for proper balloon timing (Figs. 1–52 to 1–56)
4. Check invasive line insertion sites for bleeding
5. Obtain PA, PCWP, and CVP measurements

Every 1–2 Hours

1. Assess popliteal, dorsalis pedis, and posterior tibial pulses in catheterized leg (q30min for first 2 hours following catheter insertion)
2. Assess color, temperature, and sensation in catheterized leg
3. Check insertion site dressing for bleeding
4. Assess for signs of swelling or ecchymosis at insertion site
5. Assess left brachial and radial pulses
6. Log roll patient (prevent hip flexion greater than 30 degrees in affected leg)
7. Encourage coughing and deep breathing in nonintubated patients

Every 2–4 Hours

1. Provide skin care
2. Suction patient, if intubated

Every 4–8 Hours

1. Check cardiac output; calculate cardiac index and systemic vascular resistance
2. Provide passive range of motion exercises

(continued)

Every 24 Hours

1. Assess coagulation studies for abnormalities, if ordered
2. Replace ECG electrodes
3. Change insertion site dressing using aseptic technique
4. Obtain order for chest x-ray to assess lung status and catheter placement

Ongoing

1. Have balloon timing readjusted as necessary for heart rate and rhythm changes; correctly timed counterpulsation will exhibit the following:
   A. Inflation occurs just prior to the dicrotic notch
   B. Balloon-assisted end-diastolic pressure is less than the patient's aortic end-diastolic pressure
   C. Nonaugmented systole is less than augmented systole
2. Maintain patient on strict bed rest; avoid elevating head of bed more than 30 degrees to prevent upward catheter migration
3. Maintain two sets of ECG electrodes on patient: one set attached to balloon console and one set attached to ECG monitor
4. Monitor ECG on lead that shows tallest R wave (Fig. 1–57).

Postremoval

1. Maintain direct continuous pressure over insertion site for minimum of 15 minutes followed by application of pressure dressing for 24 hours
2. Check insertion site for bleeding, swelling, or ecchymosis q30min for 2 hours, then q1h for 24 hours

OUTCOME CRITERIA

1. Restoration or maintenance of cardiac output to within patient's normal range
2. Minimal or absent complications associated with intra-aortic balloon pumping
3. Adequate perfusion maintained in leg distal to insertion site and in left arm

DOCUMENTATION

Every 15–30 Minutes
Blood pressure, heart rate, and respiratory rate

Every Hour

- Urine output
- Temperature
- Presence of correct balloon timing
- Presence or absence of bleeding from invasive line insertion sites
- PA, PCWP, and CVP measurements

Every 1–2 Hours

- Quality of popliteal, dorsalis pedis, and posterior tibial pulses in leg in which balloon is inserted
- Color, temperature, and sensation in affected leg
- Presence of any bleeding from insertion site

- Swelling or ecchymosis at insertion site
- Quality of left brachial and radial pulses
- Log rolling of patient
- Coughing and deep breathing exercises performed by nonintubated patient

Every 2–4 Hours

- Skin care
- Suctioning, amount, characteristics of secretions

Every 4–8 Hours

- Cardiac output, cardiac index, and systemic vascular resistance
- Range-of-motion exercises

Every 24 Hours

- Results of coagulation studies, if obtained
- Replacement of ECG electrodes
- Condition of insertion site at time of dressing change
- Time chest x-ray was taken

Ongoing

- Any readjustment of balloon timing
- Enforcement of bed rest and degree of head of bed elevation
- Presence of two sets of ECG electrodes
- ECG lead being monitored

Postremoval

- Name of physician removing catheter, amount of time pressure was maintained, and application of pressure dressing
- Presence or absence of swelling or ecchymosis at insertion site

SPECIAL NOTE

Contraindications

Intra-aortic balloon counterpulsation is contraindicated in the patient with moderate to severe aortic insufficiency. Augmentation of the diastolic blood pressure in these patients would cause an increase in the amount of blood regurgitated into the left ventricle during diastole.

Intrinsic Triggering

Under normal circumstances the intra-aortic balloon pulsation is triggered to inflate with the R wave of the patient's ECG. In the patient with no intrinsic heart rhythm, such as the patient on cardiopulmonary bypass, the balloon console may be set to inflate and deflate at a preset (fixed) rate, set by the machine.

(continued)

Manual Inflation

If the balloon console should fail or during periods when the console is turned on standby, such as during cardiac arrest, the balloon must periodically be inflated and deflated manually to prevent thrombus formation. The balloon should not remain deflated for more than 30 minutes.

Timing

Correct intra-aortic balloon timing for inflation and deflation is obtained from the arterial pressure tracing. The balloon is timed to inflate just prior to the dicrotic notch of the normal arterial tracing.

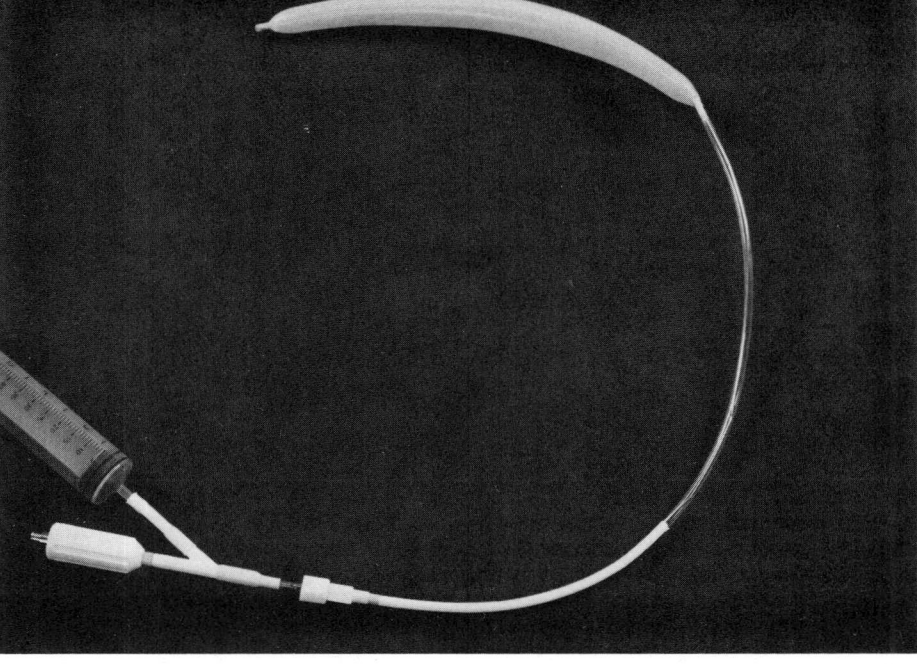

Figure 1–50. Catheter inflated.

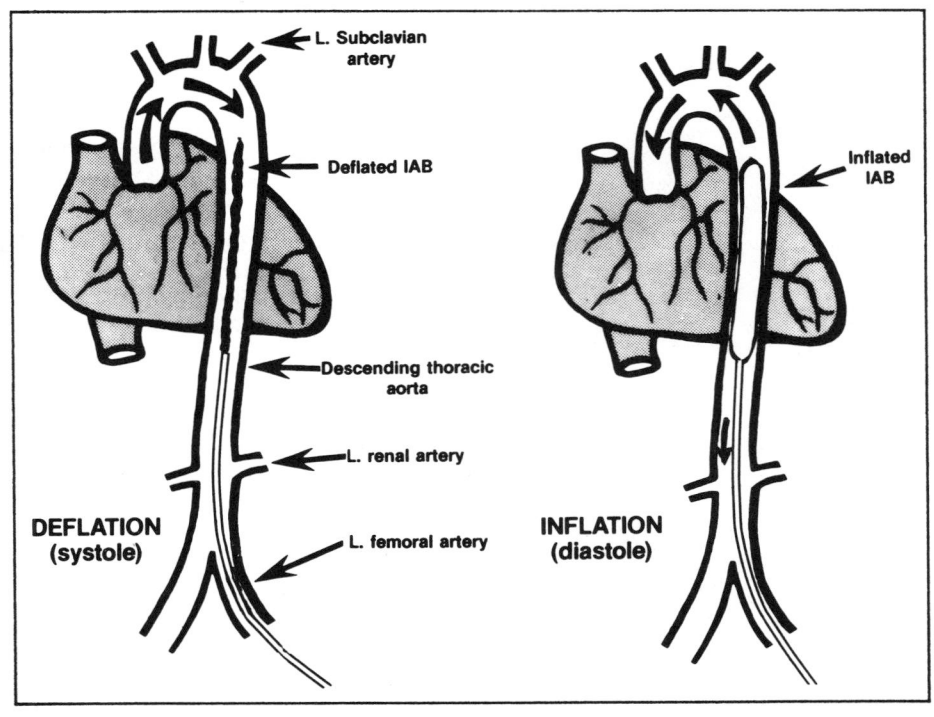

Figure 1–51. IABP placement. When the catheter is properly positioned it is located in the descending aorta with the balloon situated just distal to the left subclavian artery and above the renal arteries. *(From Bullas, J. B. Care of the patient on the percutaneous intra-aortic counterpulsation balloon. Critical Care Nurse, 1982, 2(4), 41, with permission.)*

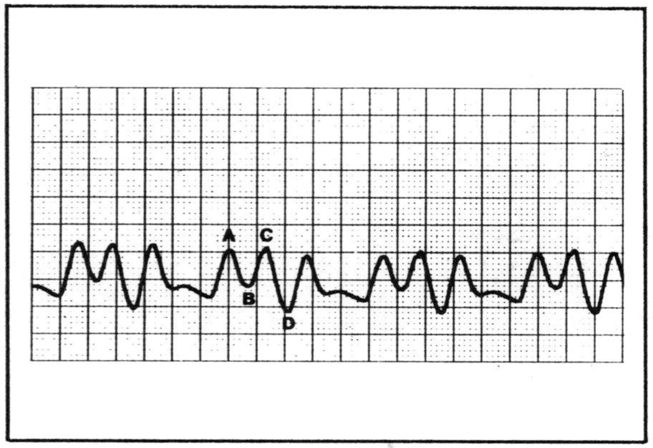

Figure 1–52. Tracing: normal timing. **A.** Patient systolic pressure. **B.** Dicrotic notch; beginning of balloon inflation. **C.** Peak diastolic pressure. **D.** Balloon assisted end-diastolic pressure.

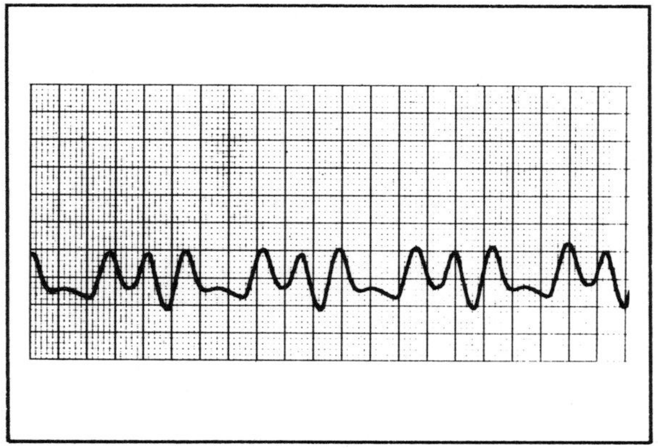

Figure 1–53. Tracing: late inflation.

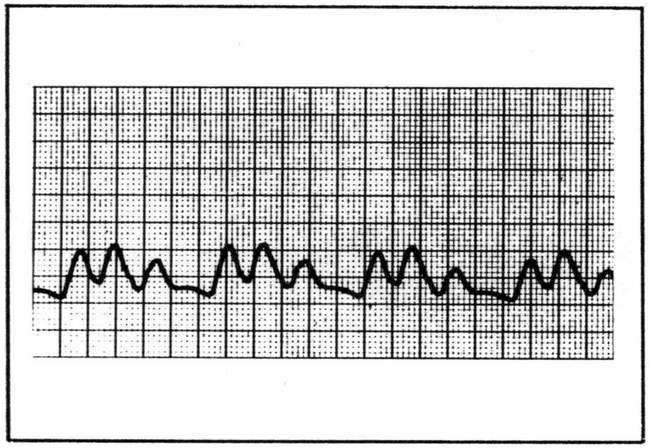

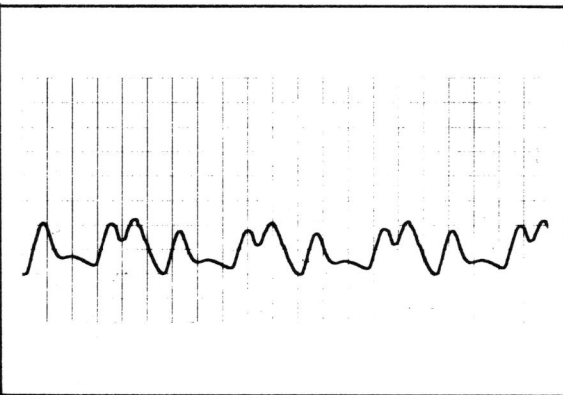

Figure 1–54. Tracing: late deflation.

Figure 1–55. Tracing: early inflation.

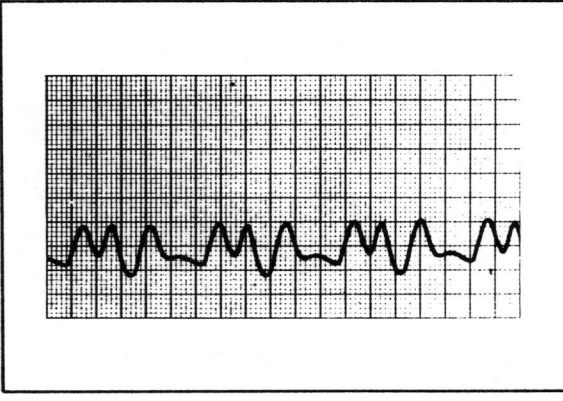

Figure 1–56. Tracing: early deflation.

Figure 1–57. Balloon triggering. Balloon inflation is *triggered* by the R wave of the ECG. The balloon should inflate at the peak of the T wave and deflate just prior to the QRS complex. *(From Bullas, J. B. Care of the patient on the percutaneous intra-aortic counterpulsation balloon. Critical Care Nurse, 1982, 2(4), 42, with permission.)*

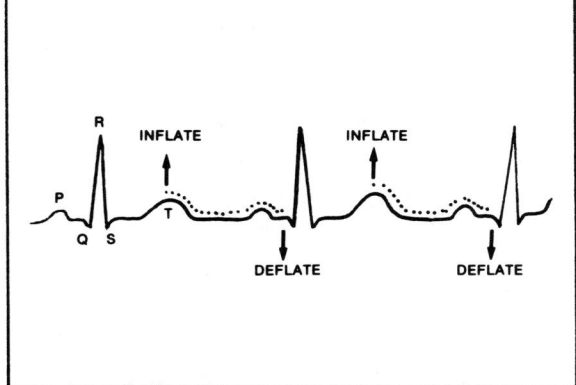

Glossary

Afterload: The resistance or impedance the ventricle must overcome in systole in order to eject its volume.

Bigeminal pulse: A pulse in which the beats occur in pairs.

Cardiac index: Cardiac output adjusted for body surface area. Normal is 2.5–4 L/min/m^2. Obtained by the following formula:

$$\frac{\text{Cardiac output}}{\text{Body surface area}}$$

Cardiac output: The amount of blood ejected from the left (or right) ventricle per minute. Cardiac output equals stroke volume times heart rate.

Cardioversion: Restoration of the heart's rhythm to normal by synchronized electrical countershock.

Defibrillation: The cessation of fibrillation of the cardiac muscle with restoration of the normal rhythm via delivery of a nonsynchronized countershock.

Dicrotic notch: A notch on the descending limb of the arterial pulse tracing associated with closure of the aortic valve.

Hypertrophy: Thickening of the walls of the heart.

Paradoxical pulse: An exaggeration of the normal variation in the pulse volume with respiration, causing a decrease or more than 10 mm Hg in systolic blood pressure during normal inspiration.

Precordium: The area on the anterior surface of the body overlying the heart and its great vessels.

Preload: Volume of blood filling the heart during diastole.

Pulse deficit: Condition in which the number of pulse beats counted at a peripheral artery is less than those counted in the same period of time at the apex of the heart.

Pulse pressure: The difference between the systolic and the diastolic blood pressure, normally 40 mm Hg.

Pulsus alternans: A pulse regular in time but with alternating pulse volume.

Pulsus bisferiens: An arterial pulse with two palpable peaks, the second stronger than the first.

Systemic vascular resistance: A measure of the impedance applied by the systemic arteriolar circuitry to systolic effort of left ventricle. Normal range is 900–1600 dynes/sec/cm^{-5}. Obtained by the following formula:

$$\frac{\text{Mean arterial pressure} - \text{CVP}}{\text{Cardiac output}} \times 80$$

Thrill: The vibration accompanying a cardiac or vascular murmur, which can be felt on palpation.

Bibliography

Alspach, J. G., & Williams, S. (Eds.). *Core curriculum for critical care nursing* (3rd ed.). Philadelphia: Saunders, 1985.

Andreoli, A., Fawkes, V., Zipes, D., & Wallace A. (Eds.). *Comprehensive cardiac care* (5th ed.). St. Louis, Mo.: Mosby, 1983.

Bates, B. *A guide to physical examination* (3rd ed.). Philadelphia: Lippincott, 1983.

Bodia, B., & Holcrast, J. Uses of the pulmonary arterial catheter in the critically ill patient. *Heart and Lung,* 1982, *11*(5), 406–416.

Bullas, J. B. Care of the patient on the percutaneous intra-aortic counterpulsation balloon. *Critical Care Nurse,* 1982, *2*(4), 40–49.

Cohen, J., Pantaleo, N., & Shell, S. What isoenzymes can tell you about your cardiac patient. *Nursing,* 1982, *12*(4), 46–49.

Finkelmeier, B., & O'Mara, S. Temporary pacing in the cardiac surgical patient. *Critical Care Nurse,* 1984, *4*(1), 108–114.

Haak, S. Intra-aortic balloon pump techniques. *Dimensions of Critical Care Nursing,* 1983, *2*(4), 196–204.

Kinney, M., Dear, C., Packa, D., & Voorman, D. (Eds.). *AACN's clinical reference for critical care nursing.* New York: McGraw-Hill, 1981.

Klein, L. Temporary AV sequential pacing. *Critical Care Nurse,* 1983, *3*(3), 36–41.

McIntyre, K., & Lewis, A. (Eds.). *Textbook of advanced cardiac life support.* Dallas, Tex.: American Heart Association, 1981.

Owen, P. The effects of external defibrillation on permanent pacemakers. *Heart and Lung,* 1983, *12*(3), 274–277.

Partridge, S. Cardiac auscultation. *Dimensions of Critical Care Nursing,* 1982, *1*(3), 152–156.

Purcell, J., Rippin, L., & Mitchell, M. Intra-aortic balloon pump therapy. *American Journal of Nursing,* 1983, *83*(5), 775–797.

Underhill, S., Woods, S., Silvarajan, E., & Halpenny, C. (Eds.). *Cardiac nursing.* Philadelphia: Lippincott, 1982.

2

PULMONARY SYSTEM

Dian Gayle Teinert

Assessment of the Pertinent Pulmonary History

RATIONALE

Obtaining a detailed health history from the patient with known or suspected pulmonary disease can be a complex process. All aspects of the patient's personal, environmental, occupational, and social history should be explored. Sources of irritants leading to pulmonary disease are numerous. The critical care practitioner must be able to obtain pertinent information in a timely, efficient manner, providing a useful framework within which to perform the physical examination. When information cannot be obtained from the patient or family in the acute setting, previous admission records may be useful in obtaining additional data.

PARAMETERS	FINDINGS	IMPLICATIONS FOR NURSING CARE
1. Family history	1. **A.** Early onset emphysema in family member **B.** Family member with asthma or allergies	1. **A.** A history of early onset emphysema in an immediate family member may be highly suggestive of alpha-antitrypsin-deficiency emphysema **B.** A history of asthma or allergies in the family may be helpful in prompt diagnosis when an acute onset of wheezing occurs. Careful assessment of the progression of wheezing and the status of breath sounds must be performed frequently. Careful attention to hydration status is indicated
2. Past health history	2. **A.** History of cardiovascular disease, such as myocardial infarction (MI) or congestive heart failure (CHF)	2. **A.** Prior history of MI or CHF may be a useful indicator in identifying an acute exacerbation of CHF or pulmonary edema. Shortness of breath when lying flat may be more closely associated with cardiac disease. Exertional dyspnea with CHF progresses over a relatively short period of time. Chest pain of cardiac origin does not vary with movement of the thorax. In CHF, dependent edema may be associated with recent progression of exertional dyspnea or orthopnea. It varies with etiology and severity of cardiac disease. In these patients, assessment of respiratory status, progression of rales and fluid balance, is of utmost importance
	B. Past pulmonary conditions	**B.** Past pulmonary infections may be associated factors in bronchiectasis. Extensive pulmonary toiletry is the most useful mechanism of support in the acutely ill patient with bronchiectasis.
	C. Progression of symptoms	**C.** Dyspnea or shortness of breath associated with chronic obstructive pulmonary disease (COPD) progresses over a long period of time. Most of the difficulty in breathing is associated with exertion and forced exhalation (pursed-lip breathing observed). Acute exacerbation of COPD produces dyspnea at rest and requires intervention. Dyspnea with asthma presents as wheezing and subsides as the bronchospasm is relieved. Careful assessment of progression of wheezing and degree of shortness of breath is critical. Acute onset of dyspnea or shortness of breath is an important indicator for assessing pneumonia, pneumothorax, hemothorax, or pulmonary embolism. Immediate response and treatment are required. Cough occurring daily over 2 or more years is indicative of chronic bronchitis. It is most pronounced upon awakening. Purulent sputum in large quantities may be associated with bronchiectasis or lung abscess, whereas viscous sputum is associated with COPD. Color, character, and amount of sputum produced are important in determining changes in condition. Hemoptysis can occur with tuberculosis, bronchogenic carcinoma, pulmonary embolism, or pulmonary abscess. Bleeding of pulmonary origin must be distinguished

		from that of a nonpulmonary source. Pulmonary blood is usually bright red and frothy. The amount of blood produced must be carefully assessed.

from that of a nonpulmonary source. Pulmonary blood is usually bright red and frothy. The amount of blood produced must be carefully assessed.

Pleuritic or chest wall pain is generally associated with inspiratory–expiratory force, coughing, or other movement involving the thorax. Sudden sharp chest pain may accompany spontaneous pneumothorax

D. Viral infection in past 1–3 weeks

D. Recent viral infection with respiratory or gastrointestinal symptoms may be associated with Guillain–Barré syndrome if accompanied by progressive muscle weakness or aches. Frequent measurement of tidal volume (V_T) and vital capacity (V_C) is critical to allow early intervention should ventilatory status deteriorate

E. Allergies

E. Allergies, specifically to inhalants, when associated with other findings, such as family history, aid in the diagnosis of asthma

F. History of peripheral vascular disease, such as phlebothrombosis

F. Pulmonary embolism is closely associated with clot formation in phlebothrombosis. Any patient with present or prior history of phlebothrombosis must be observed for acute onset of anxiety, shortness of breath (SOB), chest pain, and hemoptysis

G. Past thoracic surgeries

G. History of past pneumonectomy may be helpful in explaining absence of breath sounds on auscultation. Limited exercise tolerance related to decreased residual volume may also be present

3. Patient profile

3. A. History of smoking

3. A. Smoking history is important in identifying and differentiating emphysema from chronic bronchitis. It may be a predictor for anticipating ventilatory problems in certain patients, especially postoperatively

B. History of drug abuse

B. It is critical to determine a history of drug abuse in any patient with obvious hypoventilation, hypoxia, and central cyanosis of unexplained origin. Frequent observation for changes in respiratory rate and pattern is necessary to ensure early intervention should respiratory failure occur. Maintenance of a patent airway is of major importance in preventing respiratory failure

C. Age

C. Age is useful in distinguishing among certain disease entities, such as emphysema or alpha-antitrypsin-deficiency emphysema

4. Present problem

4. A. Thoracic trauma

4. A. Pneumothorax, hemothorax, and flail chest will compromise ventilatory status. Observation for early recognition of signs of impaired ventilatory status will be necessary to insure prompt intervention and prevention of complications

B. Thoracic or cardiovascular surgery

B. Any surgical procedure involving the chest will interfere with normal cough mechanisms and impair ventilatory efforts

C. Recent shock or major trauma

C. Any patient who has experienced shock or major trauma is predisposed to adult respiratory distress syndrome (ARDS). Acute progressive hypoxemia associated with shock or trauma is an important clue for early recognition and intervention

D. Use of high fraction of inspired oxygen (FIO_2) over prolonged period of time, usually a patient requiring ventilatory support

D. Progressive hypoxemia that occurs following use of fraction of inspired oxygen (FIO_2) greater than 40% for more than 24 hours may indicate oxygen toxicity. Once it has occurred, frequent assessment of oxygenation status by arterial blood gases is critical in identifying and treating further progression

E. Central nervous system (CNS) insult or trauma

E. CNS insult may compromise ventilatory status by altering respiratory rate and pattern. Progressive bilateral ascending paralysis is a hallmark of Guillain-Barré syndrome and may significantly compromise vital capacity and ventilatory status. Frequent monitoring of tidal volume and vital capacity is critical. Continuous ventilatory support may become necessary

Spinal cord injuries (below the level of C4) will compromise tidal volume and vital capacity, since only diaphragmatic breathing remains intact

(continued)

PARAMETERS	FINDINGS	IMPLICATIONS FOR NURSING CARE
5. Review of systems	5. **A.** Pulmonary	CNS trauma may alter respiratory rate and pattern significantly. Additionally, patients experiencing a severe head injury may develop neurogenic pulmonary edema. Frequent assessment of ventilatory status with maintenance of a patent airway is necessary for early recognition of and intervention for respiratory failure 5. **A.** Activity intolerance Airway clearance, ineffective Breathing pattern, ineffective Communication, impaired: verbal Gas exchange, impaired Tissue perfusion, alteration in: cardiopulmonary
	B. Cardiovascular	**B.** Cardiac output, alteration in: decreased Fluid volume, alteration in: excess
	C. Neuromuscular	**C.** Mobility, impaired: physical

Assessment of the Thorax by Inspection

RATIONALE   Inspection is a highly developed skill requiring acute discriminatory observation and judgment. It should be performed in a systematic manner. Visual cues provide the practitioner with instant feedback regarding changes in respiratory status. The critical care nurse should be able to identify certain observable changes in the patient without relying on laboratory data alone. Prompt recognition and intervention are the key to success in treating an acute pulmonary problem.

PARAMETERS	FINDINGS	POSSIBLE ETIOLOGIES	DOCUMENTATION
1. Respiratory rate and pattern	1. **A.** Abnormal inspiration:expiration (I:E) ratio (normal I:E ratio, 1:1½ or 1:2) **B.** Abnormal respiratory rate (RR) and pattern (normal adult, RR 15–17) **a.** Tachypnea **b.** Bradypnea **c.** Cheyne–Stokes respiration **d.** Biot's respiration **e.** Kussmaul respiration **f.** Apneustic **g.** Apnea (periodic)	1. **A.** COPD **B. a.** Pneumonia, metabolic acidosis, brainstem lesions, or respiratory distress, as observed with insufficient tidal volume (V_T), hypoxia, hypercapnea **b.** CNS depression, such as substance overdose, brainstem lesion, or metabolic alkalosis **c.** Increased intracranial pressure, meningitis, substance overdose **d.** CNS disorders **e.** Metabolic acidosis **f.** Brainstem lesions **g.** Following hyperventilation associated with anxiety–panic state	• Prolonged expiration: Respiratory rate and type of pattern (as appropriate) Additionally, level of consciousness, mental status, or other CNS assessment (i.e., decerebrate, decorticate posturing) • Description of type of abnormal chest wall movement and location of abnormality • Presence of retractions • Use of accessory muscles of respiration • Pursed-lip breathing with or without obvious dyspnea or SOB • Presence of orthopnea • Nasal flaring with accompanying signs of respiratory distress, such as anxiety, dyspnea, or SOB • Direction of tracheal shift • Changes in mental status, headache, BP, pulse, presence of yawning, presence or absence of central cyanosis • Changes in mental status, tremors, generalized seizures, headache, or asterixis
2. Chest wall movement with ventilation	2. Abnormal chest wall movement **A.** Asymmetrical **B.** Retractions **C.** Use of acessory muscles **D.** Localized expiratory bulging (paradoxical motion with ventilation)	2. **A.** Tension pneumothorax, large pleural effusion, following intubation of right or left mainstem bronchus, postpneumonectomy (normal finding), consolidation, and atelectasis **B.** COPD, asthma (associated with bronchial plugging) **C.** Increased work of breathing common during acute exacerbation of COPD **D.** Impaired integrity of chest wall with flail chest	
3. General signs and symptoms	3. Abnormal signs and symptoms **A.** Pursed-lip breathing **B.** Nasal flaring **C.** Tracheal deviation	3. **A.** COPD **B.** Respiratory distress, such as an acute exacerbation of asthma **C.** Pneumothorax (to affected side), tension pneumothorax (away from affected side), pleural effusion (away from affected side), atelectasis (to affected side)	

D. Restlessness, anxiety, apprehension, headache, confusion, disorientation, impaired judgment, hypotension, tachycardia, yawning, central cyanosis (buccal mucosa and lips)	**D.** Hypoxia as a result of COPD, pneumonia, CNS depression, neuromuscular disorders, musculoskeletal disorders, ARDS, or pulmonary edema
E. Drowsiness, tremors, confusion, generalized seizures, headache, asterixis	**E.** Hypercapnea related to hypoventilation as observed with COPD or CNS depression

POSSIBLE NURSING DIAGNOSES

- Breathing pattern, ineffective
- Airway clearance, ineffective
- Gas exchange, impaired

SPECIAL NOTE

Critical Observations

The practitioner must be aware of those critical observations requiring immediate intervention. Examples include:

1. Sudden change in respiratory rate and pattern, especially patients with any problem affecting the CNS
2. Sudden shifting of the trachea with asymmetrical movement of the chest wall; restlessness, anxiety, apprehension, hypotension, tachycardia, and cyanosis (tension pneumothorax)
3. Increasing drowsiness with confusion; asterixis and progression to generalized seizures in the patient with COPD

Assessment of the Thorax by Palpation

RATIONALE   Palpation of the thorax may have limited application in the acute care setting. It is of most help in identifying painful areas, in determining position of the trachea, and in evaluating bilateral chest expansion.

PARAMETERS	FINDINGS	POSSIBLE ETIOLOGIES	DOCUMENTATION
1. Palpation for tracheal position: Place finger in the space between the sternoclavicular joints to ascertain position of the trachea (Fig. 2–1)	1. Normal: Trachea midline position Abnormal: Shifting or deviation to one side	1. Abnormal: Shifting away from affected side Pleural effusion Tension pneumothorax Shifting to affected side Atelectasis Pneumothorax	• Position of trachea. If the position is abnormal, record any accompanying signs and symptoms of respiratory compromise
2. Palpation for bilateral chest expansion (respiratory excursion): Performed by placing both hands on chest with thumbs toward midline. As the patient inhales and exhales, watch for equal movement of both hands. Areas assessed include upper and middle anterior chest as well as posterior chest (Figs. 2–2, 2–3, and 2–4)	2. Normal: Chest excursion equal bilaterally Abnormal: Unequal chest wall movement	2. Abnormal: Decreased excursion on affected side Pneumonia Pneumothorax Intubation of right or left mainstem bronchus	• Chest excursion equal bilaterally. If unequal, record the location and extent of decrease in chest wall excursion. If abnormal, record any accompanying signs and symptoms of respiratory compromise

POSSIBLE NURSING DIAGNOSIS

• Breathing pattern, ineffective

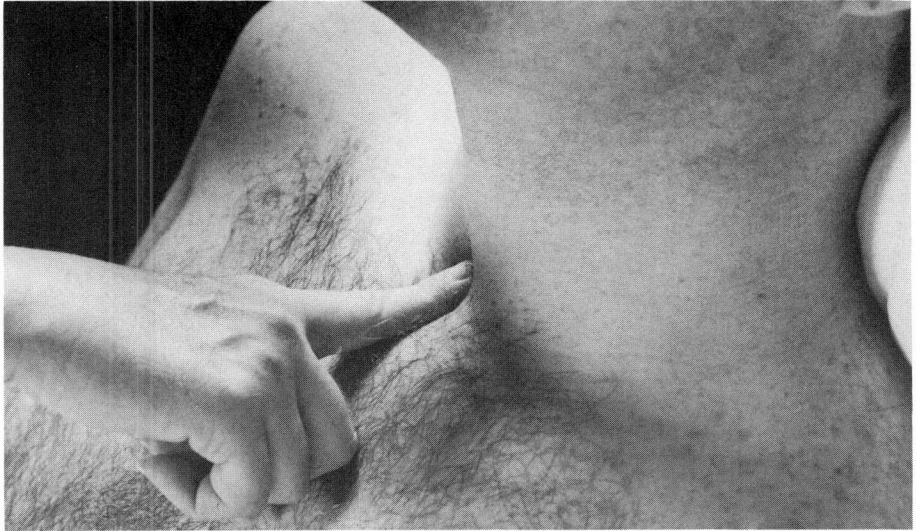

Figure 2–1. Palpation of tracheal position.

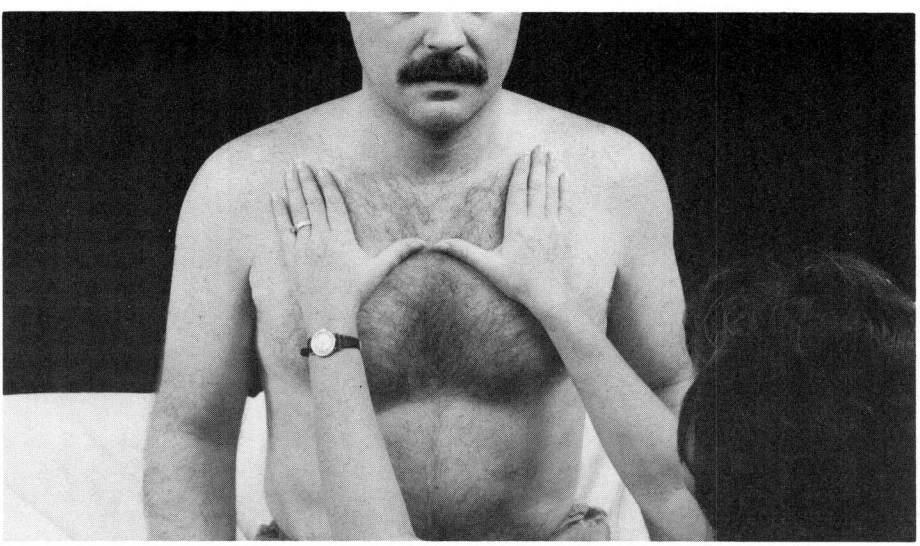

Figure 2–2. Palpation of chest excursion: anterior (upper).

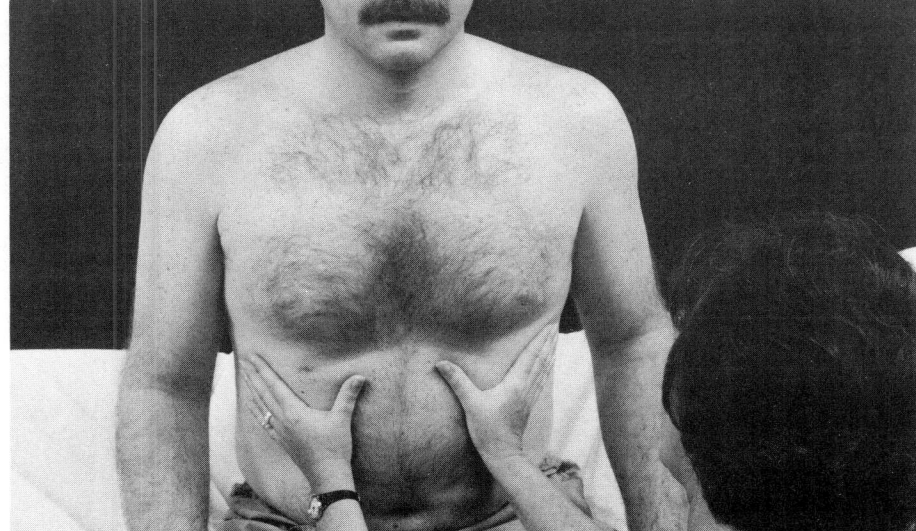

Figure 2–3. Palpation of chest excursion: anterior (midchest).

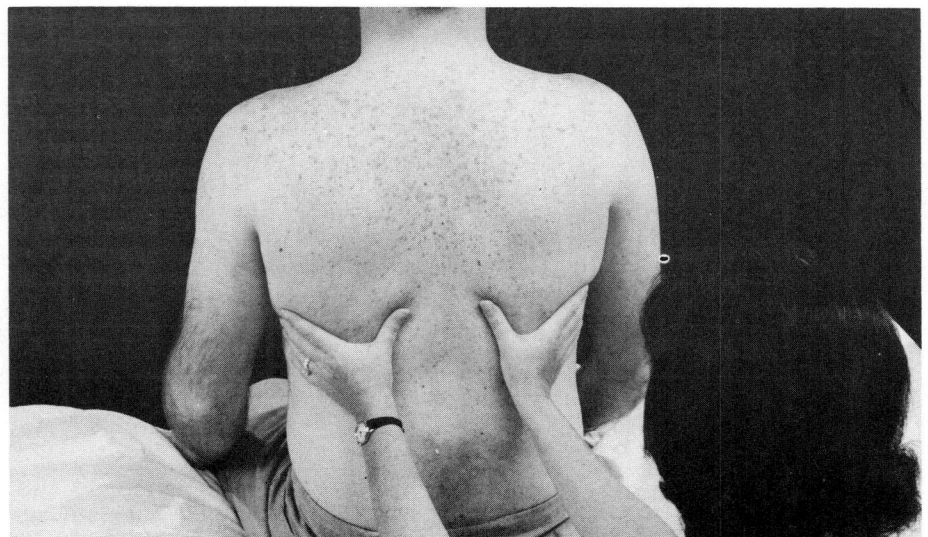

Figure 2–4. Palpation of chest excursion: posterior.

Assessment of the Thorax by Percussion

RATIONALE

Information acquired through the use of percussion of the thorax in the acute care setting is critical in identifying the presence of air or fluid in the pleural space that may compromise ventilatory function.

PARAMETERS	FINDINGS	POSSIBLE ETIOLOGIES	DOCUMENTATION
Percussion sounds (notes): produced by placing the middle finger on the surface of the chest and tapping firmly with the middle finger of the other hand. Systematic side to side comparison proceeds over the interspaces in a cephalo-caudal direction.	1. Resonance: representing air-filled spaces 2. Hyperresonance (tympany): drumlike sound representing excess air in space 3. Dullness or flatness: represents fluid or solid tissue in area and will vary with position if fluid is gravity dependent	1. Normal note over peripheral lung fields 2. Pneumothorax, emphysema 3. Hemothorax, hydrothorax, empyema, pleural effusion	• Location and quality of sound produced with percussion of the thorax (e.g., "hyperresonance on percussion of right lower to middle lobe areas of lung") • Breath sounds, type and location where heard • Accompanying signs and symptoms as applicable

POSSIBLE NURSING DIAGNOSIS

• Breathing pattern, ineffective

Assessment of the Thorax by Auscultation

RATIONALE

Auscultation of breath sounds represents the most useful assessment technique for planning and evaluating the effectiveness of nursing interventions concerned with airway clearance. Combined with inspection and critical observation, it is most useful for continually monitoring changes in ventilatory status. Breath sounds are produced by turbulent airflow through the airways and represent the single most important component of auscultation (Figs. 2–5 to 2–8).

PARAMETERS	FINDINGS	POSSIBLE ETIOLOGIES	DOCUMENTATION
1. Normal breath sounds A. Bronchial	1. A. Bronchial breath sounds are normally located in the area of the trachea and main-stem bronchus. They are loud and high-pitched, with the expiratory phase being much more pronounced than the inspiratory. Bronchial breath sounds anywhere peripheral to these locations represent an abnormality. They may be accompanied by adjacent rales	1. A. Consolidation, atelectasis	1. A,B. Description, location, and extent of bronchial or bronchovesicular breath sounds (if located peripherally) and accompanying rales, if applicable
B. Bronchovesicular	B. Bronchovesicular breath sounds are normally located in the upper airways adjacent to the sternal border. They are slightly lower in pitch and intensity than bronchial breath sounds, with the inspiration phase and the expiration phase essentially equal. If located peripherally, they are considered abnormal and may be accompanied by adjacent rales	B. Consolidation, atelectasis	
C. Vesicular	C. Vesicular sounds are normal breath sounds heard in the periphery of the lung fields. They are soft sounds, with the expiratory phase being almost silent. Absent or diminished breath sounds in any area must be noted	C. COPD, obesity, pneumothorax, pleural effusion, intubation of right or left mainstem bronchus, previous pneumonectomy	C. Area and extent of decreased, diminished, or absent breath sounds

2. Adventitious sounds
   A. Rales
	2. A. Rales, generally described as crackles, represent the presence of fluid or exudate in the terminal bronchioles or alveoli. They are generally heard on end-inspiration. They may represent the sound of collapsed terminal bronchioles or alveoli popping open
	   a. Bases and upward
	   b. Localized in one lobe, segment, or lung
		2. A. a. CHF
		
		   b. Pneumonia
			2. Description, location, extent, and progression of adventitious sounds

	c. Adjacent to area of decreased or absent breath sounds	**c.** Pneumothorax, pleural effusion
	d. Associated with bronchial breath sounds	**d.** Atelectasis, consolidation

B. Rhonchi	**B.** Rhonchi are gurgling, rattling sounds or wheezes, caused by air passing through airways that are narrowed by inflammation, spasm of smooth muscle (bronchospasm), or the presence of viscous secretions
	a. Sibilant wheezes
	    Expiratory
	    Inspiratory
	    Inspiratory and expiratory
	    Silent chest
	b. Sonorous (gurgling, rattling)
	    Expiratory
	    Clear with coughing
		B. a. Chronic bronchitis or asthma (most significant in assessment of progression during acute exacerbation of asthma). As the wheezing phase progresses and when associated with deterioration of other respiratory components, an emergency situation exists
		
		b. Consolidation, COPD, pneumonia

C. Pleural friction rub	**C.** Pleural friction rub is a grating or scratching sound caused by pleural inflammation. May be heard during inspiration or expiration	**C.** Any inflammatory process of the lung, such as tuberculosis, pneumonia, pleurisy, or lung cancer; inflammation of adjacent organs, as in hepatitis

POSSIBLE NURSING DIAGNOSES

- Airway clearance, ineffective
- Breathing pattern, ineffective

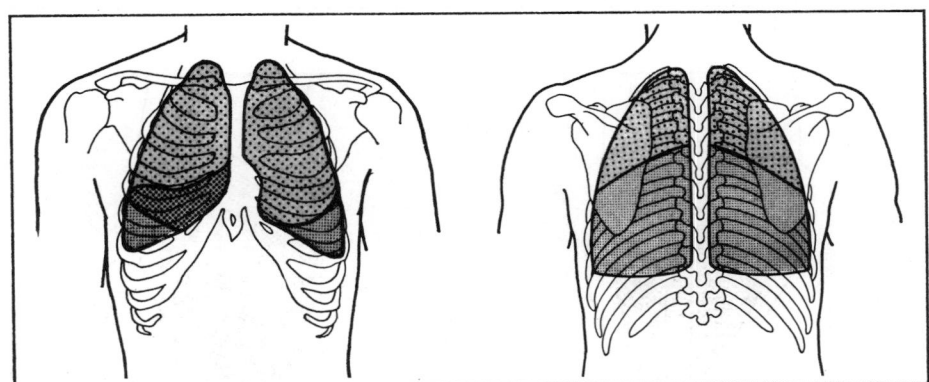

Figure 2–5. Anatomical orientation (anterior and posterior). Auscultation should be performed anteriorly, laterally, and posteriorly to allow assessment of all lobes and segments. *(From Traver, G. A. Assessment of thorax and lungs.* American Journal of Nursing, *1973, 73(3), 467, copyright 1973, American Journal of Nursing Co., with permission.)*

(continued)

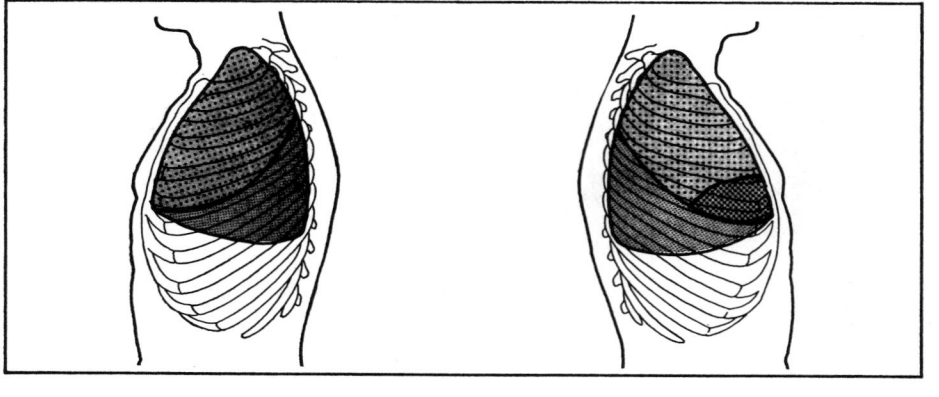

Figure 2–6. Anatomical orientation (lateral, two views). *(From Traver, G. A. Assessment of thorax and lungs. American Journal of Nursing, 1973, 73(3), 467, copyright 1973, American Journal of Nursing Co., with permission.)*

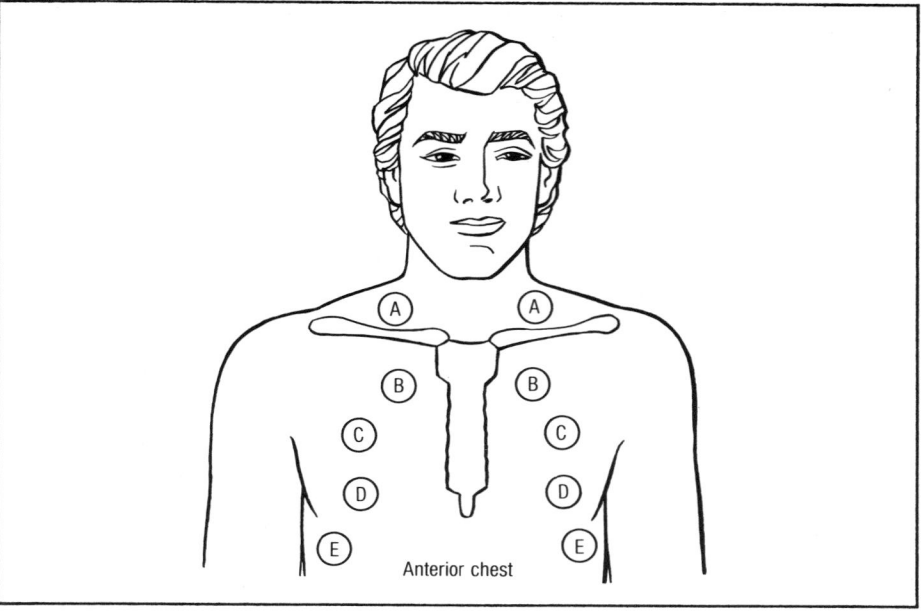

Figure 2–7. Systematic approach (anterior). Auscultation is performed systematically with a cephalocaudal approach, comparing one side of the thorax with the other. One side should be identical to the other regarding findings, if normal. *(From Norton, B. A., & Miller, A. M. Skills for professional nursing practice. Norwalk, Conn.: Appleton-Century-Crofts, 1986, p. 778, with permission.)*

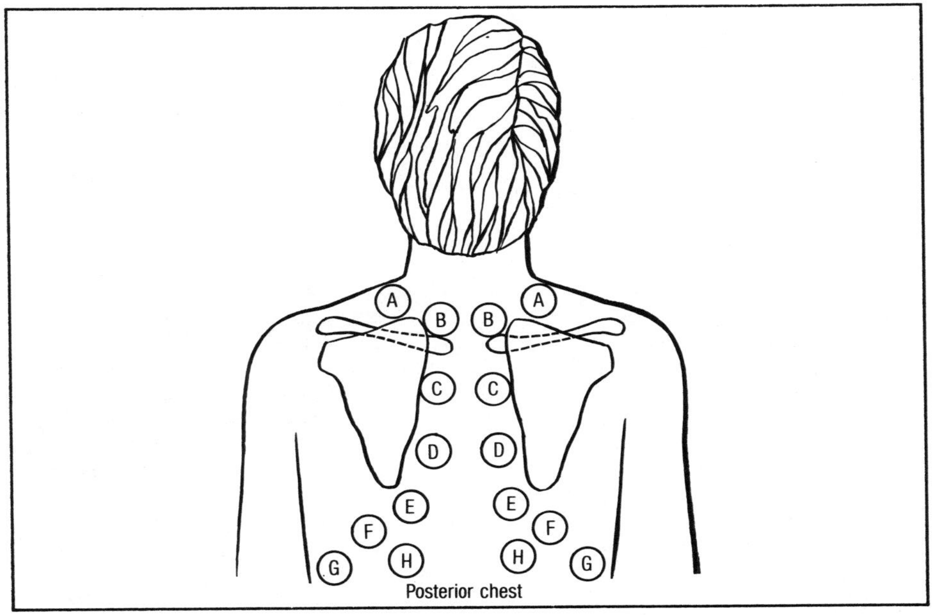

Figure 2–8. Systematic approach (posterior). *(From Norton, B. A., & Miller, A. M. Skills for professional nursing practice. Norwalk, Conn.: Appleton-Century-Crofts, 1986, p. 778, with permission.)*

Assessment of Arterial Blood Gases

RATIONALE

Arterial blood gas (ABG) analysis provides accurate parameters for assessing pulmonary gas exchange status and acid–base balance. It is an adjunct to physical assessment skills, can easily be performed at the bedside, and provides critical information regarding progress of the patient and changes in status.

PARAMETERS	FINDINGS	POSSIBLE ETIOLOGIES	DOCUMENTATION
1. Acute respiratory acidosis	1. pH below 7.35, Pa_{CO_2} above 45 mm Hg, HCO_3 base excess normal Headache, dizziness, confusion, loss of consciousness, somnolence Decreased minute volume (alteration in respiratory rate and depth), asterixis, hypertension	1. Acute alveolar hypoventilation (inadequate minute volume) produced by Respiratory failure due to an exacerbation of chronic obstructive pulmonary or restrictive lung disease Oxygen-induced respiratory depression with COPD Respiratory center depression, such as during substance overdose or head injury Inadequate mechanical ventilatory support Neuromuscular conditions: Guillain-Barré syndrome, myasthenia gravis, muscular dystrophy, spinal cord injury	1. Condition of skin (warm and dry, clammy, or diaphoretic) Level of consciousness Presence of headache, syncope, or vertigo Mental status Presence of neuromuscular irritability
2. Acute respiratory alkalosis	2. pH above 7.45, Pa_{CO_2} below 35 mm Hg, HCO_3 base excess normal Increased minute volume (alteration in respiratory rate and depth) Fatigue, headache, irritability, lightheadedness, numbness and tingling of the mouth, tongue, and extremities, muscle cramping and spasms, twitching, convulsions	2. Acute alveolar hyperventilation (minute volume exceeding normal) produced by Acute anxiety or panic states Overinflation with mechanical ventilatory support Pulmonary restrictive disorders, such as fibrosis Hypoxia (response to) Pulmonary embolism Respiratory center impairment: cerebrovascular accident, salicylate ingestion, head trauma	2. Presence of fatigue, headache, irritability, lightheadedness Numbness or tingling, muscle spasms or cramping, any twitching or convulsions
3. Compensated respiratory acidosis	3. pH near 7.35–7.45, Pa_{CO_2} above 45 mm Hg, HCO_3 base excess (increased) Decreased minute volume (over prolonged period of time) Symptoms related to degree of compensation present (variable)	3. Chronic alveolar hypoventilation COPD (specifically emphysema)	3. Presence of SOB or dyspnea Condition of skin (warm and dry, clammy, or diaphoretic) Level of consciousness Presence of headache, syncope, or vertigo Mental status Presence of neuromuscular irritability

4. Compensated respiratory alkalosis	4. pH near 7.35, $PaCO_2$ below 35 mm Hg, HCO_3 base excess decreased
	Symptoms related to degree of compensation present (variable)
		4. Prolonged alveolar hyperventilation:
		  Acute anxiety or panic states
		  Overinflation with mechanical ventilatory support
		  Pulmonary restrictive disorders, such as fibrosis
		  Hypoxia (response to)
		  Pulmonary embolism
		  Respiratory center impairment: cerebrovascular accident, salicylate ingestion, head trauma
			4. Presence of fatigue, headache, irritability, lightheadedness
			Numbness or tingling, muscle spasms or cramping, neuromuscular irritability or generalized seizures

5. Hypoxia (Fig. 2–9)	5. PaO_2 below 80, SaO_2 below 95%
	Shallow respirations
	Increased heart rate, hypotension
	Anxiety, restlessness, headache
	Cyanosis (central)
	Confusion, disorientation
	Exacerbation of angina
	Yawning
	Dyspnea
		5. Hypoxemia, acute or chronic
		  Respiratory failure due to an exacerbation of chronic obstructive pulmonary or restrictive lung disease
		  Oxygen-induced respiratory depression with COPD
		  Respiratory center depression, such as during substance overdose or head injury
		  Inadequate mechanical ventilatory support
		  Neuromuscular conditions: Guillain-Barré syndrome, myasthenia gravis, muscular dystrophy, spinal cord injury
		  Alterations in PaO_2 will occur earlier with hypoventilation than will CO_2 retention and acidosis
			5. Any SOB or dyspnea
			Presence or absence of central cyanosis
			Any chest pain
			Mental status
			Any headaches
			Presence of yawning
			
			Note: Documentation for all respiratory conditions should include the following:
			  ABG results
			  Respiratory rate and pattern
			  Vital signs (temperature, pulse, and blood pressure)

POSSIBLE NURSING DIAGNOSIS

- Gas exchange, impaired

SPECIAL NOTE

Compensation

Chronic respiratory acidosis or alkalosis may be partially or completely compensated. Symptomatology correlates with pH. As the pH is returned to near normal, symptomatology will be minimized

COPD

Oxygen-induced hypoventilation in the patient with COPD occurs as follows:
1. The body compensates over time for chronic CO_2 elevation by not responding to CO_2 elevation with increased ventilatory effort. The kidney has had time to compensate for the acidosis by increasing HCO_3 levels and by normalizing the pH. Decreased pH due to increased CO_2 normally stimulates increased ventilation
2. Respirations are stimulated by hypoxic drive only

(continued)

3. Oxygen therapy given to patient raises O_2 to normal level, reducing hypoxic drive. Hypoventilation results, leading to increased CO_2 retention (acute, severe hypercapnea) and respiratory acidosis

This represents a life-threatening situation to the nonintubated, nonventilator-supported patient. Prevention is the best treatment. Maintenance of low-flow oxygen therapy to the COPD patient is recommended.

In situations where cardiac or respiratory arrest has occurred or when the patient is ventilator supported, the danger of oxygen-induced hypoventilation is no longer a consideration and should not prevent use of high-concentration oxygen therapy, such as 100% FIO_2.

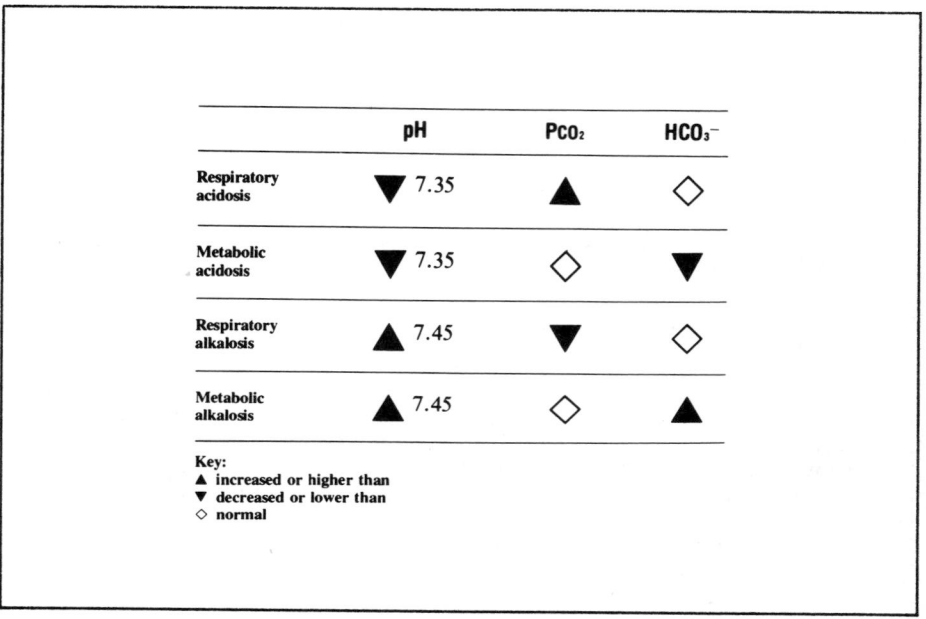

Figure 2–9. Comparison of arterial blood gas findings. *(From Shrake, K. The ABCs of ABGs. Nursing 79, 1979, 9(9), 29, copyright 1979, Springhouse Corporation, with permission.)*

Care of the Patient Requiring Percutaneous Puncture for Arterial Blood Gas Sampling

NURSING DIAGNOSES	RATIONALE	DEFINING CHARACTERISTICS	EXPECTED OUTCOME
Injury, potential for	ABG analysis is performed to provide the health care team with the information necessary to adequately assess gas exchange status and acid–base balance in the acutely ill patient. Arterial blood may be obtained on an intermittent basis through percutaneous arterial puncture. Injury resulting from improper technique or inadequate observation of puncture sites can have serious consequences. The practitioner, therefore, should be aware of and alert for early signs of complications.	Pain, numbness, coldness, tingling, or paresthesia of the involved extremity Loss of peripheral pulses distal to occlusion of the artery Swelling and discoloration at injection site Bleeding at injection site Decreased blood pressure, increased pulse rate Decreased hemoglobin and hematocrit	No injury will result from ABG puncture

NURSING INTERVENTIONS

1. Confirm and verify the physician's order
2. Review chart for evidence of coagulopathy or administration of anticoagulant medications
3. Collect equipment
4. Select the site for puncture. Radial and brachial artery sites are recommended over the femoral site. The radial and brachial arteries are relatively small arteries compared to the femoral, and pressure control following puncture is enhanced by their close proximity to bone
5. If the radial artery site is used, collateral circulation should be evaluated by Allen's test prior to performing arterial punctures.
6. Position the extremity as follows:
   A. Radial artery: Dorsiflex the wrist over a small folded towel or gauze roll (Fig. 2–10)
   B. Brachial artery: Hyperextend the arm over a pillow for support (Fig. 2–11)
   C. Rotate wrist or arm to a position where the pulse can most easily be palpated
7. Cleanse the site with povidone–iodine or alcohol
8. Fix the area of maximum pulsation between two fingers
9. Using a heparinized syringe equipped with a short-beveled, 22-gauge needle, puncture the artery at the following angle (Fig. 2–12).
   A. Radial: 45 degrees
   B. Brachial: 60 degrees
10. Entry should be firm and steady, avoiding any probing maneuvers under the skin
11. When blood is seen pulsating in the syringe, the artery has been entered. Allow syringe to fill passively, with 3–5 ml of blood (Fig. 2–13)
12. Withdraw the needle and apply firm pressure to the site for a minimum of 5 minutes. If the patient is on anticoagulant therapy or has a bleeding dyscrasia, pressure must be held longer. A pressure bandage may be applied, if necessary

13. If the syringe is prelabeled and the rubber plug and ice are nearby, it is possible to maintain pressure and carry out the following process with one hand:
    A. Remove all the air bubbles from the syringe and seal the needle with the rubber plug
    B. Immediately place the sample on ice to be transported for analysis. If a second person is available, he or she may either apply pressure or handle the specimen
14. Check the puncture site and extremity for swelling, hematoma formation, bleeding, circulation, and sensation q5min for a minimum of 30 minutes following the procedure

OUTCOME CRITERIA

1. No injury will result from ABG puncture
    Pain, numbness, coldness, tingling, or paresthesia of involved extremity will be absent
    No change in peripheral pulses distal to puncture site will occur
    No swelling or discoloration will occur at the site of puncture
    No bleeding will occur from the site of puncture
    No change in blood pressure or pulse will occur
    No change in hemoglobin or hematocrit related to bleeding from arterial puncture site will occur
2. Any complications that occur will be minimized by prompt identification and intervention

DOCUMENTATION

- Quality of collateral circulation per Allen's test (if appropriate)
- Time the ABGs were drawn and sent to the laboratory
- Location of arterial puncture
- Application of pressure to the site for 5 minutes or more (be specific as to length of time)
- Results (preferably on flow sheet, if available)
- Notification of physician of results of test
- Initiation of any interventions for bleeding or occlusion
    Time
    Method
    Frequency
    Response

SPECIAL NOTE

Technique

Air bubbles remaining in the syringe with the arterial blood for any significant amount of time will affect the Pao_2. The Pao_2 will change also if the arterial blood is not chilled.

Blood gas kits are available containing preheparinized syringes. If a kit is not available, a syringe can be heparinized by drawing up a small quantity of 1:1000 U heparin (e.g., 0.1–0.2 ml) in the syringe, moving the plunger up and down to coat the sides, and then discarding the remaining heparin from the syringe. It is important to discard the remaining heparin to avoid affecting the pH of the blood sample.

When a plastic syringe is used or when cardiac output is low, blood will not push the plunger of the syringe upward. Pulsation may be seen in the hub. If it is felt that the artery has been entered, the plunger can be gently raised to withdraw blood. There are times when it is difficult to determine if a venous or arterial sample has been obtained, such as in the presence of severe reduction of cardiac output.

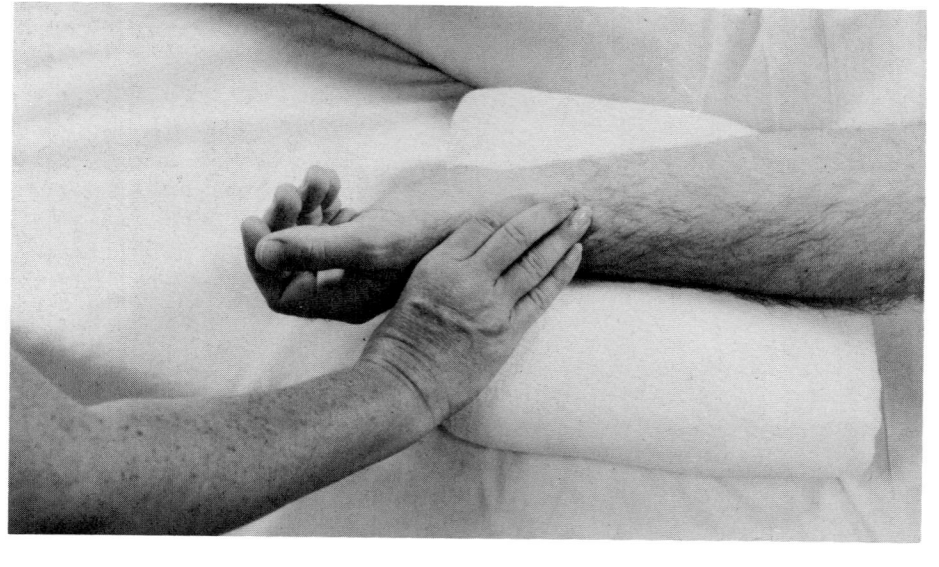

Figure 2–10. Position for radial artery.

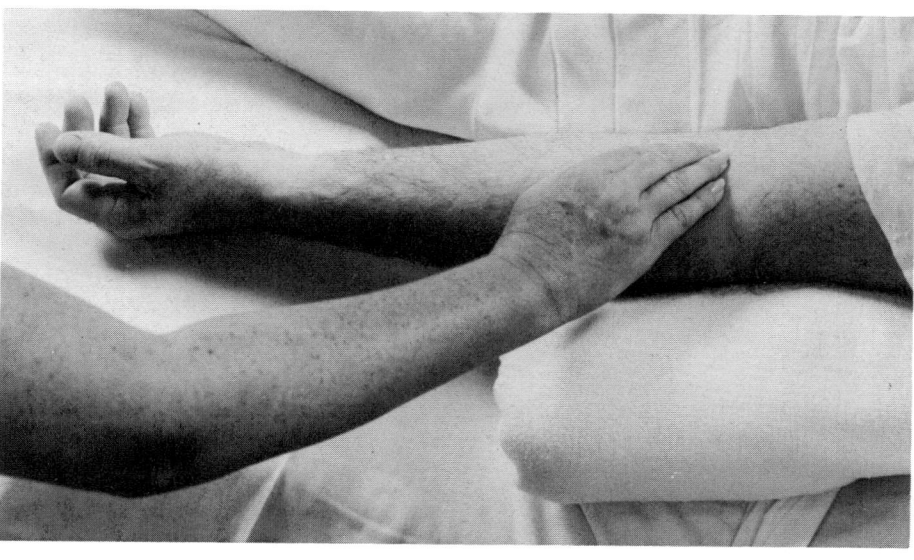

Figure 2–11. Position for brachial artery.

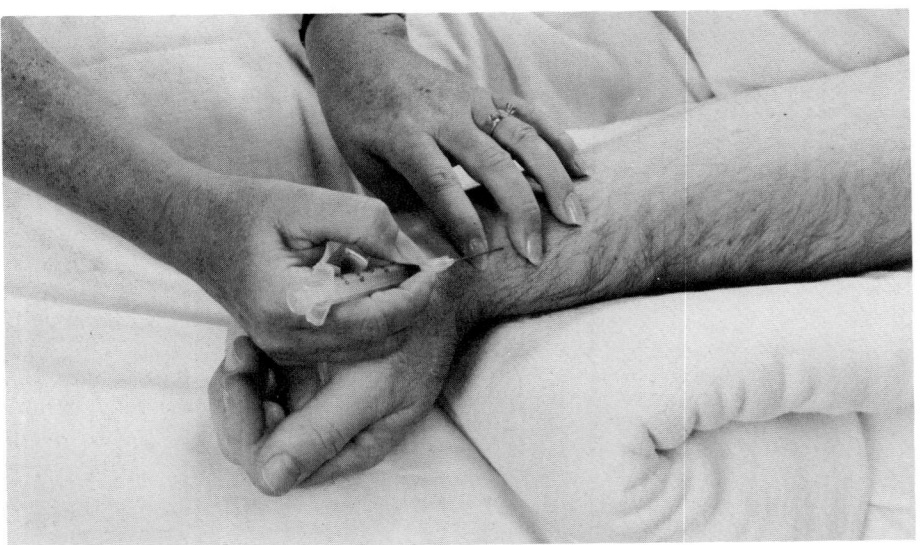

Figure 2–12. Insertion of the needle, bevel up at a 30 degree angle.

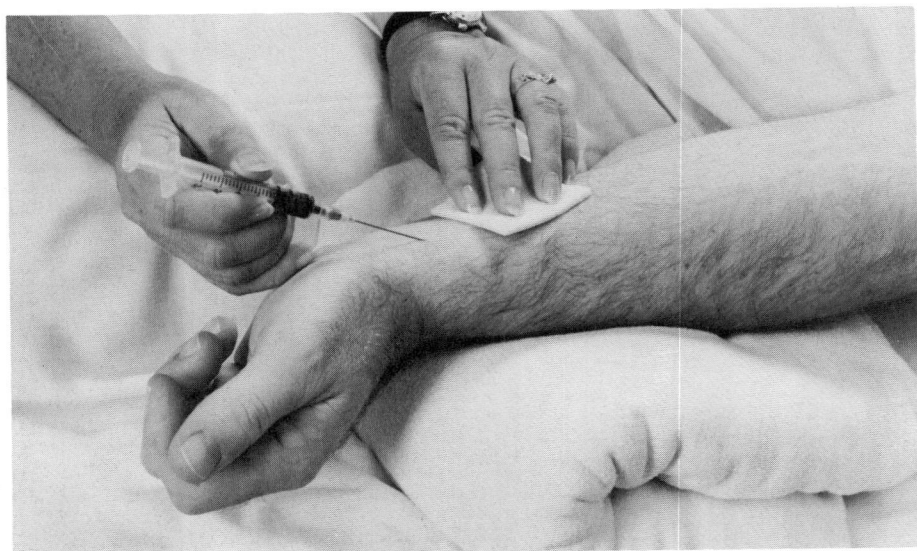

Figure 2–13. Backflow of blood into syringe.

Care of the Patient Requiring Oxygen Therapy

NURSING DIAGNOSES	RATIONALE	DEFINING CHARACTERISTICS	EXPECTED OUTCOME
1. Gas exchange, impaired	1. Supplemental oxygen therapy is indicated when gas exchange is impaired by low FIO_2, alveolar hypoventilation, ventilation–perfusion abnormality, or diffusion impairment resulting in hypoxemia. Tissue level gas exchange status is affected by Hgb level, Hgb affinity or lack of affinity for oxygen, and cardiac output. Supplemental oxygen will be required if Hgb level is inadequate, if affinity for oxygen has been altered, or if cardiac output is inadequate	1. Hypoxia Decreased PaO_2 and SaO_2 Hypoventilation (decreased respiratory rate or depth) Central cyanosis Decreased blood pressure, increased heart rate Dyspnea Exacerbation of angina Changes in mental status (anxiety, restlessness, confusion, disorientation) Headache Yawning	1. Gas exchange will be maintained at an optimal level
2. Injury, potential for	2. The appliances used to provide oxygen to the patient vary with respect to flow rates used and amount of oxygen that can be delivered. Although there are differences in appliances, there are general principles that should be applied in maintaining safe oxygen delivery at all times. Complications related to oxygen therapy should not be minimized. These complications may include hypoventilation produced in the patient with chronic CO_2 retention (hypoxic stimulus for breathing eliminated), atelectasis (nitrogen eliminated and surfactant lost causing the collapse of alveoli), and oxygen toxicity (prolonged administration of FIO_2 greater than 0.40 more than 24 hours). Nursing interventions should be planned to provide maximum benefits with the fewest complications (Figs. 2–14 to 2–20)	2. Increasing hypoxemia and hypercapnea leading to CO_2 narcosis and acute acidemia Progressive decrease in PaO_2 with increase in FIO_2 Decreased or absent breath sounds accompanied by rales Central cyanosis Dyspnea, tachypnea Inspiratory pain Changes in mental status or level of consciousness (restlessness, inability to concentrate, lethargy, coma) Headache Fatigue, lethargy, malaise Paresthesias Anorexia, nausea, vomiting Cough	2. No complications related to oxygen therapy will occur

NURSING INTERVENTIONS

1. Observe type, concentration, and flow rate of oxygen therapy and verify for accuracy with physician's orders
2. Maintain proper humidification
   A. Monitor fluid level in humidifier or nebulizer
   B. Replace sterile water as necessary
   C. Monitor temperature of humidified air (should be same as patient's body temperature)
3. Monitor ABG as ordered (recommended frequently with FIO_2 greater than 0.40 and with changes in condition)

4. Assess pulmonary status frequently (a minimum of every hour or more often if indicated) as follows:
   A. Airway patency
   B. Respiratory rate and pattern
   C. Presence, absence, or progression of SOB or dyspnea
   D. Presence or absence of central cyanosis (i.e., buccal)
   E. Cough
   F. Sputum production (amount, color, character, odor)
   G. Any subjective complaints of pain or discomfort
   H. Mental status, level of consciousness
5. Perform pulmonary toiletry as necessary
6. Maintain oxygen device on patient as consistently as possible

OUTCOME CRITERIA

1. ABG will return to or be maintained at optimal level
2. Complications related to oxygen therapy are prevented or minimized as evidenced by:
   ABG maintained at optimal level
   Normal mental status
   Absence of central cyanosis
   Normal breath sounds, absence or clearing of adventitious sounds

DOCUMENTATION

- Type of device, concentration, and flow rate of oxygen therapy every shift or with each change in therapy
- ABG results with time drawn, site, and condition of site
- Pulmonary status
   Respiratory rate and pattern
   Presence, absence, or progression of SOB or dyspnea
   Mental status, level of consciousness
   Airway patency
   Cough (effective, ineffective)
   Sputum production (amount, color, character, odor)
   Presence or absence of central cyanosis (lips, tongue)
   Comfort level
   Breath sounds (present, absent, bilateral)
   Adventitious sounds (if present, location, quality, changes)
- Pulmonary toiletry
   Performance
   Results: sputum amount, color, character, odor
   Efficacy (clearing of rhonchi)
- Patient's cooperation with oxygen therapy. If patient displays a lack of cooperation, document as, for example, "Patient continually removes nasal cannula"

SPECIAL NOTE

Airway Patency

Clearing of secretions and maintaining a patent airway are necessary if oxygen therapy is to be effective. Pulmonary toiletry consists of a series of interventions for the purpose of mobilizing secretions to clear the airways. Any one or combination of the following methods may be used:

(continued)

1. Humidification with or without bronchodilator medication
   A. Handheld nebulizer or intermittent positive pressure breathing (IPPB)
   B. If the patient has a tracheostomy or endotracheal tube, instillation of 5 ml sterile saline, accompanied by deep lung inflations (i.e., sigh–ventilator or ventilation–self-inflating bag) will help to loosen secretions prior to suctioning
2. Suctioning via nasotracheal or orotracheal route or via endotracheal or tracheostomy tube if present
3. Chest percussion and postural drainage
4. Assistance with coughing

Chest PT

Chest physiotherapy may be used as part of an intensive, systematic pulmonary toiletry program for those patients with copious secretions with or without accompanying atelectasis. Modified positioning for postural drainage may be necessary if ventilatory status is easily compromised or other conditions contraindicate, such as unstable cardiovascular status (Figs. 2–21 and 2–22).

Interrupting Therapy

Interruption of oxygen therapy causes wide fluctuations in oxygenation and should be avoided. Oxygen at 2 L/min per nasal cannula may be used to maintain therapy during meals for those patients who are taking oxygen per mask and are able to eat.

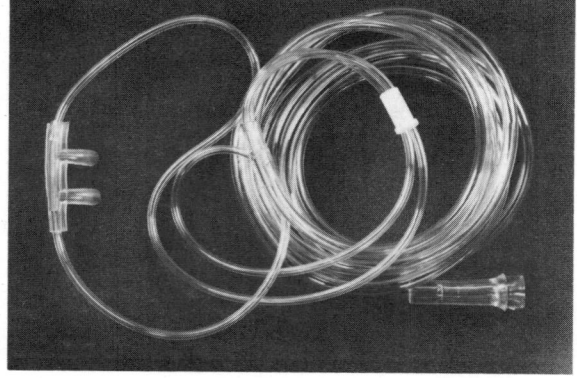

Figure 2–14. Nasal cannula.

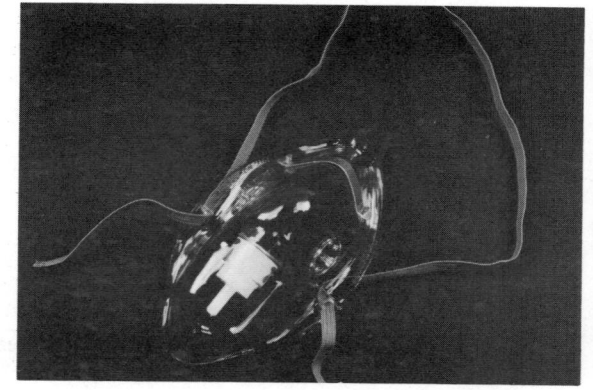

Figure 2–15. Green face mask.

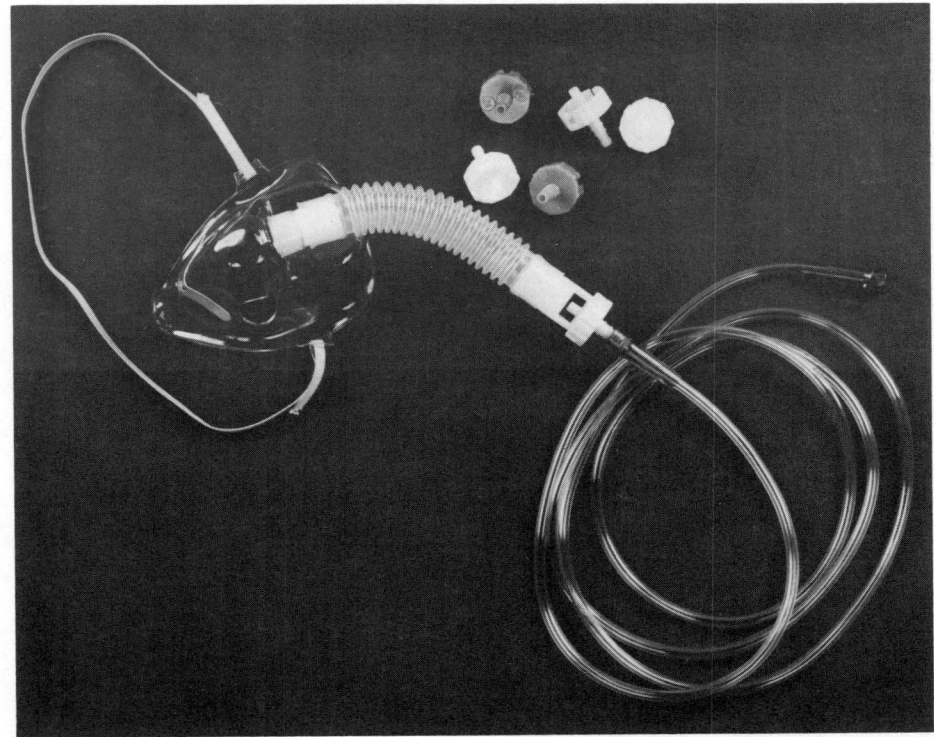

Figure 2–16. Venturi mask.

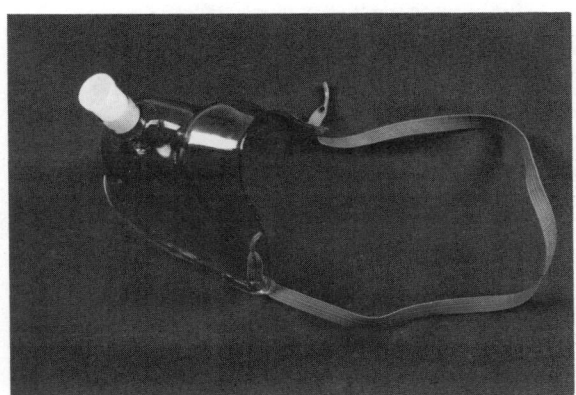

Figure 2–17. Face tent (shield).

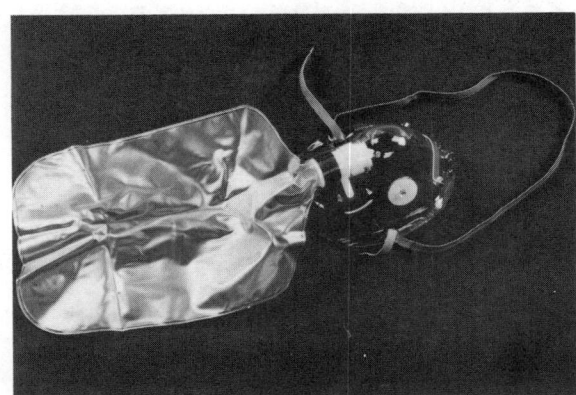

Figure 2–18. Partial rebreathing mask (nonrebreathing mask).

(continued)

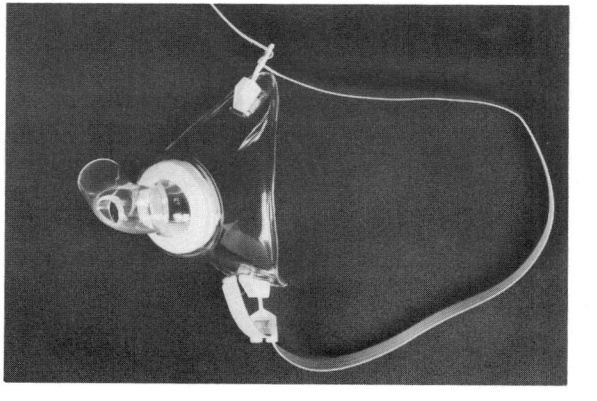

Figure 2–19. Trach collar or mask.

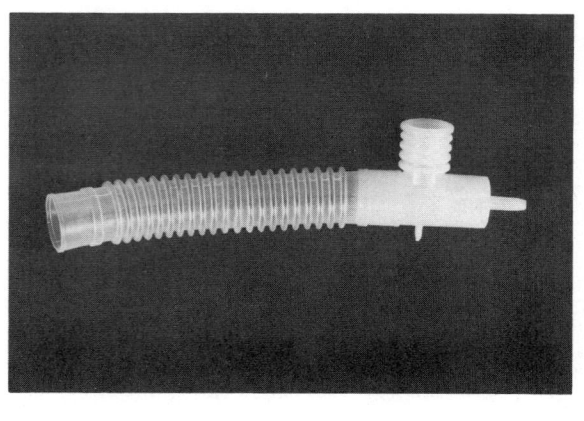

Figure 2–20. T-tube (trach).

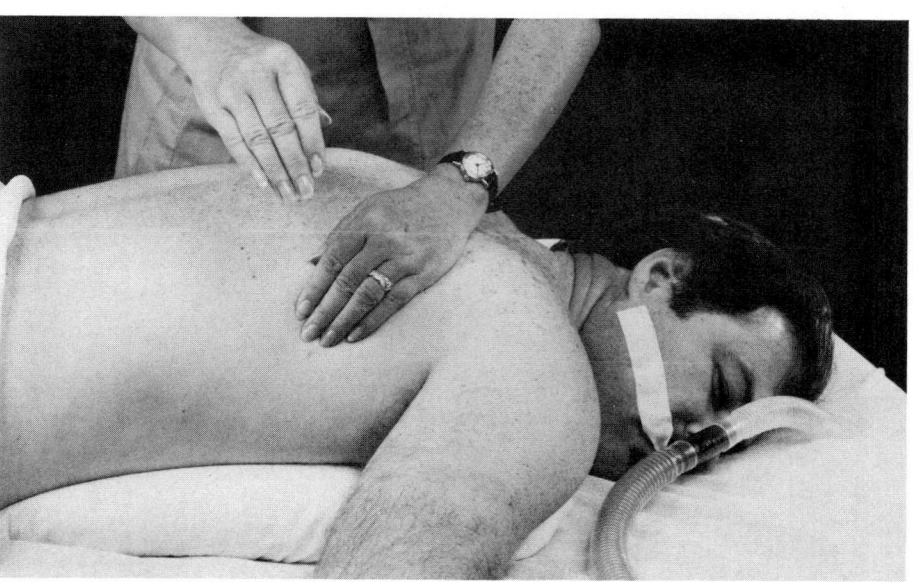

Figure 2–21. Posterior segment: right upper lobe.

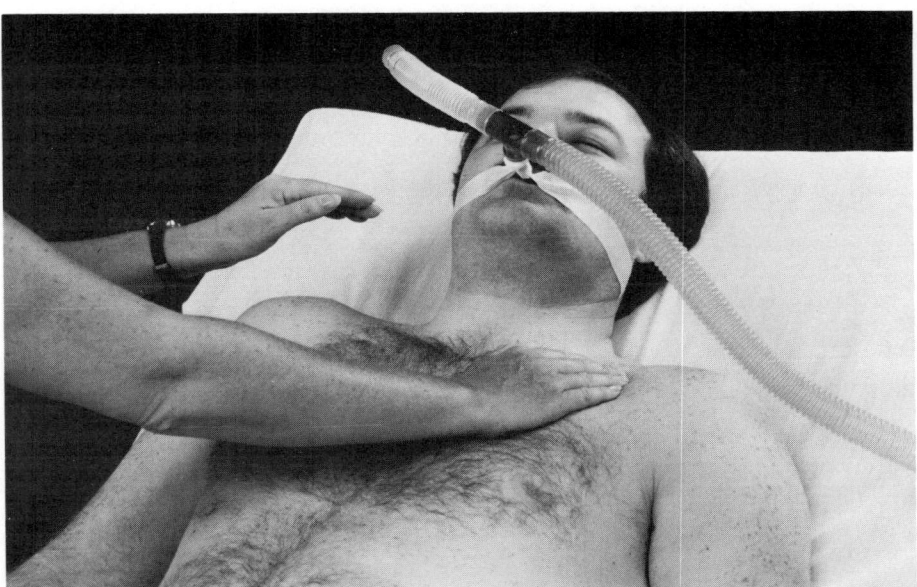

Figure 2–22. Apical segments: upper lobes.

Care of the Patient Requiring Assistance with Airway Management

NURSING DIAGNOSES	RATIONALE	DEFINING CHARACTERISTICS	EXPECTED OUTCOME
1. Airway clearance, ineffective	1. In the unconscious patient, occlusion of the posterior oropharynx by a flaccid tongue is the most common cause of airway obstruction. When this situation occurs, the first response is to open the airway by tilting the head backward and raising the mandible. In patients with cervical spine injuries, a simple chin lift may be employed. This measure is only temporary. Devices that will assist in maintaining patency include the oral and nasal airway. Ventilatory support can be provided, if necessary, with mouth-to-mouth resuscitation, a bag-valve-mask apparatus, or with a positive pressure device. When ventilatory support is required, an esophageal obturator airway, endotracheal tube, or tracheostomy tube may be inserted by specially trained personnel to reestablish and maintain airway patency	1. Snoring respirations Unconsciousness Occlusion of posterior oropharynx by flaccid tongue Ineffective or absent cough mechanism Rhonchi	1. The airway is maintained patent and is as free of obstructing substances as possible
2. Injury, potential for	2. Patients unable to clear secretions must often be assisted to do so with nasopharyngeal or oropharyngeal suctioning. Repeated suctioning, especially nasopharyngeal, can cause trauma to the mucosa and ultimately bleeding. Realizing this, the practitioner can prevent injury by suctioning through a nasopharyngeal airway, thus protecting the nasal mucosa. It is important to note that the nasal airway is also useful for maintaining a patent airway in patients with facial or jaw fractures	2. Need for frequent nasotracheal suction Nasal bleeding	2. No trauma occurs to the nasal mucosa

NURSING INTERVENTIONS

1. Assess respiratory rate and pattern, breath sounds, ABG, presence or absence of central cyanosis, and level of consciousness frequently
2. If the patient is unconscious, the tongue flaccid, occluding the posterior oropharynx, and the respiratory rate and pattern altered (i.e., uneven snoring respirations), an artificial airway may be needed to allow adequate ventilation

3. Insert an oropharyngeal or oral airway as follows:
   A. Open the mouth
   B. Insert the airway over the tongue, with the end pointed toward the roof of the mouth (Fig. 2–23)
   C. Advance the airway slowly, turning it over as it is moved toward the back of the throat (Fig. 2–24)
   D. An alternate method of insertion would be to hold the tongue down with a tongue blade while directly inserting the oral airway
   E. Gagging may occur but is usually temporary. Careful attention, should vomiting occur, will prevent aspiration. If gagging is excessive, remove the airway immediately
   F. Anchor the airway by placing strips of tape across the flanged edges
   G. A side-lying position will minimize aspiration, should vomiting occur
   H. Perform mouth care q8h or more frequently as necessary. Observe integrity of skin around mouth. Reposition airway as necessary to prevent pressure
   I. Suction oropharynx as needed to maintain airway patency
4. If the patient requires frequent nasotracheal or nasopharyngeal suctioning, a nasopharyngeal airway may be used to prevent nasal trauma. Insert as follows:
   A. Select a tube of proper length by measuring from the end of the patient's nose to the earlobe. Mark the proper distance on the tube, if necessary. The diameter of the tube should be slightly larger than the nostril. This will allow a close fit
   B. Lubricate the tube with water or lubricant
   C. Gently insert the tube into the nostril while pressing the tip of the nose upward. Advance the tube, following the natural curvature of the nasopharynx, until fully inserted
   D. Check placement by having the patient exhale through the nose. Air will move freely through the tube. Observe the tip of the tube behind the uvula, using a tongue blade to depress the tongue
   E. If the tube is left in place, humidification should be provided to maintain patency
   F. The tube should be suctioned thoroughly prior to removal. If it is difficult to remove, lubricate the areas around the tip of the nose and gently rotate

OUTCOME CRITERIA

1. Adequate airway clearance will be maintained providing optimal ventilation and ABGs
2. Patient's nasal mucosa will remain free of trauma, with no bleeding noted

DOCUMENTATION

- Respiratory rate and pattern (presence of uneven snoring respirations), breath sounds, (present, absent) adventitious sounds, ABGs, presence or absence of central cyanosis, and level of consciousness
- Insertion and maintenance of artificial airway (oropharyngeal or nasopharyngeal)
- Positioning of patient
- Mouth care performed and condition of oral mucosa
- Suctioning: Frequency, amount of secretions, color, character, and odor
- Patient's ability to maintain a patent airway
- Humidification and oxygen therapy, if applicable (type, flow rate, concentration)
- Any evidence of nasal bleeding (amount, character, time, and nature of occurrence)

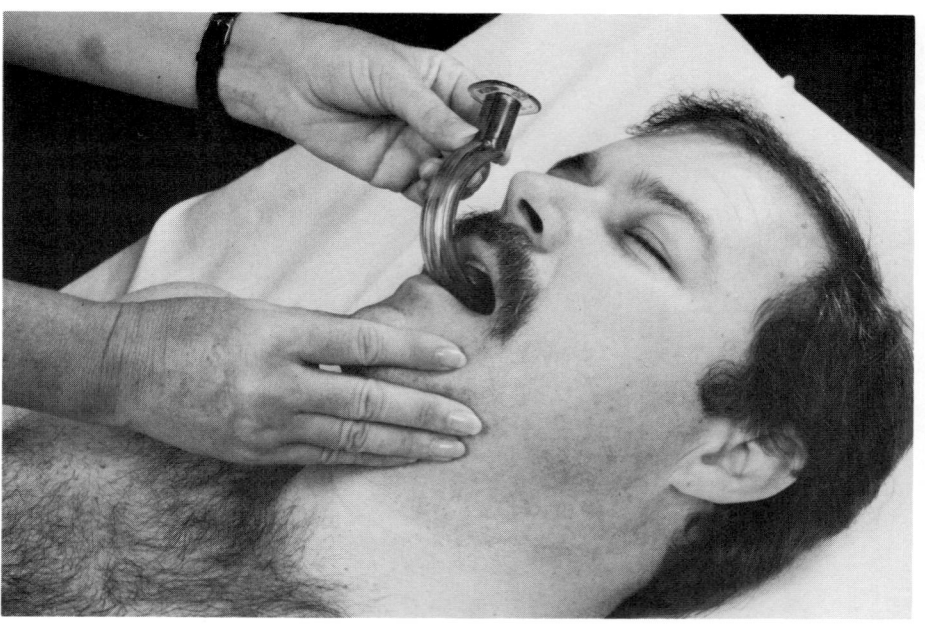

Figure 2–23. Airway insertion.

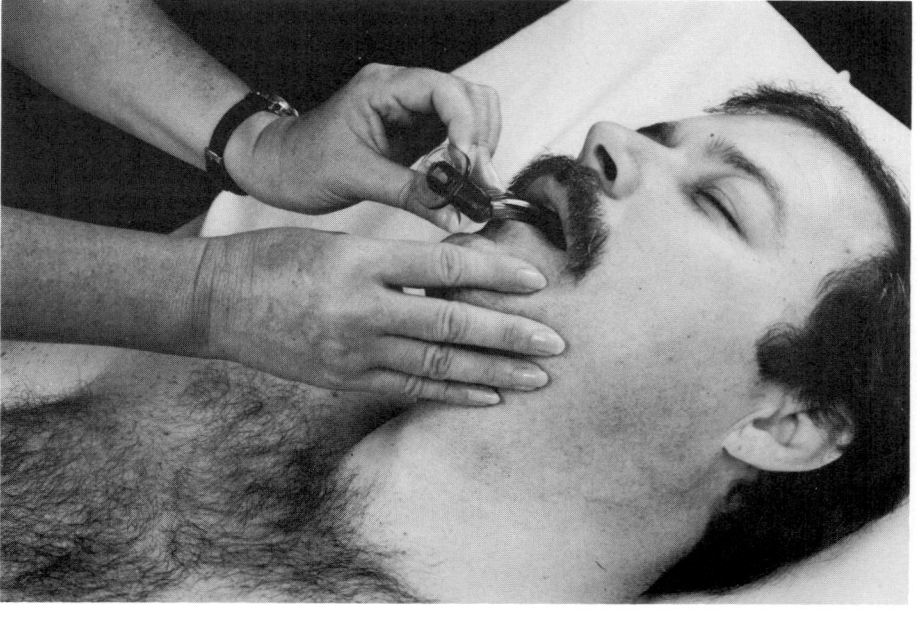

Figure 2–24. Oropharyngeal airway in place.

Care of the Patient Requiring Endotracheal Intubation

NURSING DIAGNOSES	RATIONALE	DEFINING CHARACTERISTICS	EXPECTED OUTCOME
1. Breathing pattern, ineffective	1. Breathing pattern may be affected by respiratory center impairment, neuromuscular impairment, musculoskeletal impairment, and alterations in lung tissue compliance	1. Shortness of breath, dyspnea Arterial blood gas abnormalities Altered respiratory rate and pattern	1. An effective breathing pattern will be maintained
2. Gas exchange, impaired	2. Gas exchange may be impaired by low FIo_2, alveolar hypoventilation, ventilation–perfusion abnormalities, and diffusion impairment	2. Arterial blood gas abnormalities Central cynanosis Shortness of breath, dyspnea Mental status changes, such as anxiety, restlessness, confusion, depression, lethargy, fatigue, headache, or changes in sleep pattern, may vary according to character of alteration of blood gases Abnormal respiratory rate and pattern	2. Respiratory gas exchange will be maintained at an optimal level
3. Airway clearance, ineffective	3. Airway clearance may be affected by the presence of an upper airway obstruction or by the inability to clear secretions	3. Unconscious Uneven, snoring respirations Flaccid tongue occluding posterior oropharynx Ineffective or absent cough reflex Rhonchi, wheezes, decreased breath sounds, bronchial breath sounds, rales (atelectasis) Stridor with dyspnea, increased respiratory rate and effort Anxiety Decreased V_T ABG abnormalities Central cyanosis	3. Airways will be patent and free of obstructing substances
4. Communication, impaired	4. Placement of an endotracheal tube creates a physical barrier, preventing air from passing over the vocal cords. Speech is impossible	4. Inability to speak with endotracheal tube in place	4. Patient will communicate effectively with staff and significant others
5. Injury, potential for	5. Endotracheal intubation is a life-sustaining measure and yet may potentially produce several complications. Among the common complications are tracheal stenosis–necrosis, oral mucosal ulceration, and pulmonary infection. Endotracheal tubes may be inserted via the nasal route or the oral route. Nasotracheal intubation is generally reserved for elective situations, although it is more comfortable for the patient. Orotracheal intubation is the more common procedure	5. Blood-tinged sputum Areas of ulceration on tongue or lips Change in character or volume of sputum	5. No complications associated with endotracheal intubation will occur

Preintubation

1. Hyperoxygenate the patient prior to intubation, if possible
2. Select appropriate size (Fig. 2–25)
3. Check endotracheal tube cuff for leaks

During Intubation

1. Assure that oxygen therapy is not interrupted for prolonged periods of time. Do not interrupt CPR for more than 15–20 seconds. If intubation is unsuccessful, hyperoxygenate and attempt again
2. Have suction available should vomiting occur
3. Suction nasopharynx as needed

Postintubation

1. Low-pressure cuffed tubes should be used at all times. Inflate cuff using the minimal leak technique. If this technique is used, periodic deflation is not considered necessary. If the cuff is inflated using a pressure manometer, inflate to a maximum of 20 mm Hg or 25 cm H_2O pressure; measure pressures q4–8h and reinflate as necessary
2. Ensure proper tube placement by:
   A. Auscultation of the chest for bilateral breath sounds
   B. Inspection and palpation of the chest for bilateral excursion
   C. Note movement of air through the tube with respirations
   D. Chest x-ray documentation of tube position (Fig. 2–26)
3. If orally intubated, place a bite block or oral airway in the mouth to prevent biting of the tube and to provide a route for oropharyngeal suctioning
4. Tape the tube securely
5. Check tube placement (auscultate for bilateral breath sounds, observe chest excursion) frequently
6. Provide humidification (i.e., T-tube)
7. Trim excess length from the tube so that only 1 inch extends from the mouth or nose. This avoids kinking of the tube and obstruction
8. Move the tube from one side of the mouth to the other every 8 hours to avoid pressure areas on the tongue or lips. Perform mouth care q8h or more often, as needed. Note any areas of ulceration on the tongue or lips
9. Perform pulmonary toiletry as necessary to maintain airway patency (indicator: rhonchi on auscultation). Note any blood-tinged sputum
10. Assess ventilatory status frequently (e.g., rate and pattern of respirations, arterial blood gases, mental status, cyanosis)
11. Provide patient with a Magic Slate or blackboard to communicate with staff and significant others. If the patient is unable to read or write, develop a code for communication (e.g., nodding of the head, finger code)
12. Position the call signal within the patient's reach at all times
13. When the patient is able to maintain an adequate airway, ventilation, and blood gases without mechanical support, he may be extubated per physician's order
    A. Elevate head of the bed 45 degrees
    B. Suction the endotracheal tube and oropharynx or nasopharynx thoroughly
    C. Ventilate the patient using a self-inflating bag
    D. Deflate the cuff on the endotracheal tube
    E. Remove the tube during peak inflation with the bag
    F. Monitor and observe the following
       a. ABG 30 minutes postextubation
       b. Ventilatory status
       c. Presence or absence of stridor or SOB or dyspnea

(continued)

OUTCOME CRITERIA

1. Respiratory rate and pattern will be adequate
2. ABG will be within normal limits
3. Rhonchi and wheezes will decrease or clear. Breath sounds will be improved
4. Communication with staff and significant others will take place
5. Character of sputum will remain unchanged
   Trauma to oral cavity and mucosa will be promptly recognized and treated
   Volume of sputum will be decreased

DOCUMENTATION

- Intubation with hyperoxygenation
- Cuff inflated or deflated and technique used. If pressure manometer used, amount of pressure maintained
- Postplacement of tube
   Bilateral breath sounds
   Bilateral chest excursion
   Patency of tube
   Chest x-ray shows placement above carina
- Reassessment of tube placement at least q2h and more frequently if necessary
- Oxygen–humidification therapy (i.e., type, percentage, flow rate)
- Mouth care and condition of oral mucosa q4h
- Pulmonary toiletry performance and results (i.e., sputum production, amount, color, character, and odor)
- Patient's ability to communicate and the methods used
- Extubation of patient and critical observations following extubation
   ABG 30 minutes postextubation
   Ventilatory status (i.e., chest excursion, breath sounds, mental status, presence or absence of cyanosis)
   Presence or absence of stridor, SOB or dyspnea

SPECIAL NOTE

Minimal Leak

Minimal leak technique on low-pressure cuffed endotracheal or tracheostomy tubes is carried out as follows (Fig. 2–27):

1. Place the diaphragm of the stethoscope next to the trachea
2. Insert air through the balloon port until no air leak is heard
3. Withdraw enough air to create a minimal leak on peak inspiration. Slight air turbulence should be heard

Suctioning

Special considerations in performing pulmonary toiletry on the intubated patient include:

1. Hyperoxygenate with 100% O_2 prior to suctioning and between each entry to suction
2. Normal saline (sterile) may be injected through the tube followed by ventilations with a self-inflating bag to loosen secretions, if needed
3. Aseptic technique must be utilized when suctioning
4. Suction should be applied for no longer than 10–15 seconds

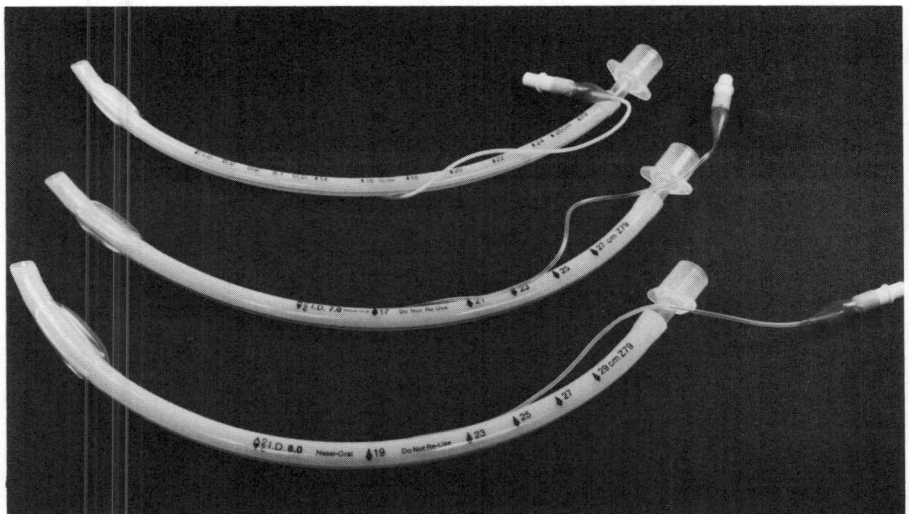

Figure 2–25. Sizes of endotracheal tubes.

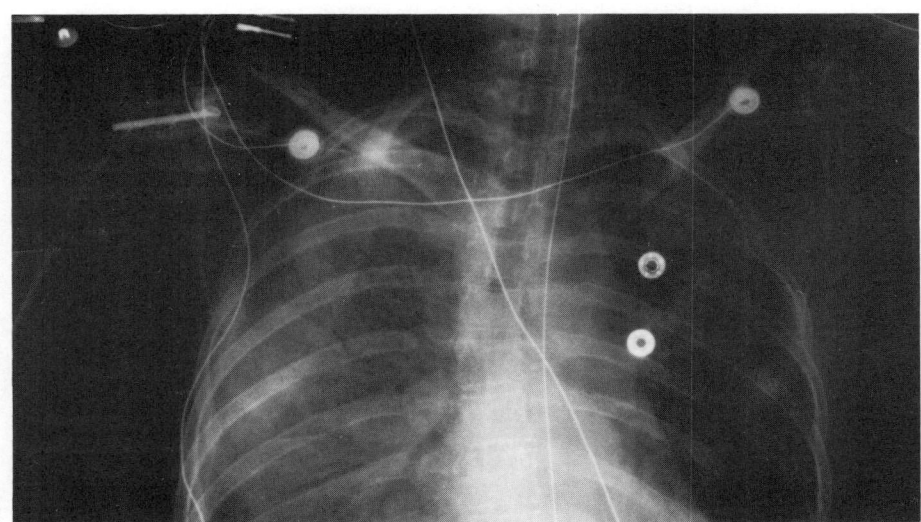

Figure 2–26. Chest x-ray documentation of tube position.

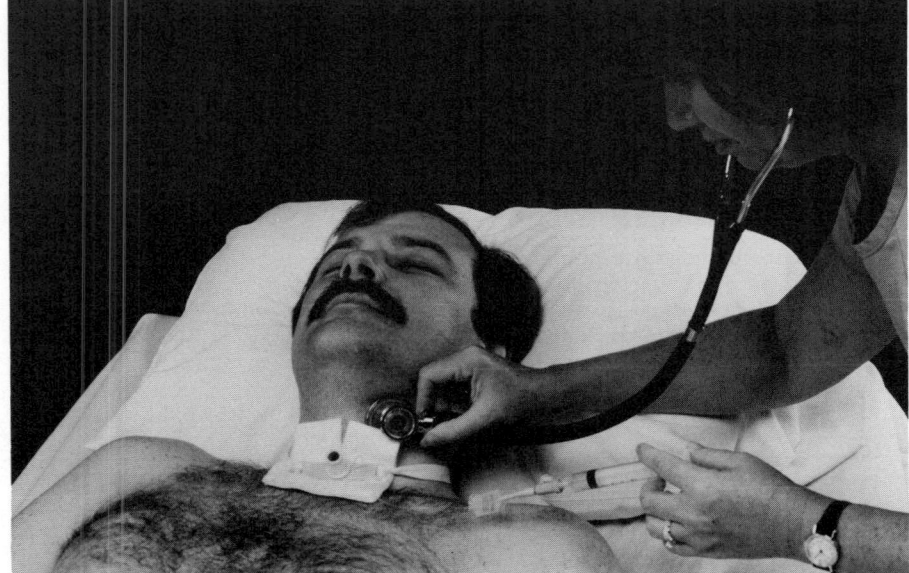

Figure 2–27. Minimal leak technique.

Care of the Patient with a Tracheostomy

NURSING DIAGNOSES	RATIONALE	DEFINING CHARACTERISTICS	EXPECTED OUTCOME
1. Breathing pattern, ineffective	1. Breathing pattern may be affected by respiratory center impairment, neuromuscular impairment, musculoskeletal impairment, and alterations in lung tissue compliance	1. Shortness of breath ABG abnormalities Altered respiratory rate and pattern	1. An effective breathing pattern will be maintained
2. Gas exchange, impaired	2. Gas exchange may be impaired by low FIO_2, alveolar hypoventilation, ventilation–perfusion abnormalities, and diffusion impairment	2. ABG abnormalities Central cynanosis Shortness of breath Mental status changes, such as anxiety, restlessness, confusion, depression, lethargy, fatigue, headache, or changes in sleep pattern, may vary according to character of alteration of blood gases Abnormal respiratory rate and pattern	2. Gas exchange will be maintained at an optimal level
3. Airway clearance, ineffective	3. Airway clearance may be affected by the presence of an upper airway obstruction (e.g., edema, lesions) or by an inability to clear secretions	3. Unconscious Uneven, snoring respirations Flaccid tongue Ineffective or absent cough reflex Rhonchi, wheezes, decreased breath sounds, bronchial breath sounds, rales (atelectasis) Stridor with dyspnea and increased respiratory rate and effort Anxiety Decreased V_T ABG abnormalities Central cyanosis	3. Airway is patent and free of obstructing substances
4. Communication, impaired	4. If the cuff on a cuffed tracheostomy tube is inflated, the patient will not be able to speak due to the physical barrier preventing passage of air upward through the vocal cords. With a deflated cuff, a fenestrated or uncuffed tube, the patient can be taught to speak around the tube	4. Inability to speak with tracheostomy tube in place	4. Effective communication with staff and significant others occurs
5. Injury, potential for	5. Common complications associated with tracheostomy tubes include tracheal stenosis–necrosis, tracheal wound infection, bleeding from the tracheal wound, innominate artery erosion, pulmonary infection, and subcutaneous emphysema (Figs. 2–28 and 2–29)	5. Blood-tinged sputum, purulent drainage or bleeding from tracheal wound, frank blood in tracheostomy, change in character or volume of sputum, or subcutaneous crepitus	5. No complications associated with tracheostomy occur

1. Immediately postoperative, observe closely for extensive bleeding from wound (look behind neck for gravity-dependent drainage)
2. If the patient is being mechanically ventilated or to prevent aspiration, inflate cuff using the minimal leak technique or a cuff pressure manometer
3. Ensure tube placement by
   A. Auscultation of chest for bilateral breath sounds
   B. Inspection and palpation for bilateral chest excursion
   C. Noting movement of air through the tube
   D. Chest x-ray documentation of position of the tube
4. Perform tracheostomy care q8h and more frequently if needed
   A. Remove soiled dressing
   B. Using sterile technique, cleanse the site with hydrogen peroxide, removing any secretions
   C. Saline-soaked sponges may be applied around the site if additional loosening of encrusted secretions is required
   D. If the tracheostomy tube has an inner cannula, remove and clean:
      a. Immerse in hydrogen peroxide and clean with a brush or pipe cleaner
      b. Rinse in sterile water
      c. Reinsert into tracheostomy tube
   E. Tracheostomy ties should be changed whenever they become encrusted with drainage or secretions:
      a. Tie the ties in a knot, never a bow
      b. Tie the ties snugly but allow enough space for two fingers to be inserted between the ties and the neck
   F. Place the new dressing around the tube
5. Perform pulmonary toiletry as necessary to maintain airway patency
6. Assess ventilatory status frequently
7. Provide patient with a Magic Slate or blackboard for communication with staff and significant others. If the patient is unable to read or write, develop a code of communication (e.g., nodding of head, finger code)
8. Maintain the call signal within the patient's reach at all times
9. If the cuff is deflated, the patient can learn to speak by inhaling, placing a finger over the end of the tube, and then speaking on exhalation
10. Maintain an obturator and an extra tracheostomy tube at the bedside at all times. A tracheal dilator should be at the bedside for at least the first 24 hours after the procedure

OUTCOME CRITERIA

1. Maintenance or return of adequate respiratory rate, pattern, and V_T will continue to be maintained
2. Maintenance or return to optimal ABG levels
3. Decrease or clearing of rhonchi, wheezes, and improved breath sounds
   Prevention of the development of bronchial breath sounds and rales
4. Patient able to communicate with staff and significant others
5. Patient will be able to speak around tube if cuff is deflated
6. Patient will be able to speak adequately if a speaking tracheostomy tube is used
7. Patient sustains minimal or no complications as evidenced by
   Minimal or no blood-tinged sputum
   Absence of inflammation and purulent drainage at tracheal wound site
   Character and volume of sputum decreases or remains unchanged
   Freedom from or early detection of subcutaneous emphysema
   Any signs of complications are recognized and treated promptly

(continued)

DOCUMENTATION

- Any bleeding around tracheostomy site
- Cuff inflated or deflated (if deflated, patient tolerance of)
- Tube placement status
    Bilateral breath sounds
    Bilateral chest excursion
    Position of tube above carina determined by x-ray
- Tracheostomy care performed and observations regarding drainage around tube (color, consistency, volume)
- Pulmonary toiletry
    Performance
    Sputum (amount, color, character, odor)
- Ventilatory status
- Ability of patient to communicate with staff or significant others and method used

SPECIAL NOTE

Communication

Talking tracheostomy tubes are now available in some institutions and should be used whenever possible. Special care for a talking tracheostomy tube includes (Fig. 2–30):

1. Daily flushing of air vent:
    A. Tracheostomy cuff must be inflated during procedure and the inner cannula must be in place
    B. Remove the speaking air supply and connection from the transparent tube
    C. Flush the air supply tube back and forth with 10 ml of saline
    D. Remove the saline when finished
    E. Reattach the connector and apply suction to remove residual saline
2. Assisting the patient to speak:
    A. Attach 6–8 L/min (up to a maximum of 12 L) of humidified oxygen or compressed air to the air supply vent
    B. To speak, the patient must place a finger over the large part of the vent. This allows the air supply to travel up through the vocal cords and the patient to speak

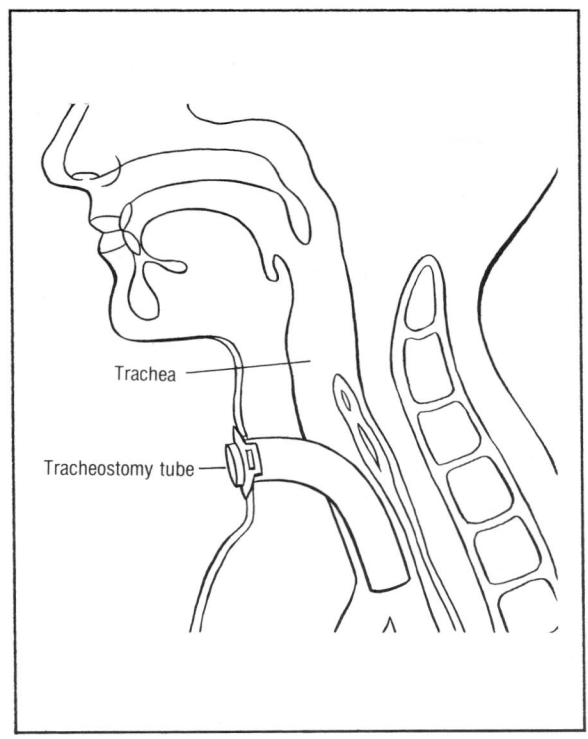

Figure 2–28. Anatomical position of tracheostomy tube. *(From Norton, B. A., & Miller, A. M. Skills for professional nursing practice. Norwalk, Conn.: Appleton-Century-Crofts, 1986, p. 801, with permission.)*

In the diagram: Trachea, Tracheostomy tube

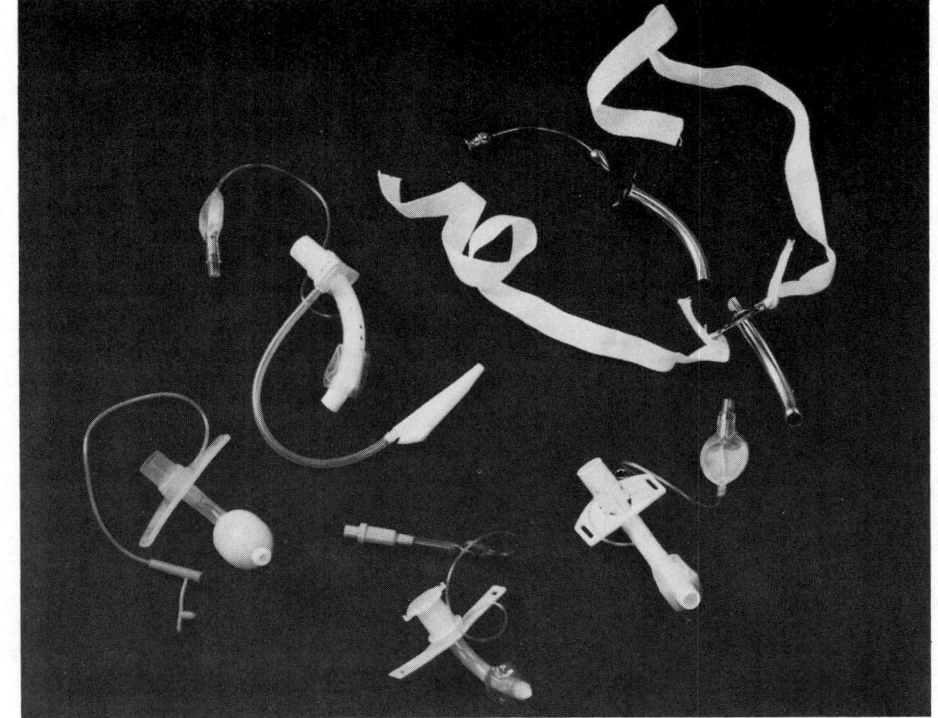

Figure 2–29. Types of tracheostomy tubes may vary, but principles of care do not.

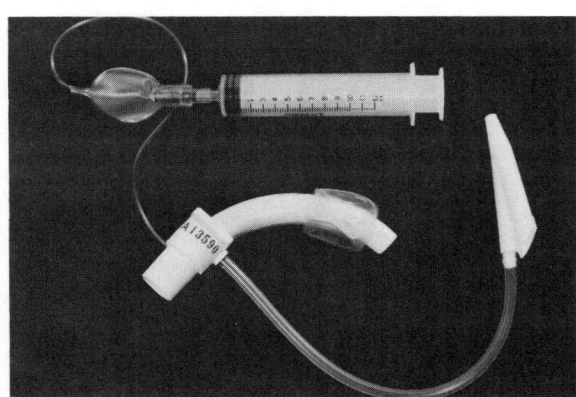

Figure 2–30. Communitrach.

Care of the Patient Requiring Continuous Ventilatory Support

NURSING DIAGNOSES	RATIONALE	DEFINING CHARACTERISTICS	EXPECTED OUTCOME
1. Breathing pattern, in-effective	1. Breathing pattern may be affected by respiratory center impairment, neuromuscular impairment, musculoskeletal impairment, and alterations in lung tissue compliance	1. Shortness of breath ABG abnormalities Altered respiratory rate and pattern	1. An effective breathing pattern is maintained
2. Gas exchange, impaired	2. Gas exchange may be impaired by low FIO_2, alveolar hypoventilation, ventilation–perfusion abnormalities, or diffusion impairment	2. ABG abnormalities Central cyanosis Shortness of breath Mental status changes, such as anxiety, restlessness, confusion, depression, lethargy, fatigue, headache, changes in sleep pattern, may vary according to character of alteration of blood gases	2. Gas exchange is maintained at an optimal level

3. Injury, potential for	3. Complications attributed to continuous ventilatory support are generally related to artificial airways (i.e., endotracheal or tracheostomy tubes), oxygen administration (i.e., oxygen toxicity), or positive pressure ventilators (i.e., barotrauma and impaired cardiac output).
	    Barotrauma and impaired cardiac output occur most often with the use of positive end expiratory pressure (PEEP). Artificial airway complications and oxygen toxicity have been previously discussed, and therefore this section addresses barotrauma specifically
		3. Barotrauma or spontaneous pneumothorax may be recognized by the following signs and symptoms
		   Abnormal breath sounds (decreased or absent)
		   Asymmetrical chest excursion
		   Tracheal shifting
		   Changes in vital signs (e.g., tachycardia hypotension)
		   Changes in arterial blood gas values
		   Subcutaneous emphysema
		   Decreased cardiac output
			3. No injury associated with continuous ventilatory support will occur

NURSING INTERVENTIONS

1. Maintain a patent airway by
   A. Proper endotracheal or tracheostomy tube positioning
   B. Proper inflation of endotracheal–tracheostomy cuff
   C. Adequate pulmonary toiletry
2. Maintain adequate ventilatory support by
   A. Monitoring ventilatory settings every hour
      V_T
      I:E ratio
      Sensitivity
      FIO_2
      Peak inspiratory airway pressure

Sigh
Humidity and temperature
Rate
Alarm system
B. Monitoring patient response to ventilatory support
ABG
Presence or absence of central cyanosis
Respiratory rate and pattern (patient ventilatory effort synchronous with ventilator)
Level of consciousness
Mental status
Breath sounds
Symmetry of chest excursion
Vital signs
ECG
Cardiac output
C. Monitoring the patient for possible injury (i.e., barotrauma)
Symmetry of chest excursion
Breath sounds
Tachycardia
Central cyanosis
Hypotension
Decreased cardiac output
Subcutaneous emphysema
Tracheal position
D. Prevent injury or barotrauma by
Monitoring and maintaining PEEP or PEEP with IMV as ordered
Maintaining good pulmonary toiletry
E. Monitoring for return of adequate breathing pattern and gas exchange to begin weaning from ventilatory support

OUTCOME CRITERIA

1. Adequate respiratory rate, pattern, and V_T will be maintained
2. Adequate respiratory rate, pattern, and V_T will return
3. Maintenance or return to optimal ABG levels
4. Signs and symptoms of barotrauma will be promptly detected and treated

DOCUMENTATION

- Airway patency
  Tube position
  Cuff inflation
  Pulmonary toiletry status
- Ventilator settings (usually recorded on a flowsheet)
- Patient response to ventilatory support, including signs of complications
  ABG
  Presence or absence of central cyanosis
  Respiratory rate and pattern (patient: machine ratio)
  Level of consciousness
  Mental status (e.g., anxious, confused)

(continued)

Breath sounds (bilateral)
Chest excursion (symmetrical, nonsymmetrical)
Vital signs (pulse, BP)
Cardiac rate and rhythm
Cardiac output
Presence or absence of subcutaneous emphysema
Tracheal position

SPECIAL NOTE

Monitoring

Many institutions have respiratory therapists who routinely monitor ventilatory settings and record them on a flowsheet. It remains a nursing responsibility to know the settings and whom to notify should a problem arise.

Weaning

Methods and protocols for weaning patients from continuous ventilatory support vary from institution to institution. General considerations in weaning include:

1. Ventilatory function adequate to maintain acceptable ABG (i.e., V_T, V_C)
2. Muscle strength adequate to support ventilatory function
3. Patient not requiring FIO_2 greater than 0.40 or PEEP
4. Patient maintaining a patent airway

During weaning, the following parameters must be monitored closely:

1. ABG
2. V_T, V_C
3. Respiratory rate and pattern
4. Increased SOB, dyspnea
5. ECG
6. Anxiety level
7. Diaphoresis

Types of Ventilators

Continuous ventilatory support can be provided by a variety of methods. Positive pressure devices are most commonly used and can be categorized as follows (Figs. 2–31 and 2–32):

- Assist: Responds to and augments patient's inspiratory effort
- Control: Unresponsive to patient's effort, ventilates according to preset intervals
- Assist–control: Operates on both modes, assistance and control
- Volume cycled: Inspiratory phase ends when preset volume is reached
- Time cycled: Change over from inspiratory phase to expiratory phase is determined by preset timing
- Pressure cycled: Inspiratory phase ends when preset pressure is reached
- Combined: Some ventilators have more than one cycling capability (e.g., time and pressure). Cycling will be dependent upon which parameter is reached first (Fig. 2–33)

Devices used to augment ventilatory support provided by positive pressure include PEEP, CPAP, and IMV.

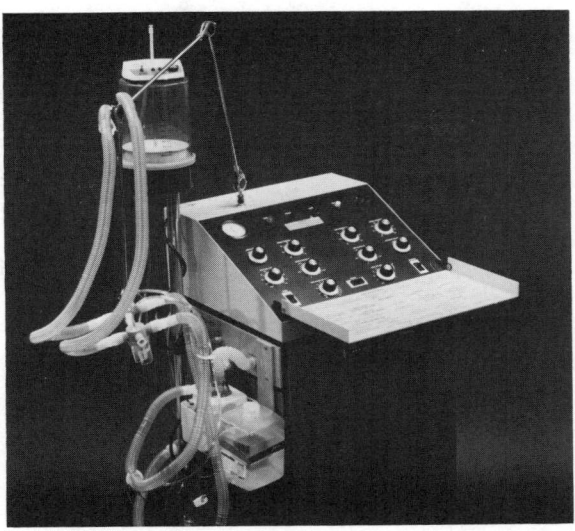

Figure 2–31. MA-1 ventilator.

bird
MARK 7
respirator
OFF
AIR-MIX

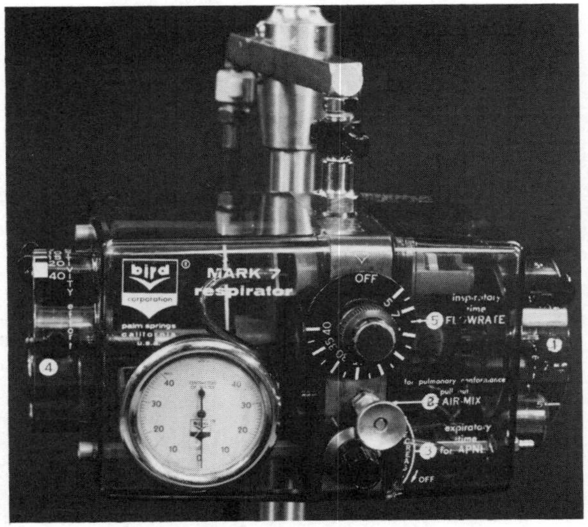

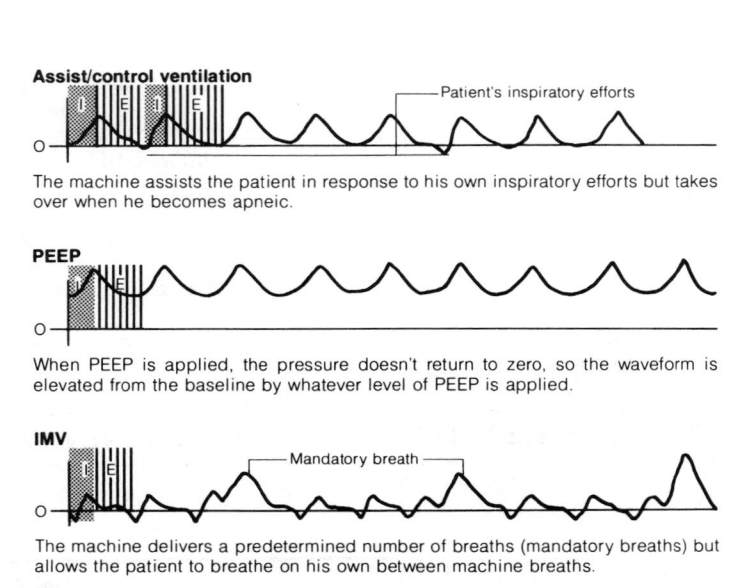

Figure 2–32. Bird ventilator.

These drawings show how a normal breathing pattern is modified by patient-ventilator systems. The horizontal line O represents the baseline pressure of zero, I represents inspiration, and E represents expiration.
Spontaneous (normal) breathing
I
E
O
1 minute
Inspiration creates a negative pressure (below the baseline), while expiration creates a small positive pressure (above the baseline).
Controlled ventilation
Mechanical sigh
I
E
O
The machine does everything; the waveform moves from zero pressure to the maximum inspiratory pressure and back to zero.
Assisted ventilation
I
E
O
The machine cycles on in response to the patient's inspiratory efforts (small negative pressure), which triggers the respirator to deliver a preset volume (positive pressure).
Assist/control ventilation
Patient's inspiratory efforts
I
E
I
E
O
The machine assists the patient in response to his own inspiratory efforts but takes over when he becomes apneic.
PEEP
I
E
O
When PEEP is applied, the pressure doesn't return to zero, so the waveform is elevated from the baseline by whatever level of PEEP is applied.
IMV
Mandatory breath
I
E
O
The machine delivers a predetermined number of breaths (mandatory breaths) but allows the patient to breathe on his own between machine breaths.

Figure 2–33. Ventilatory wave patterns. *(From Fuchs, P. Understanding continuous mechanical ventilation.* Nursing 79, *1979, 9(12), 29, copyright 1979, Springhouse Corporation, with permission.)*

Care of the Patient Requiring Chest Tubes

NURSING DIAGNOSES	RATIONALE	DEFINING CHARACTERISTICS	EXPECTED OUTCOME
1. Breathing pattern, in-effective	1. Conditions interfering with breathing pattern requiring insertion of a chest tube include pleural air or fluid interfering with lung expansion. Pneumothorax (air) or hemothorax (blood) represent the most common occurrences necessitating chest tube insertion. Pneumothorax is the more common of the two. Pneumothorax can occur as either closed (simple), tension, or open (communicating). The need for intervention is usually associated with the size or severity of the pneumothorax	1. Pneumothorax Decrease or absence of breath sounds in affected area Rales adjacent to affected area Sudden, sharp pain in chest Shortness of breath, dyspnea Central cyanosis Anxiety Air-percussion note hyperresonant Tracheal shifting (with tension pneumothorax to unaffected side) Nonsymmetrical excursion Abnormal ABGs Changes in respiratory rate and pattern Hemothorax Decrease or absence of breath sounds Shortness of breath, dyspnea Nonsymmetrical excursion Changes in respiratory rate and pattern Fluid-percussion note flat	1. Effective breathing pattern is maintained
2. Injury, potential for	2. The most common complications that occur are infection, hemorrhage, and tension pneumothorax	2. Fever, purulent drainage around chest tube insertion site or from tube Bloody drainage from tube or around insertion site Sudden SOB, dyspnea, cyanosis, anxiety, tracheal shifting, nonsymmetrical excursion of chest, abnormal ABGs, increased respiratory rate and heart rate, and decreased BP	2. No complications associated with chest tubes will occur

NURSING INTERVENTIONS

Observations
1. Changes in breath sounds
2. Adventitious sounds
3. Sudden chest pain
4. Shortness of breath
5. Dyspnea
6. Central cyanosis
7. Anxiety
8. Percussion note: Hyperresonant or flat

9. Tracheal shifting
10. Asymmetrical chest excursion
11. Sudden unexplained abnormal ABG (acute hypoxemia)
12. Changes in respiratory rate and pattern

Preinsertion

Patient should be placed in upright or semi-upright position (lung tissue will fall free from the chest wall).

During Insertion

Upon connection to drainage system, bubbling in the waterseal chamber indicates escape of air from the chest.

After Insertion

1. Maintain chest tube drainage system as prescribed
   A. Systems available include traditional waterseal (i.e., one, two, or three bottle) or disposable units (waterseal or waterless) (Figs. 2–34 to 2–38)
   B. Maintain all water levels at proper prescribed levels (20 cm H_2O pressure is maximum recommended)
   C. Maintain pressure settings or adjustments as prescribed
   D. Monitor amount of chest drainage hourly until stable and then q8h thereafter
   E. Observe for air bubbles in system (air leak). If previous bubbling has ceased, check breath sounds for full lung reexpansion
   F. Maintain intact occlusive dressing at insertion site
   G. Tape all tubing connections tight and free from leaks
   H. Maintain drainage tubing in a loop secured to the bed (do not allow to hang down on side of bed)
   I. Strip tubing as necessary to maintain free drainage. Beginning near the insertion site, pinch the tubing with one hand while stripping with the other toward the drainage system. Stripping in sections from top downward is recommended
   J. Chest tube should not be clamped for any reason. Tension pneumothorax could develop. When transporting patient maintain chest tube to gravity drainage by simply discontinuing suction without disconnecting the patient from the waterseal or waterless unit
2. Assess the patient frequently for
   A. Changes in breath sounds
   B. Changes in respiratory rate and pattern
   C. Adventitious sounds
   D. Changes in level of comfort (e.g., pain at insertion site)
   E. Changes in SOB, dyspnea
   F. Central cyanosis
   G. Changes in anxiety level
   H. Changes in percussion note
   I. Tracheal shifting
   J. Changes in chest excursion
   K. Changes in ABG
   L. Fever
   M. Changes in color or character of chest drainage, such as purulence, bleeding, or in amount of chest drainage, such as abrupt cessation
   N. Bleeding through chest tubes or around insertion site
3. Mark chest drainage level a minimum of once q8h or more often if necessary. Immediately following chest tube insertion, this may be indicated every hour or more often

(continued)

OUTCOME CRITERIA

1. Maintenance or return of adequate respiratory rate, pattern, and V_T
2. Lung will be fully reexpanded
3. Complications associated with chest tube therapy will be promptly detected and treated

DOCUMENTATION

Preinsertion Assessment

- Presence or absence of bilateral breath sounds
- Adventitious sounds
- Chest excursion (symmetrical, nonsymmetrical)
- Rate and pattern of respirations
- Percussion note: Hyperresonant? flat?
- Any chest pain or discomfort
- Any SOB or dyspnea
- Presence or absence of central cyanosis
- Mental status, level of consciousness
- Tracheal position (midline, shifted)

Following Chest Tube Insertion

- Type of system
- Amount of negative pressure
- Amount and character of chest tube drainage
- Presence or absence of air leak
- Dressing intact and character of any drainage around dressing
- Dressing changes, if necessary
- Tube stripping, if necessary
- Assessment of
    Breath sounds: Bilateral?
    Respiratory rate and pattern
    Adventitious sounds
    Level of comfort
    SOB, dyspnea
    Presence or absence of central cyanosis
    Mental status, level of consciousness
    Tracheal position
    Chest excursion: Bilateral?
    ABG
    BP

SPECIAL NOTE

Stripping

Chest tube stripping should only be performed as necessary to maintain drainage. Stripping results in transmission of excessive negative pressure within the system and can damage lung tissue adjacent to chest tube suction ports.

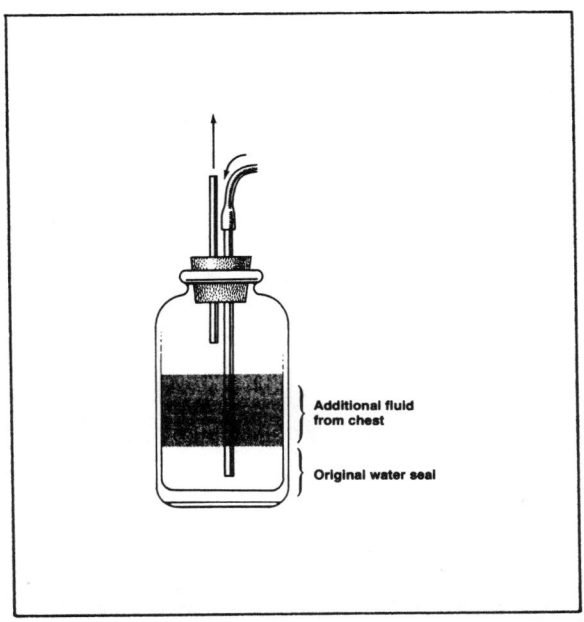

Figure 2–34. One bottle concept. *(Figures 2–34 to 2–36 are from Bricker, P. L. Chest tubes: The crucial points you mustn't forget. RN, 1980, 43(11), 24, with permission.)*

Additional fluid from chest

Original water seal

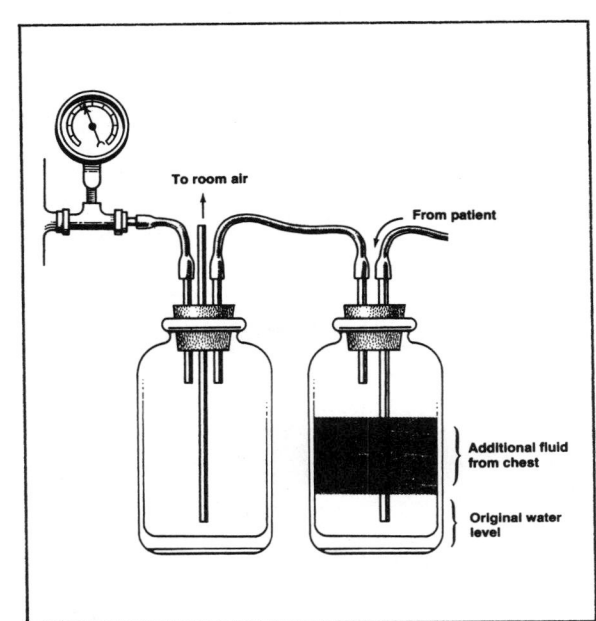

To room air

From patient

Additional fluid from chest

Original water level

Figure 2–35. Two bottle concept.

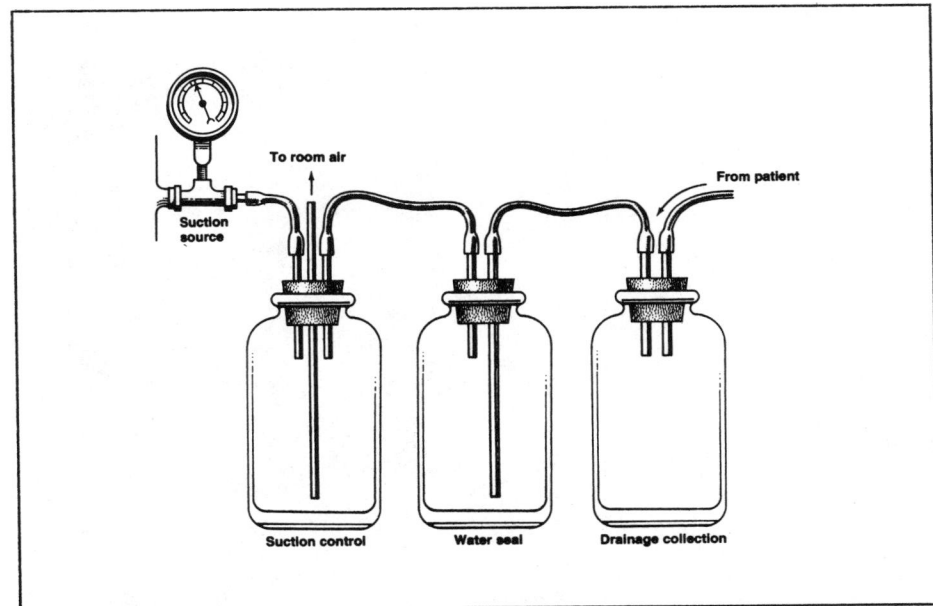

Suction source

To room air

From patient

Suction control

Water seal

Drainage collection

Figure 2–36. Three bottle concept.

(continued)

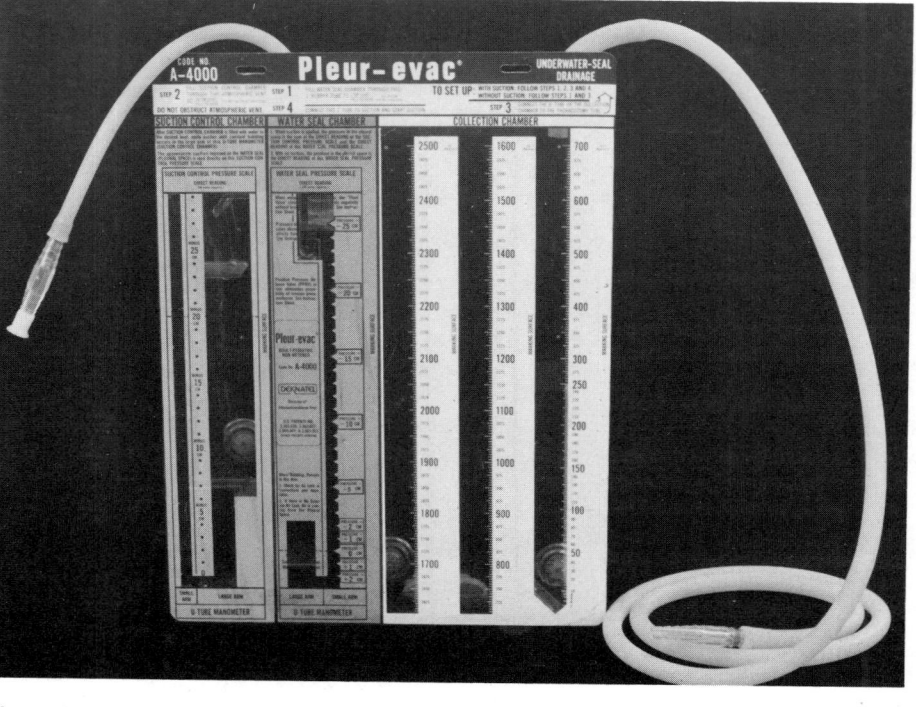

Figure 2–37. Pleurevac system.

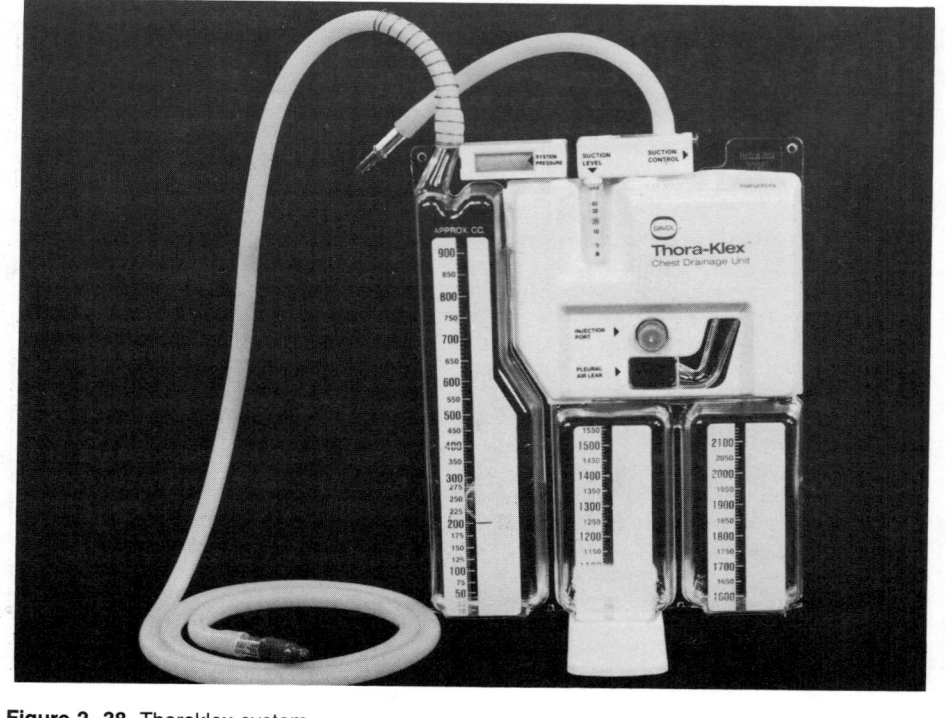

Figure 2–38. Thoraklex system.

Care of the Patient Requiring the Roto Rest Kinetic Treatment Table

NURSING DIAGNOSIS	RATIONALE	DEFINING CHARACTERISTICS	EXPECTED OUTCOME
Airway clearance, ineffective	The Roto Rest* table can serve as a useful adjunct in the treatment of any patient needing postural drainage and mobilization of secretions. Immobilized patients in the supine position are unable to clear secretions from the airways due to the postural effects on airway diameter (reduced), pooling of secretions in dependent areas, and often ineffective or absent cough mechanism. Pneumonia and atelectasis will develop if adequate mobility is not maintained. Special mobility problems requiring interventions may include obesity, neurological conditions, burns, trauma, or spinal cord injury (Fig. 2–39).	Ineffective or absent cough reflex Immobility Rhonchi, wheezes, decreased or absent breath sounds, rales (atelectasis)	Airways are maintained patent and free of obstructive substance

NURSING INTERVENTIONS

1. Explain the use of the table to the patient and family
2. Place the patient on the Roto Rest table after verifying the physician's order and electrical safety report
3. Secure all clamps, safety belts, and hatches prior to initiating electrical rotation settings on the bed, and check to see that they are secure at least q8h
4. Set the controls for side to side rotation
5. Assess ventilatory status frequently
   Rate and pattern of breathing
   Presence or absence of bilateral breath sounds
   Presence or absence of adventitious sounds
6. Perform pulmonary toiletry as indicated after assessment of ventilatory status
7. Assess mental status (i.e., anxiety level) frequently. Patient may need to be removed from bed if unable to tolerate
8. Observe for pain associated with rotation of bed. Reposition patient, if necessary (should be pain-free—refers to spinal cord injury patients)
9. For those patients with rib fractures, rotation of the bed can be modified to avoid pressure on the painful area

---

The Roto Rest Kinetic Treatment Table is a product of Kinetic Concepts, Inc., San Antonio, Texas.

OUTCOME CRITERIA	1. Rhonchi and wheezes will decrease or clear
	2. Breath sounds will be improved
	3. Bronchial breath sounds and rales will be detected promptly and treated

DOCUMENTATION

- Time patient placed on Roto Rest table
- Application of clamps, safety belts, and hatches. Note time checked for security
- Control settings and changes
- Ventilatory status
    Rate and pattern of breathing
    Presence or absence of bilateral breath sounds
    Presence, absence, or changes in adventitious sounds
- Pulmonary toiletry performance
    Time
    Method
    Results (i.e., sputum production)
- Mental status

SPECIAL NOTE

Rotation

Once the bed has been balanced, it will automatically rotate at a preset time interval. Rotation is usually 60 degrees but the table can be set at a modified rotation of 30 degrees for those patients unable to tolerate full rotation.

Physiological Benefits

The Roto Rest Kinetic Treatment Table is designed to assist immobile patients in maintaining minimum requirements for physiological mobility. Although the pulmonary benefits are addressed in this chapter, it is important to emphasize other physiological benefits as well. These include:

Cardiovascular: Prevention of venous thrombosis secondary to stasis, reduction in postural hypotension
Gastrointestinal: Stimulation of peristalsis reducing the incidence of constipation and other complications related to immobility
Musculoskeletal: Stabilization of fractures, reduction in flexion contractures and decalcification of bone
Genito-urinary: Reduced incidence of urinary stasis and renal calculi
Skin: Reduced incidence of decubiti

Precautions

Use of the bed in those patients with unstable fractures of the cervical spine who have not developed complications related to immobility is contraindicated.

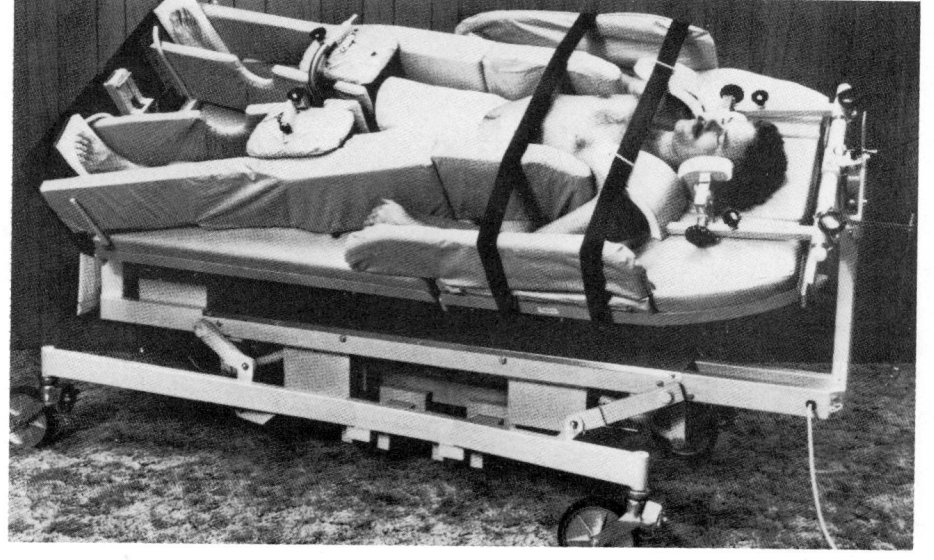

Figure 2–39. Roto Rest Kinetic Treatment Table.

Care of the Patient Requiring Continuous Monitoring of Mixed Venous Oxygen Saturation

NURSING DIAGNOSES	RATIONALE	DEFINING CHARACTERISTICS	EXPECTED OUTCOME
Gas exchange, impaired	Continuous monitoring of Svo_2 is necessary to termine changes in oxygen transport (cardiopulmonary function) or oxygen consumption at the cellular level. Adequate tissue perfusion is supported when the Svo_2 remains between 60 and 80%. Those conditions that will decrease Svo_2 include: 1. Decreased arterial oxygen saturation (e.g., interruption of ventilatory support, suctioning, alterations in Hgb-binding capacity of oxygen, progression of primary cause of hypoxia) 2. Decreased cardiac output (e.g., hypovolemia, cardiogenic shock, arrhythmias, hypotension) 3. Increased tissue oxygen consumption (e.g., increased muscular activity, increased metabolic activity) 4. Decreased hemoglobin (e.g., anemia)	1. $Sao_2 < 95\%$ Central cyanosis Dyspnea Changes in mental status (e.g., anxiety, restlessness, headache, confusion, disorientation) Increased heart rate Hypotension Exacerbation of angina 2. Dehydration Blood loss Cardiac failure Peripheral cyanosis Pulmonary congestion Dyspnea, tachypnea Orthopnea Arrhythmias Dizziness Anginal pain Hypotension Increased or decreased central venous pressure (CVP) Increased pulmonary capillary wedge pressure Weight gain 3. Shivering Clinical seizure activity Thyrotoxicosis Hyperthermia 4. Anemia Bleeding	Optimal gas exchange and tissue oxygenation will be maintained.

NURSING INTERVENTIONS

The following steps must be followed when monitoring the Svo_2 with the Oximetrix catheter.

1. Connect the optical module and connecting cable of the catheter to the oximeter
2. Calibrate the oximeter
   A. Draw a sample of blood from the distal port and determine oxygen saturation per co-oximeter
   B. Compare co-oximeter results with oximeter
   C. If difference is greater than 4%, recalibrate
3. Recalibrate oximeter at least once q24h and any time the catheter has been disconnected from the computer
4. Press the event marker to mark the recording paper whenever performing procedures or initiating therapy that may affect the Svo_2
5. Document the event on the recording paper (i.e., brief description)
6. Set the low alarm at 50, with the exception of any patient whose Svo_2 is chronically below 50
7. The alarm must be kept on at all times. If it alarms during a procedure (i.e., suctioning), the procedure should be altered or discontinued (always hyperoxygenate patient with 100% O_2 prior to suctioning and limit time of suctioning)
8. ABG should be determined if the Svo_2 drops below 55% or varies 15% from the baseline value

OUTCOME CRITERIA

1. Changes in Svo_2 will be promptly identified and treated
2. Gas exchange status is maintained at baseline Svo_2 or improved

DOCUMENTATION

- Vital signs
- Mental status
- Presence or absence of central or peripheral cyanosis
- Presence or absence of peripheral edema
- Breath sounds
- Presence of any pain: location, quality, extent
- Cardiac rhythm
- CVP, pulmonary artery pressure (PAP), and pulmonary capillary wedge pressure (PCWP), as applicable
- Weight
- Intake and output
- Svo_2 readings prior to each PCWP reading and with each significant change in patient status or intervention

SPECIAL NOTE

Implications for Practice

Continuous monitoring of mixed venous oxygen saturation (Svo_2) is accomplished by reflection spectrophotometry using a fiberoptic catheter in the pulmonary artery (Oximetrix catheter). In addition to providing pulmonary artery pressure and cardiac output readings, this catheter provides oxygen saturation determinations (Fig. 2–40).

Nursing interventions interrupting or altering ventilatory status, redistributing ventilation–perfusion relationships in the lung, or increasing patient activity may significantly decrease SvO_2 in patients with poor cardiac compensation. Nursing care should be planned to minimize these effects.

(continued)

Continuous monitoring of Svo_2 during patient activity is important in preventing complications. Additionally, continuous Svo_2 determinations are a useful parameter by which to titrate vasoactive drugs. Continuous monitoring of Svo_2 greatly reduces the need for traditional repeated measurement of ABG following ventilation setting changes.

Transport

Do not disconnect the catheter from the connecting cable for transport of the patient; disconnect the connecting cable from the computer.

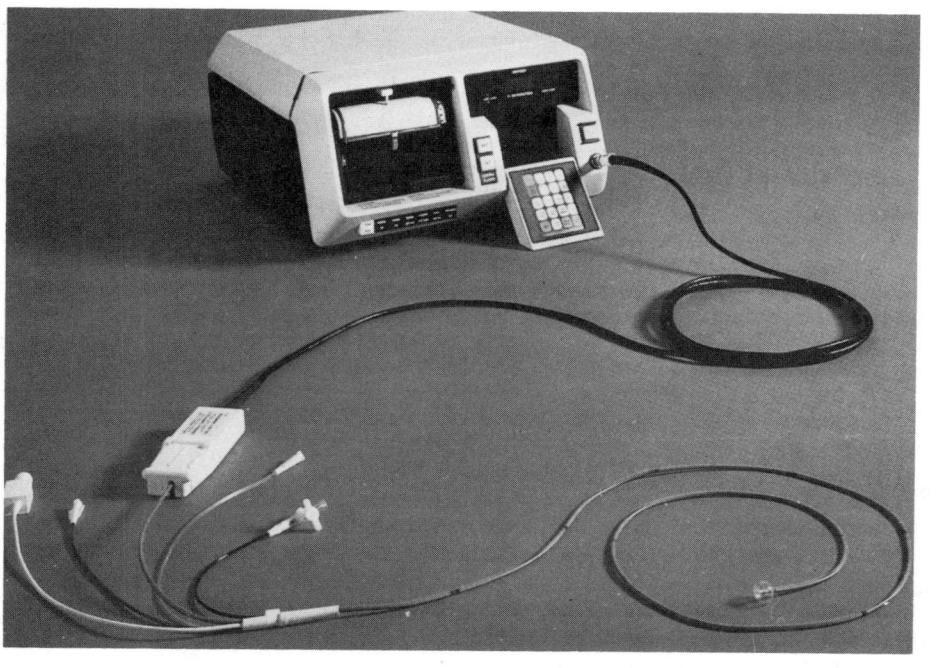

Figure 2–40. Oximetrix monitoring equipment.

Glossary

Alveolar arterial oxygen tension difference (AaDo$_2$): Represents the difference between alveolar and arterial oxygen tension with 100% inspired oxygen concentration.

Apnea: The absence of breathing.

Apneustic: An abnormal form of ventilatory pattern consisting of prolonged inspirations alternating with short expiratory movements.

Arterial blood gases (ABG): A clinical expression for the determination of the partial pressures of oxygen and CO_2 in the blood, commonly including other parameters relating to acid–base status.

> **pH:** Symbol for the logarithm of the reciprocal of the hydrogen ion (H) concentration (increase in pH = decrease in H+, decrease in pH = increase in H+) (normal pH 7.35–7.45).
>
> **Pao$_2$:** Partial pressure of oxygen in the arterial blood (normal 80–100 mm Hg).
>
> **Paco$_2$:** Partial pressure of CO_2 in the arterial blood (normal 35–45 mm Hg).
>
> **Sao$_2$:** Arterial oxygen saturation, represents the percentage of hemoglobin saturated with oxygen (normal 95% or more).
>
> **HCO$_3$:** Arterial content of bicarbonate ion, reflection of metabolic status with regard to acid–base balance (normal 22–26 (mEq/L).
>
> **Base excess:** Represents the amount of buffer base (mEq/L) exceeding or below the normal (normal −2 to +2).

Asterixis: Flapping tremor, an abnormal flapping tremor consisting of involuntary jerking movements, especially in the hands. Can occur with hypercapnea.

Barotrauma: Refers to injury resulting from pressure. May be commonly associated with mechanically ventilated patients (high positive pressures used for ventilation) and may include pneumothorax, pneumomediastinum, and subcutaneous emphysema.

Biot's respiration: Abnormal pattern of breathing characterized by abrupt and irregular alternating periods of apnea and constant rate and depth of breathing.

Bradypnea: Abnormal slowness of respiration, specifically a slow respiratory frequency.

Cheyne–Stokes respiration: Abnormal repeating pattern of breathing with gradual progressive increase in depth and sometimes rate to a maximum, followed by a gradual decrease ending in apnea.

Chronic obstructive pulmonary disease (COPD): Commonly includes chronic bronchitis, emphysema, and asthma. Group of diseases in which obstruction of the airways occurs as a result of the disease process.

Continuous positive airway pressure (CPAP): Positive airway pressure is applied during inspiration and expiration. Airway pressure never reaches zero. May be applied to spontaneous breathing or to a mechanical ventilator.

Fraction of inspired oxygen (FIo$_2$): Represents the fraction of inspired air that is oxygen. This may be expressed as a decimal or a percentage, with a maximum value of 1.00 or 100%, respectively.

$$FIo_2 = \frac{AaDo_2 + 100 \text{ mm Hg}}{760 \text{ mm Hg (atmospheric–barometric pressure)}}$$

Friction rub (pleural): Coarse scratching sound produced by inflammation of the pleural surface.

Hypercapnea: Hypercarbia, the presence of an abnormally large amount of carbon dioxide in the circulating blood. Increased arterial carbon dioxide tension.

Hypoxia: Subnormal oxygenation of arterial blood, short of anoxia.

Inspiratory: expiratory ratio (I:E ratio): Ratio of inspiratory phase time to expiratory phase time during ventilation. In order to support adequate ventilation, should normally be 1:1½ or 1:2.

Intermittent mandatory ventilation (IMV): Method commonly used to support weaning from continuous mechanical ventilation. Allows intermittent delivery of a predetermined volume of air to the patient. With the exception of the intermittent volume delivered, inspiratory effort is initiated by the patient.

Oxygen toxicity: Pathological condition in the lungs resulting from breathing high partial pressures of oxygen. The condition is not well understood. Major changes that result include decreased lung compliance and an increase in AaDo$_2$.

Positive end expiratory pressure (PEEP): Utilized with continuous ventilatory support to enhance gas exchange at the alveolar level. Commonly used in the treatment of severe ARDS and oxygen toxicity. Positive pressure (greater than atmospheric) is maintained during end expiration at the opening of the airway to minimize collapsing of the alveoli.

Pulmonary function parameters:

> **Tidal volume (Vτ):** Volume of air that is inspired or expired in a single breath during regular breathing. Generally measured as a normal exhaled breath following a normal inhalation (normal 500 ml; will vary according to body size).
>
> **Minute volume (Vϵ):** Volume of air moved per minute. Generally computed by multiplying Vτ by respiratory rate per minute (normal 6000 ml/min; will vary according to body size).
>
> **Vital capacity (Vc):** The greatest volume of air that can be exhaled from the lungs after a maximum inspiration (normal 4800 ml; will vary).

Rales: Crepitant, fine bubbling or crackling sound produced by the presence of a very thin secretion in the smaller bronchial tubes.

Respiratory acidosis: Caused by retention of CO_2, due to inadequate alveolar ventilation (alveolar hypoventilation), with decrease in blood pH unless compensated by renal retention of bicarbonate.

Respiratory alkalosis: Resulting from abnormal loss of CO_2 produced by alveolar hyperventilation, with concomitant reduction in arterial plasma bicarbonate concentration. Blood pH may be elevated depending on degree of renal compensation.

Respirometer: A device for measuring exhaled pulmonary volumes.

Rhonchi: An adventitious breath sound occurring during inspiration or expiration, heard on auscultation of the chest, caused by air passing through bronchi that are narrowed by inflammation, spasm of smooth muscle, or the presence of mucus in the lumen (sonorous: high-pitched, whistling, squeaky quality; sibilant: wheeze).

Roto Rest Kinetic Treatment Table: A device that automatically turns the patient from side to side while maintaining immobility of the spinal cord.

Sigh: Ventilator setting that allows intermittent delivery of a predetermined volume of air, generally larger than the tidal volume. Felt to be useful in expanding alveoli that may have become atelectatic in poorly ventilated areas of the lung.

Stridor: A high-pitched noisy respiration. A sign of respiratory obstruction, especially in the trachea or larynx.

Subcutaneous emphysema: The presence of air or gas in the subcutaneous tissues. Identified by the presence of crepitus (crackling on palpation of the skin) and tissue edema.

System pressure: Pressure usually measured in cm of H_2O, reached during the inspiratory phase of mechanical ventilation.

Bibliography

Alspach, J. G., & Williams, S. (Eds.). *Core curriculum for critical care nursing* (3rd ed.). Philadelphia: Saunders, 1985.

Beland, I., & Passos, J. *Clinical nursing: Pathophysiological and psychosocial approaches* (4th ed.). New York: Macmillan, 1981.

Carrieri, V., Murdough, C., & Janson-Bjerklie, S. A framework for assessing pulmonary disease categories. *Focus on Critical Care,* 1984, *11,* 9–16.

Duncan, C., & Erikson, R. Pressures associated with chest tube stripping. *Heart and Lung,* 1982, *11,* 166–176.

Gershan, J. Effect of positive end expiratory pressure on pulmonary capillary wedge pressure. *Heart and Lung,* 1983, *12,* 143–144.

Grosmaire, E. Use of patient positioning to improve PaO_2—A review. *Heart and Lung* 1983, *12,* 650–653.

Guzman, L., & Norton, L. Minimizing cuff-related laryngeal-tracheal complications. *Focus* 1982, *2,* 23–25.

Holloway, N. M. *Nursing the critically ill adult* (2nd ed.). Menlo Park, Calif.: Addison-Wesley, 1984.

Jung, R., & Newman, J. Minimizing hypoxia during endotracheal airway care. *Heart and Lung,* 1982, *11,* 208–212.

Kaye, W. Invasive monitoring techniques: Arterial cannulation, bedside pulmonary artery catheterization, and arterial puncture. *Heart and Lung,* 1983, *12,* 395–427.

King, C. Examining the thorax and respiratory system. *RN,* 1982, *8,* 55–63.

Kinney, M., Dear, C., Packa, D., & Voorman, D. *AACN's clinical reference for critical care nursing.* New York: McGraw-Hill, 1981.

Mackenzie, C. Compromises in the choice of orotracheal or nasotracheal intubation and tracheostomy. *Heart and Lung,* 1983, *12,* 485–492.

Millar, S., Sampson, L., Soukup, M., & Weinberg, S. *Procedures in critical care—The AACN manual* (2nd ed.). Philadelphia: Saunders, 1985.

Nett, L. Respiratory care today and tomorrow. *Heart and Lung,* 1982, *11,* 58–60.

Robinson, J. & Russo, P. (Eds.). *Nursing photobook—Providing respiratory care.* Springhouse, Pa.: Intermed Communications, 1979.

3

NEUROLOGICAL SYSTEM

Ann Lorene Quinn

Assessment of the Pertinent Neurological History

RATIONALE   Although protected by the skull and vertebral column, the major components of the central nervous system (CNS) remain susceptible to injury. The results of CNS insult, particularly at the cellular level, may have grave consequences for both the patient and family. Assessment of the pertinent history permits evaluation of events prior to hospitalization, identification of the client at risk, and consequently, analysis of available information for implementation of appropriate care. Should neurological impairment render the patient unable to give a history, family and significant others become invaluable resources for the critical care nurse.

PARAMETERS	FINDINGS	IMPLICATIONS FOR NURSING CARE
1. Family history	1. **A.** Hereditary disorders, such as craniosynostosis and neuro-fibromatosis **B.** Familial predispositions, such as intracranial berry aneurysms or seizure disorders	1. **A.** Craniosynostosis and neurofibromatosis are autosomal dominant disorders carrying a risk factor of 50% per pregnancy. Special consideration may be in order for the patient and family newly diagnosed. In addition, a genetic counseling referral may be helpful **B.** High stress levels associated with admission to a critical care environment may result in rupture of a previously undiagnosed aneurysm. Irritative cortical lesions may manifest as seizure activity if aggravated by altered electrolyte status, cardiac dysfunction, or respiratory distress

2. Past health history	2. **A.** Previous neurological dysfunction requiring medical or surgical management
	  a. CNS tumors
	    Gliomas
	    Astrocytomas
	    Meningiomas
	    Neurofibromas
	  b. Congenital or developmental anomalies
	    Arnold–Chiari malformation
	    Dandy–Walker syndrome
	    Arteriovenous malformations of the neuroaxis
	  c. Neurological disorders
	    Completed cerebrovascular accident (CVA)
	    Parkinsonian disease
	    Various movement disorders and demyelinating diseases, such as multiple sclerosis (MS)
	B. Previous neurological trauma
	  a. Head injury
	    Concussion or contusion
		2. **A. a.** Following initial diagnosis and resection, these tumors have a high incidence of recurrence. Psychosocial needs of these patients and their families should be carefully assessed
		
		  b. Family members skilled in the care of relatives with the consequences of these disorders can be valuable resources to the health care team for planning nondisruptive, individualized care
		
		  c. Sequelae associated with the presence of neurological disorders may interfere with or mask development of new neurological dysfunction
		
		B. a. Head injuries not related to present admission may have produced multiple problems Postconcussive syndrome with alterations in memory, ability to concentrate, and emotional liability

Evulsion of brain mass
Hematomas (epidural, subdural, intracerebral)
Skull defects
b. Spinal cord injury
Paraplegia
Quadriplegia
C. Previous cardiovascular dysfunction
  a. Coronary artery disease
  b. Cardiac dysrhythmias

  c. Valvular heart disease

  d. Cardiac valvular prosthesis

  e. Hypertension

D. Previous respiratory dysfunction, such as hemothorax or pneumothorax, pneumonia, adult respiratory distress syndrome (ARDS), pulmonary edema, and respiratory arrest
E. Previous hematological dysfunction
  a. Hypovolemic shock
  b. Congenital bleeding or clotting dyscrasias
  c. Acquired bleeding or clotting dyscrasias

3. A. Pharmacological agents

  B. Tobacco

  C. Alcohol

  D. Diet

Severe closed head injury with static disorders of cognition and personality
Destructive intracranial lesions with fixed focal motor deficits

b. The patient who survives spinal cord injury is faced with major life readjustments. Attention to individualized routines will greatly reduce the potential complications of chronicity so easily developed by this patient population
C. a. Known atherosclerotic occlusive disease identifies the patient at risk for developing cerebrovascular insufficiency

b. Cardiac dysrhythmias not only compromise cardiac output but also reduce systemic arterial blood flow. This results in lowered cerebral blood flow and perfusion pressure, a condition that may be detrimental to the patient's neurological status
c. Patients with diagnosed valvular heart disease are predisposed to bacterial endocarditis, a condition in which vegetation develops on the valve leaflets. Dislodged vegetations may present as microemboli and cause transient ischemic attacks (TIA). Additionally, intracranial seeding may result in micotic aneurysms
d. Patients requiring anticoagulant therapy for artificial cardiac valvular prostheses are at risk for developing intracranial bleeding if their prothrombin time is not monitored closely and kept within a therapeutic range
e. Cerebrovascular disease is a complication of hypertension. Vessels are weakened through a process of fibrotic change and are, therefore, more easily ruptured
D. The brain consumes oxygen at a rate 20 times greater than skeletal muscle. Respiratory dysfunction may contribute to the development of cerebral ischemia as a result of diminished arterial oxygen saturation during inadequate ventilation

E. a. When the amount of functional hemoglobin available to transport oxygen to the brain is diminished, level of consciousness may be depressed. Cerebral perfusion pressure may drop, with subsequent cerebral ischemia
b. Identifies patient at risk for cerebral hemorrhage

c. Patients with leukemia and those receiving pharmacological agents known to produce clotting dyscrasias are at risk for cerebral hemorrhage
3. A. Pharmacological agents have the potential for altering level of consciousness, cerebral metabolism, and cerebral perfusion. Use of marijuana has been associated with neurological dysfunction. Other classes of drugs, such as anticonvulsants, anticoagulants, oral contraceptives, and barbiturates, may impact the CNS. All medications identified should be noted on the nursing care plan
B. Nicotinic acid constricts arterioles and may decrease already compromised cerebral blood flow (CBF). Smoking, therefore, is a risk factor in cerebrovascular disease
C. Alcohol can be toxic with respect to quantity and quality consumed, severity of withdrawal, and associated malnutrition. Effects include alterations in level of consciousness, cerebral perfusion, and cerebral metabolism
D. Identification of preexisting conditions requiring dietary regulation should alert the nurse to the potential sequelae of noncompliance. New medication regimes may require

---

3. Patient profile

(continued)

PARAMETERS	FINDINGS	IMPLICATIONS FOR NURSING CARE
	E. Occupation	dietary modification, e.g., bioavailability of anticonvulsants is influenced by the integrity of the gastrointestinal tract, and levodopa use is adversely affected by dietary intake of vitamin B and pyridoxine **E.** Certain occupations predispose employees to potential neurological dysfunction. Those participating in contact sports and members of protective agencies are at greatest risk. In addition, workers subjected to industrial exposure of chlordeconce or organomercurial fungicides may develop neurological deficits. The brain has been identified as the organ most sensitive to certain pollutants. Commonly used neurotoxic substances, such as lead-based compounds, methylmercury, chlorinated hydrocarbon insecticides, or dichlorodiphenyltrichloroethane (DDT) may produce alterations in level of consciousness, cerebral perfusion, and cerebral metabolism
	F. Travel history	**F.** Travel to particular areas may result in neurological sequelae if the patient has been exposed to pesticides used by the agriculture industry, bites from a venomous snake, a rabid animal, a disease-bearing insect, or parasitic infestation (various routes of entry)

4. Present problem	**4. A.** Trauma	**4. A.** Severe trauma may affect the CNS in several ways
		  a. Hypovolemia may result in ischemia
		  b. Long bone fractures may result in fat emboli
		  c. With altered circulatory perfusion, intracranial autoregulation may become dysfunctional
		  d. Altered metabolism may result in metabolic encephalopathies
		  e. Impaired ventilation may result in ischemia

	B. Infection	**B.** Contaminants from various sites and causes may be transmitted to the CNS resulting in meningitis, encephalitis, brain abscess, or subdural empyema. Patients at risk include those with facial or skull fractures, dural tears with CSF leaks, or chronic sinusitis
	C. Decreased perfusion	**C.** Altered cerebral perfusion potentiates the risk for development of cerebral ischemia. Patients sustaining severe hypotensive insults, such as cardiopulmonary arrest or hemorrhage, require frequent neurological assessment to ensure early detection of deteriorating status
	D. Decreased oxygenation	**D.** In the adult, 25% of inspired oxygen is utilized by the brain. Decreased oxygenation, associated with ineffective ventilation, places the patient at risk for cerebral ischemia
	E. Alterations in metabolism	**E.** Neuronal cellular metabolism depends upon a precise chemical balance. Alterations in serum concentrations of fluids, electrolytes, glucose, and nitrogen resulting from disruption of other organ systems may adversely affect the CNS
	F. Surgical intervention	**F.** The effects of general anesthesia upon the CNS are not completely understood. Complications may range from mild to severe. The use of extracorporeal perfusion during open-heart surgery may produce postperfusion syndrome. Surgery involving manipulation of the brain or spinal cord may result in transient neurologic deficits
5. Review of systems	**5. A.** CNS and peripheral nervous system	**5. A.** Level of consciousness, alteration in Communication, impaired verbal Injury, potential for Mobility impaired, physical Self-care deficit (specify level: feeding, bathing–hygiene, dressing–grooming, toileting) Sensory perceptual alteration Thought processes, alteration in
	B. Cardiovascular	**B.** Cardiac output, alteration in: decreased Tissue perfusion, alteration in

	C. Pulmonary	**C.** Airway clearance, ineffective Breathing patterns, ineffective Gas exchange, impaired
	D. Endocrine	**D.** Fluid volume deficit, potential Urinary elimination, alteration in, pattern

Assessment of the Basic Vital Signs: The Neurological Component

RATIONALE

The components of the basic vital signs—temperature, pulse, respiration, and blood pressure—can be indicators of neurological function. Whereas irreversible neurologic dysfunction may result in abnormal vital signs, impending and, thus, potentially reversible CNS damage may be detected by prompt recognition of vital sign trends. Initiation of aggressive interventions may avert a catastrophic neurological event.

PARAMETERS	FINDINGS	POSSIBLE ETIOLOGIES	DOCUMENTATION

1. Temperature	1. Hypothermia
	   Shivering (increased pulse and basal metabolic rate)
	   Vasoconstriction
	   Piloerection
	   Decreased heart rate
	  Hyperthermia
	   Perspiration
	   Peripheral vasodilatation (radiation of heat)
	   Hyperventilation
	   Dehydration
	   Increased heart rate and basal metabolic rate
		1. Hypothermia
		   Injury to the posteromedial region of the hypothalamus
		   Spinal shock
		   Metabolic or toxic coma
		   Drug overdose
		   Environmental or iatrogenic causes
		  Hyperthermia
		   Destructive lesion in the preoptic area of hypothalamus
		   CNS or peripheral nervous system infection
		   Subarachnoid hemorrhage
			• Temperature q2h. Sudden change will be reported immediately and will necessitate increasing the frequency of assessment to every hour. Temperature elevation alters cerebral metabolism, resulting in potential exacerbation of any current neurological dysfunction. The temperature is recorded numerically on the critical care flow sheet, emphasizing the route symbolically, e.g., 98.6/0 or 100.8/R
			   A Axillary
			   O Oral
			   R Rectal
			   C Core

2. Pulse (rhythmic component)	2. Significant sinus arrhythmia Sinus arrest Junctional escape	2. Dysrhythmias associated with neurological dysfunction include alterations in both rhythm and conduction. The specific mechanism is not always known. Sinus tachycardia and eventual sinus bradycardia are associated with the Cushing reflex and increased intracranial pressure (IICP) following subarachnoid hemorrhage. IICP may cause ischemia to that area of the brainstem (medulla) controlling vasomotor activity. A sympathetic response is then elicited causing the systolic blood pressure to rise and a widening pulse pressure to occur. Elevation of BP stimulates the baroreceptors in the carotid arteries and aortic arch, resulting in vagal stimulation and consequently a bradycardic response	• Pulse q1h. Dysrhythmias are to be documented with a rhythm strip and reported immediately. Dysrhythmias put the patient at risk for developing cerebral ischemia
3. Respiration	3. Cheyne–Stokes respirations Central neurogenic hyperventilation Apneustic breathing Cluster breathing Ataxic breathing	3. Cheyne–Stokes respirations are associated with bilateral cerebral hemispheric lesions and with lesions in the basal ganglia (Fig. 3–1) Central neurogenic hyperventilation is associated with a lesion in midbrain or upper pons	• Respirations q1h. Gradual or sudden changes in breathing patterns should be reported immediately. Ventilatory support should be documented.

		Apneusitic breathing is associated with a lesion in middle or lower pons
		Cluster breathing is associated with a lesion in lower pons and upper medulla
		Ataxic respirations are associated with a lesion in the medulla
			Abnormal breathing patterns are documented narratively
			  Cheyne–Stokes: An alteration of crescendo hyperpnea and decrescendo apnea
			  Central neurogenic hyperventilation: A pattern of rapid, regular, and deep respirations
			  Apneusis: A prolonged inspiratory phase with a pause at the peak
			  Cluster: Irregular with clusters of breathing alternating with periods of apnea
			  Ataxic: No pattern, erratic and unpredictable

4. Blood pressure (BP)	4. Hypotension Hypertension Widening pulse pressure	4. Hypotension can be associated with systemic shock, neurological deterioration, or a lesion in the brainstem at the level of the medulla Hypertension can be associated with increased intracranial pressure or dysfunction of baroreceptors Widening pulse pressure can be reflective of inadequate cerebral perfusion pressure (CPP), IICP, or activation of the Cushing reflex	• Blood pressure q1h. Trends or sudden changes should be reported immediately. In the presence of neurological dysfunction, autoregulation may be impaired. With the inability to maintain a constant CBF over a variable range of systemic arterial pressures, autoregulation fails and the brain has the potential to develop cerebral ischemia

POSSIBLE NURSING DIAGNOSES

- Breathing patterns, ineffective
- Cardiac output, alteration in: decreased
- Gas exchange, impaired
- Injury, potential for
- Tissue perfusion, alteration in: cerebral

SPECIAL NOTE

Direct and Indirect Measurement

Correlation of intra-arterial blood pressures with cuff pressures should be performed during initial assessment. Calibration of the arterial line should be performed q24h with rezeroing of the arterial line at least q8h.

(continued)

Core Temperature

Core temperatures can be obtained from the thermodilution port of a pulmonary artery catheter as well as from a thermotic sensor on an indwelling urethral catheter. Core measurements are more reflective of the patient's true temperature (Figs. 3–2 and 3–3).

Autonomic Dysreflexia

Autonomic dysreflexia: A chronic, *critical* complication for patients with spinal cord injuries above the sixth thoracic vertebrae. Characteristics include a sudden, *severe* rise in BP, headache, flushing, and diaphoresis above the level of injury. Autonomic dysreflexia is triggered by a noxious stimulus, usually a distended bladder or bowel, below the level of the spinal cord lesion. This lesion interferes with the normal transmission of the sympathetic impulse within the autonomic nervous system. Proper attention to bladder and bowel function by the critical care nurse is *essential* in preventing this life-threatening phenomenon.

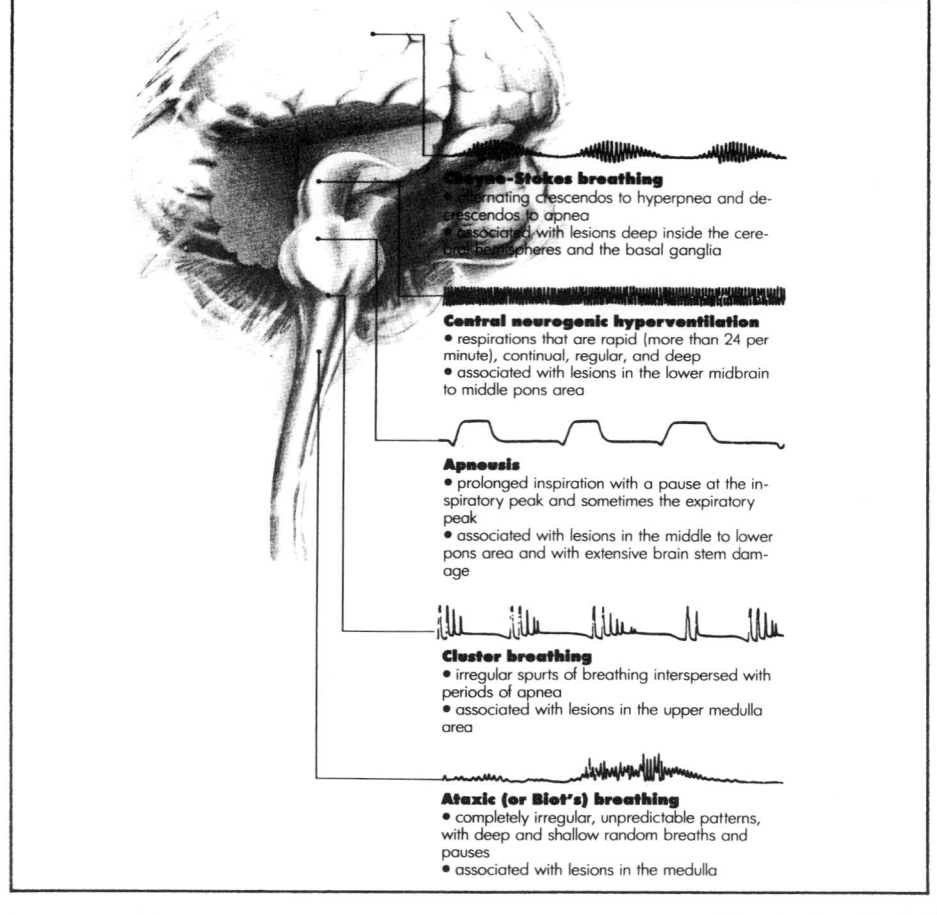

Cheyne-Stokes breathing
- alternating crescendos to hyperpnea and decrescendos to apnea
- associated with lesions deep inside the cerebral hemispheres and the basal ganglia

Central neurogenic hyperventilation
- respirations that are rapid (more than 24 per minute), continual, regular, and deep
- associated with lesions in the lower midbrain to middle pons area

Apneusis
- prolonged inspiration with a pause at the inspiratory peak and sometimes the expiratory peak
- associated with lesions in the middle to lower pons area and with extensive brain stem damage

Cluster breathing
- irregular spurts of breathing interspersed with periods of apnea
- associated with lesions in the upper medulla area

Ataxic (or Biot's) breathing
- completely irregular, unpredictable patterns, with deep and shallow random breaths and pauses
- associated with lesions in the medulla

Figure 3–1. Identified respiratory patterns may reflect the level of intracranial lesions. *(From Johnson, L. If your patient has increased intracranial pressure, your goal should be: No surprises.* Nursing 83, *1983, 13(6), 62, copyright 1983, Springhouse Corporation, with permission.)*

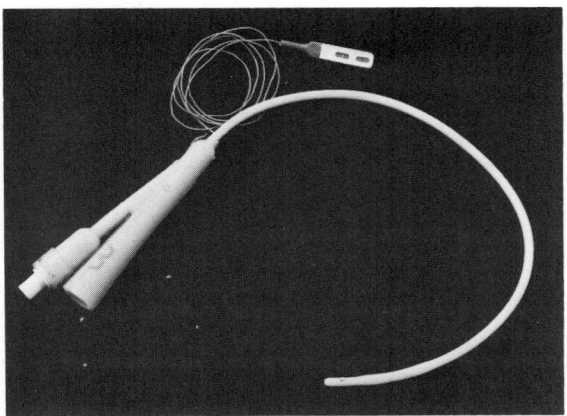

Figure 3–2. Core thermotic urethral catheter. *(Courtesy of Mon-A-Therm, Inc., St. Louis, Mo.)*

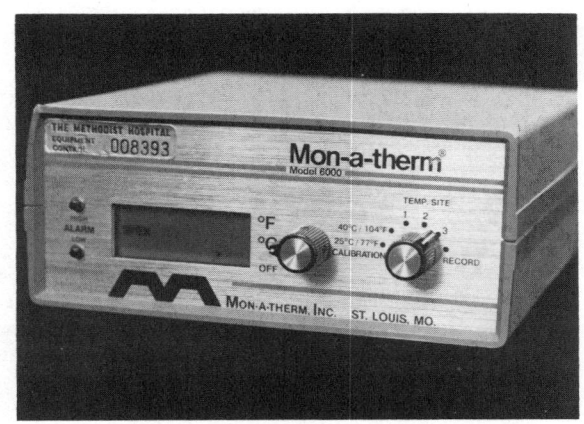

Figure 3–3. Display monitor. *(Courtesy of Mon-A-Therm, Inc., St. Louis, Mo.)*

Assessment Parameters of the Glasgow Coma Scale

RATIONALE

The Glasgow coma scale, devised by Teasdale and Jennett at the University of Glasgow in 1974, has become an international standard for broad assessment of neurological status. The Glasgow coma scale assesses neurological function as a circuit: input received–transmission begun–integration completed–production of output elicited. Stimulus is received by the peripheral nervous system, transmitted to the CNS, and back again for a response. This tool has received wide acceptance because of its proven simplicity, reliability, and low variability with various levels of staff expertise. Three parameters are evaluated—eye opening, motor response, and verbal response—and they are scored numerically.

PARAMETERS	FINDINGS	POSSIBLE ETIOLOGIES	DOCUMENTATION
1. Eye opening	1. **A.** Score of 4: Spontaneous (Fig. 3–4) **B.** Score of 3: To verbal stimulus (Fig. 3–5) **C.** Score of 2: To painful stimulus; consistent use of proximal nailbed pressure to be used by all examiners (Figs. 3–6 and 3–7) **D.** Score of 1: No eye opening (Fig. 3–8)	1. **A.** Reticular activating system functioning with appropriate level of wakefulness **B.** Patient lethargic possibly due to fatigue, analgesics, narcotics, anesthesia, postictal state, beginning evidence of increased intracranial pressure, or hypoxia **C.** Patient with definite decrease in level of consciousness resulting from alteration in cerebral perfusion and metabolism (trauma, infection, neoplasm, cardiovascular anomaly, metabolic imbalance, toxic or pharmacologic agents) **D.** Rule out previous neurological disorder, specifically, myasthenia gravis. Otherwise indicative of profound decrease in level of consciousness—alteration of cerebral perfusion and cerebral metabolism associated with increased intracranial pressure, expanding mass effect, hypoxia or diminished cerebral perfusion	• Record Glasgow coma scale score q1h. A score for each finding of the three parameters will be documented. The level of stimulus required to elicit the response and whether the response was sustained or sporadic should also be noted. Narrative documentation by the nurse, supporting the scores, provides both a consistent method for assessment and a continuing record of trends in the patient status. Any extenuating circumstances that would influence the scoring of the Glasgow coma scale will be reflected.
2. Motor response	2. **A.** Score of 6: Follows command appropriately (Fig. 3–9) **B.** Score of 5: Purposely pushes away (Fig. 3–10) **C.** Score of 4: Semipurposeful withdrawal (Fig. 3–11)	2. **A.** Reticular activating system functioning with appropriate level of wakefulness **B.** Patient lethargic, may not comprehend the given command due to impaired integration of language. Evidence of minimal neurological dysfunction. Alteration in level of consciousness, cerebral perfusion, and cerebral metabolism **C.** Evidence of alteration in level of consciousness from a neurological dysfunction. Disruption of motor pathway in central nervous	Neuromuscular blockade: Interferes with motor response Presence of endotracheal tube: Interferes with verbal response Periorbital edema: Interferes with eye opening response

	D. Score of 3: Flexion to pain (Fig. 3–12)	system (mass effect, neoplasm, cerebral ischemia, cerebrovascular anomaly, trauma) **D.** Indicates severe alteration in level of consciousness or disruption of motor pathway at the pontine level in the brainstem (trauma, herniation of brain, IICP, cerebrovascular anomaly, neoplasm)
	E. Score of 2: Extension to pain (Fig. 3–13)	**E.** Indicates increasingly severe alteration in level of consciousness or disruption of motor pathway at the medullary level in the brainstem (trauma, herniation of brain, IICP, cerebrovascular anomaly, neoplasm)
	F. Score of 1: No response to pain	**F.** Indicates complete blockage of motor pathway at lower brainstem–high cervical area (akinetic mutism, profound coma, absence of cerebral perfusion, trauma, cerebral ischemia, neoplasm, cardiovascular anomaly, pharmacologically induced coma)
3. Verbal response	**3. A.** Score of 5: Oriented and content appropriate	**3. A.** Able to comprehend, correlate, and communicate appropriately
	B. Score of 4: Disoriented and converses	**B.** Evidence of minimal dysfunction in frontal lobe (hypoxia, trauma, altered perfusion, hydrocephalus, neoplasm, cerebrovascular anomaly, early indication of IICP, sleep deprivation, pharmacologic toxicity)
	C. Score of 3: Incomplete words and phrases	**C.** Indicative of dysfunction in primary speech centers, Broca's and Brodman's area (dominant hemisphere compression from edema, trauma, alterations in cerebral perfusion, neoplasm, cerebrovascular anomaly)
	D. Score of 2: Unintelligible sounds	**D.** Indicative of severe dysfunction in speech center or major alteration in level of consciousness (dominant hemisphere lesion, trauma, IICP, cerebrovascular anomaly, neoplasm)
	E. Score of 1: No verbal response	**E.** Indicative of increasingly severe dysfunction in speech centers or major alteration in level of consciousness (dominant hemisphere lesion, trauma, IICP, cerebrovascular anomaly, neoplasm)

POSSIBLE NURSING DIAGNOSES

- Level of consciousness, alteration in: decreased
- Communication, impaired: verbal
- Mobility, impaired: physical
- Self-care deficit (specify level: feeding, bathing–hygiene, dressing–grooming, toileting)
- Sensory–perceptual alterations

(continued)

SPECIAL NOTE

Using the Glasgow Coma Scale

Glasgow scale scores are related but not necessarily interdependent or mutually exclusive. For example, a Glasgow coma scale score of 15 is indicative of spontaneous eye opening, clear and appropriate speech, and motor response that is performed voluntarily and to command. In comparison, a score of 7 may be indicative of a patient in a semicomatose state and a score of 3 of brain death.

Expressly documenting extenuating circumstances is a vital nursing responsibility. This step will eliminate the possibility of treating the score and not the patient, e.g., patient receiving a neuromuscular blockade may score 3 but may actually be awake and alert; patient with an endotracheal tube cannot speak and will score 1 on verbal response but may be awake and following commands; patient with bilateral periorbital edema severe enough to prohibit eye opening would consequently be marked lower even though he is awake, alert, and may move all extremities to command (Fig. 3–14).

Serial Assessments

Status of cerebral function, when monitored by serial assessments with the Glasgow coma scale, will more fully indicate an alteration in the level of consciousness than will a single assessment finding. The rapidity of neurological deterioration can be startling! Do not be afraid to recheck in 1–2 minutes. Trust your observations when made; nervous system changes may occur from minute to minute.

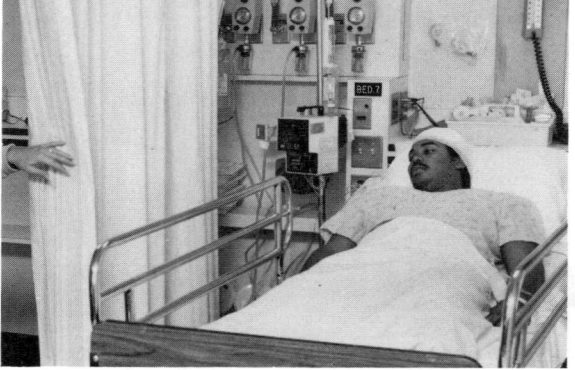

Figure 3–4. Spontaneous eye opening.

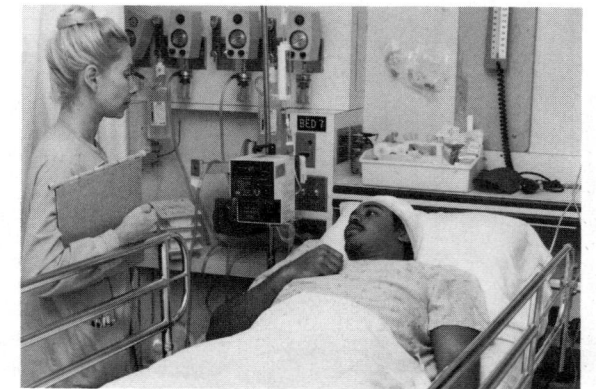

Figure 3–5. Eye opening to verbal stimulus.

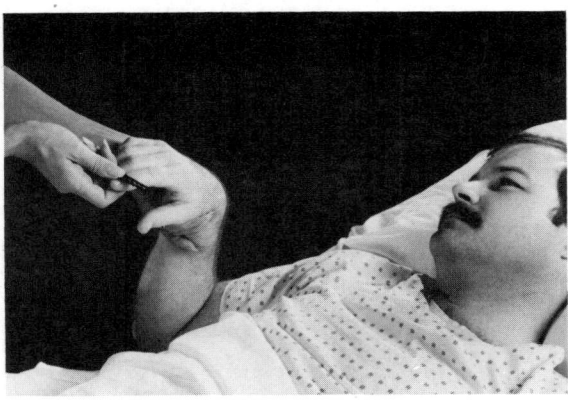

Figure 3–6. Eye opening to painful stimulus.

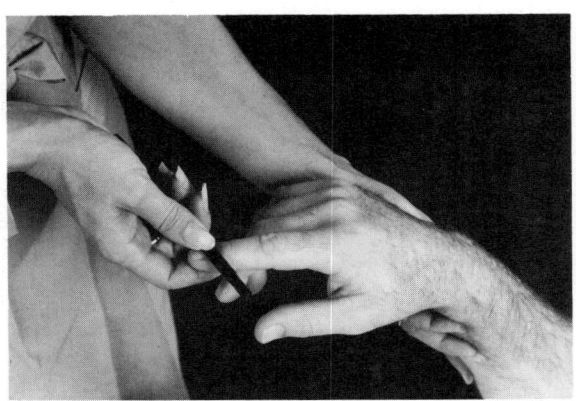

Figure 3–7. Application of painful stimulus.

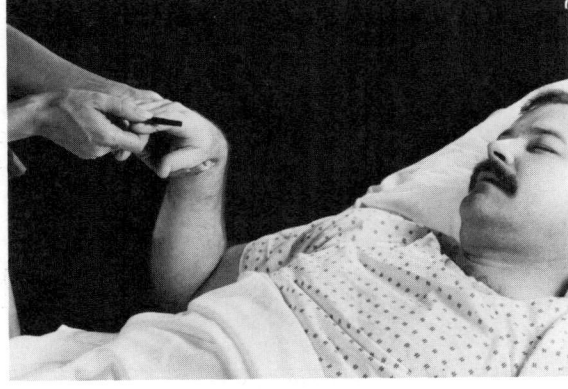

Figure 3–8. No eye opening to painful stimulus.

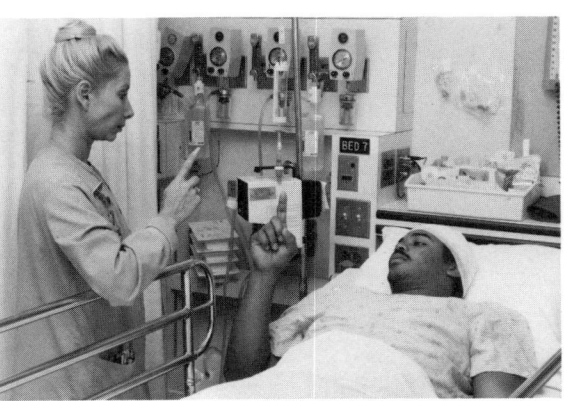

Figure 3–9. Obeys commands.

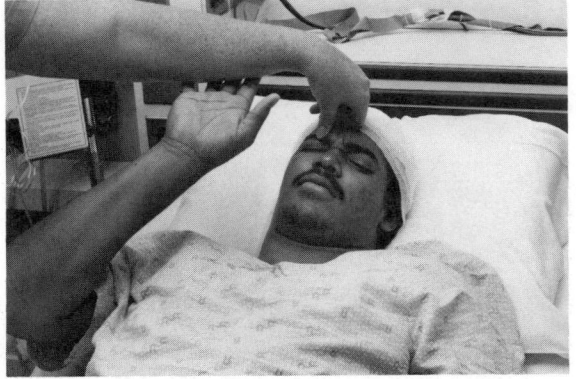

Figure 3–10. Localizes to pain.

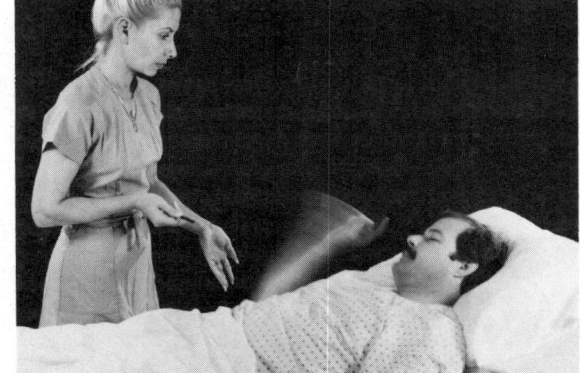

Figure 3–11. Semipurposeful withdrawal.

(continued)

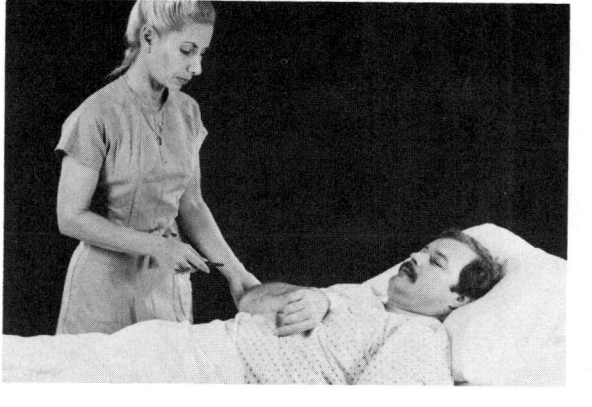

Figure 3–12. Decortication.

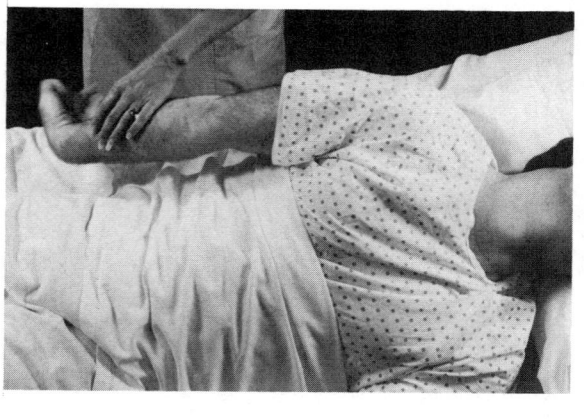

Figure 3–13. Decerebration.

GLASGOW COMA SCALE			
Eyes	Open	Spontaneously	4
		To verbal command	3
		To pain	2
	No response		1
Best motor response	To verbal command	Obeys	6
	To painful stimulus*	Localizes pain	5
		Flexion—withdrawal	4
		Flexion—abnormal (decorticate rigidity)	3
		Extension (decerebrate rigidity)	2
		No response	1
Best verbal response**		Oriented and converses	5
		Disoriented and converses	4
		Inappropriate words	3
		Incomprehensible sounds	2
		No response	1
Total			3-15

Figure 3–14. Glasgow coma scale.

Assessment of the Eye: The Neurological Component

RATIONALE

Neurological assessment of the eye evaluates three functions—pupillary reflex, extraocular movements, and visual field integrity. Findings necessarily give information regarding integrity of the circuit: input–transmission–integration–output. Cranial nerves II, III, IV, and VI are assessed. In addition, lesions along the visual pathway may be detected. The complexity of neuro-ophthalmology has been simplified here to avoid confusion.

PARAMETERS	FINDINGS	POSSIBLE ETIOLOGIES	DOCUMENTATION

1. Direct pupillary reflex	1. Pupils equal in size and constrict briskly to light (Fig. 3–15)
	  A. Anisocoria: The pupils are unequal in size but react normally to light and accommodation unless so predisposed by disease (Fig. 3–16)
	  B. Third nerve palsy (oculomotor nerve): One pupil is dilated, fixed, and nonreactive to light. Ipsilateral ptosis may accompany this disorder (Fig. 3–17)
	  C. Dilated and fixed: Both pupils are fixed, dilated, and nonreactive to light (Fig. 3–18)
		1. A. Congenital or manifestation of a disturbance in the ophthalmic pathway. Anisocoria is the most common abnormal eye sign; found in 17% of the population as a congenital defect. In these instances, anisocoria is not considered pathological
		  B. Lesion along the CN III (oculomotor) pathway
		
		  C. Midbrain lesion; significant brainstem site of major neurological dysfunction. Sympathomimetic drugs (atropine sulfate) may, however, produce the same response
			• Pupil size and response to direct and consensual light every hour
			  Numerical size of the pupil is recorded in millimeters
			  Symbolic reaction of pupillary response is recorded:
			    + Brisk
			    ± Sluggish
			    − Nonreactive
			• An acceptable acronym for normal pupillary response is PERRLA: *Pupils equal, round, and react to light and accommodation*

2. Accommodation pupillary reflex	2. Pupils constrict with near fixation and internal rotation
	  A. Pupils do not constrict with near fixation and internal rotation
	  B. Argyll–Robertson pupil: Pupils are small and irregular in shape bilaterally. Reaction to light is by accommodation only (Fig. 3–19)
		2. A. Central lesion of oculomotor nerve (CN III)
		
		  B. Pathological effect from syphilis, diabetes, brain tumors, and alcohol abuse. Interruption of pathway from pretectal region to Edinger–Westphal nucleus
			• If extraocular movements are intact, e.g., "EOM full and intact." If not, indicate deficit, e.g., "EOM intact except for upward gaze"
			• Any visual field defect, e.g., patient unable to see objects to the right (indicative of right homonymous hemianopsia)

3. Extraocular movements (EOM)	3. Ability to move the globe of the eye in all six directions (Figs. 3–20 and 3–21)
	  A. Nystagmus: Involuntary directional movement of the eye
	
	  B. Ophthalmoplegias: Signs of cranial nerve (CN) III, IV, VI palsies
	    a. CN III (oculomotor) (third nerve palsy)
	      Constriction and dilation of pupil
	      Elevates the eye lid
	      Allows the eye to move up, down, and in
		3. A. Lesion along neural pathways of CN III, IV, VI
		    Lesion in brainstem or cerebellum
		    Lesion in vestibular system
		    Lesion in visual perception system
		  B. Lesions of central or peripheral CN III, IV, VI
			Note: Ophthalmic prostheses are to be noted narratively as such and *not* indicated as a nonreactive pupil.

	b. CN IV (trochlear) (fourth nerve palsy) Allows the eye to move down and in **c.** CN VI (abducens) (sixth nerve palsy) Allows the eye to move outward **C.** External ophthalmoplegia: Ptosis, dilated pupil, and outward deviation of the eye **D.** Sixth nerve palsy (abducens nerve): Diplopia and inward deviation of the eye (Fig. 3–22)	**C.** Oculomotor nerve palsy along peripheral pathway **D.** Lesion along abducens (CN VI) pathway
4. Visual field integrity (Figs. 3–23 and 3–24)	**4. A.** Unilateral defect: Visual field integrity affected in one eye **B.** Bitemporal defect: Visual field integrity affected in lateral (temporal) region of both eyes **C.** Homonymous defect: Visual field integrity affected in the same half (right or left) of both eyes **D.** Upper field defect: Visual field integrity affected in the upper half of both eyes **E.** Lower field defect: Visual field integrity affected in the lower half of both eyes	**4. A.** Lesion of the optical nerve anterior to the optic chiasm **B.** Lesion of the optic chiasm **C.** Lesion posterior to the optic chiasm **D.** Lesion in the inferior portion of the optic nerve **E.** Lesion in the superior portion of the optic nerve

POSSIBLE NURSING DIAGNOSES

- Injury, potential for
- Self-care deficit (specify level: feeding, bathing–hygiene, dressing–grooming, toileting)
- Sensory perceptual alterations

SPECIAL NOTE

Time of Onset

Visual impairment affects multiple activities of daily living. If onset is gradual, the deficit may go unnoticed as compensatory functions are developed. In the critical care setting, sudden onset of visual impairment should be investigated promptly. Aggressive intervention may reverse or minimize dysfunction

Cold Calorics

Cold calorics is a procedure performed on comatose patients to elicit the presence of the oculovestibular reflex and to establish that the vestibular cerebellar pathway is intact. The procedure elicits a response from the vestibular system by the stimulation of cold water running through the external auditory canal. Eyes deviate away from the external auditory canal being stimulated and exhibit horizontal nystagmus. Failure to elicit a response may be indicative of irreversible neurological dysfunction. Results of this procedure may be used as a criterion for determining brain death, when in addition to the patient having negative barbiturate levels and being normothermic, cold caloric testing is serially performed (usually over 3 days)

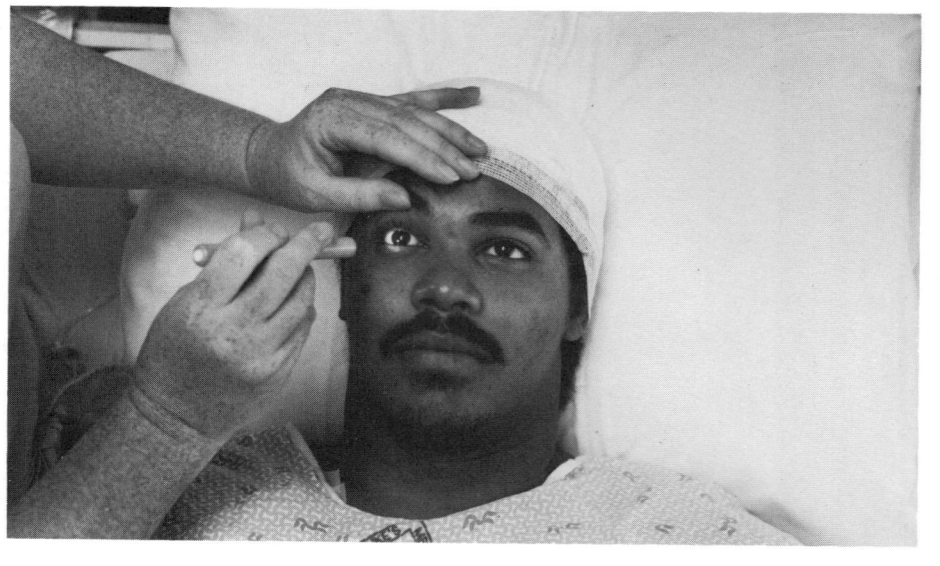

Figure 3–15. Assessment of direct pupillary response to light.

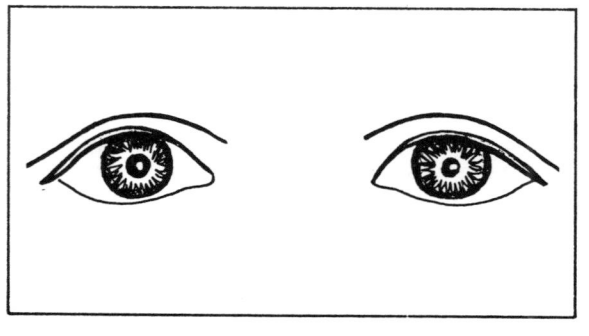

Figure 3–16. Anisocoria.

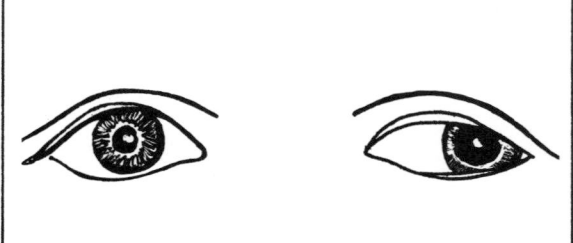

Figure 3–17. Ptosis and dilated pupil (ipsilateral) (third nerve palsy).

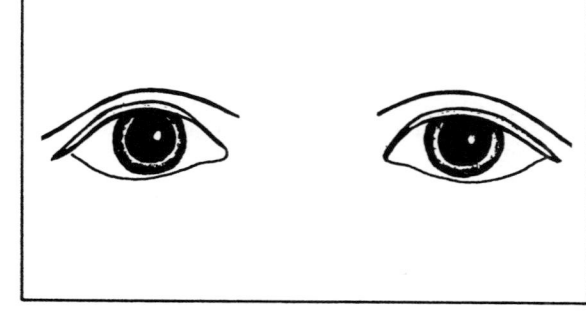

Figure 3–18. Dilated, fixed pupils.

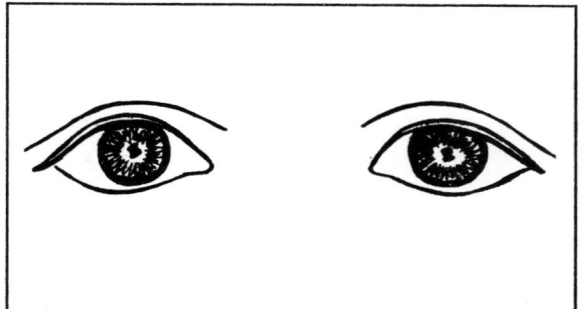

Figure 3–19. Bilaterally small pupils; irregularly shaped.

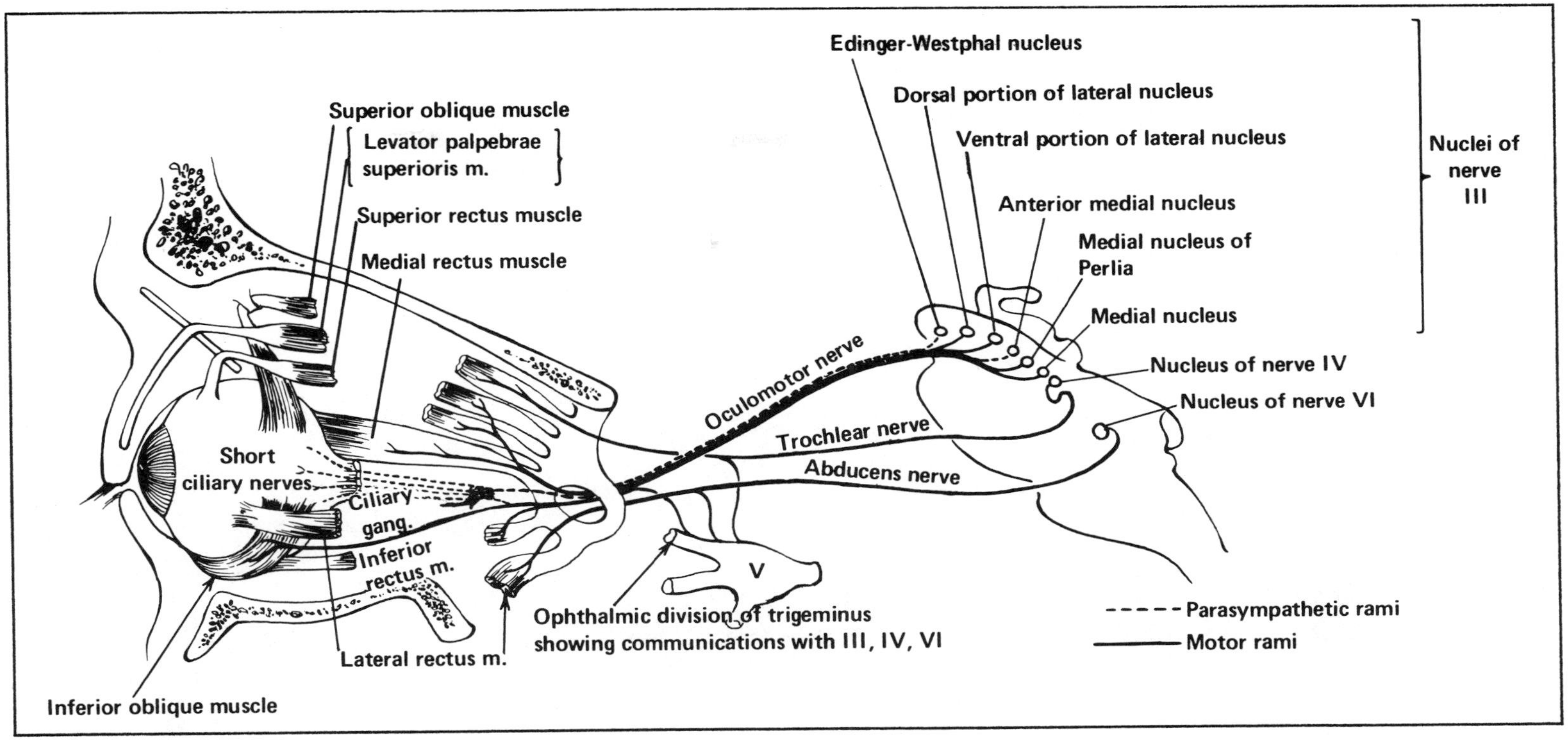

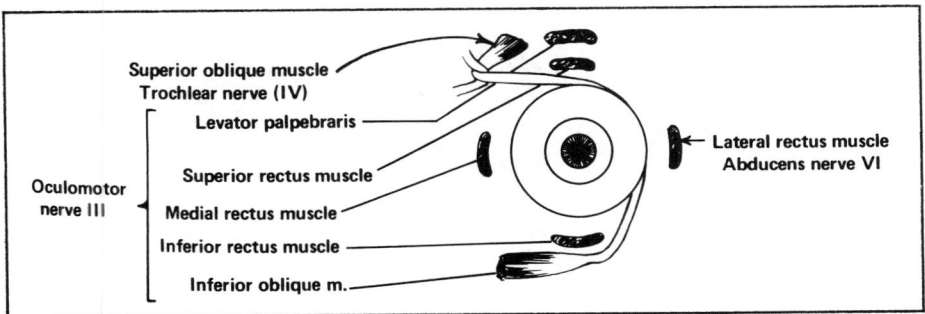

Figure 3–20. Extraocular muscle enervation by cranial nerves III, IV, and VI (lateral). *(From Chusid, J. G. Correlative neuroanatomy and functional neurology (19th ed.). Los Altos, Calif.: Lange, 1985, p. 116, with permission.)*

Figure 3–21. Extraocular muscle enervation by cranial nerves III, IV, and VI (AP). *(From Chusid, J. G. Correlative neuroanatomy and functional neurology (19th ed.). Los Altos, Calif.: Lange, 1985, p. 116, with permission.)*

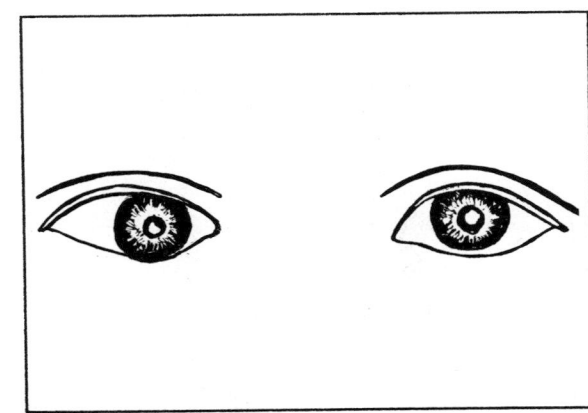

Figure 3–22. Sixth nerve palsy.

(continued)

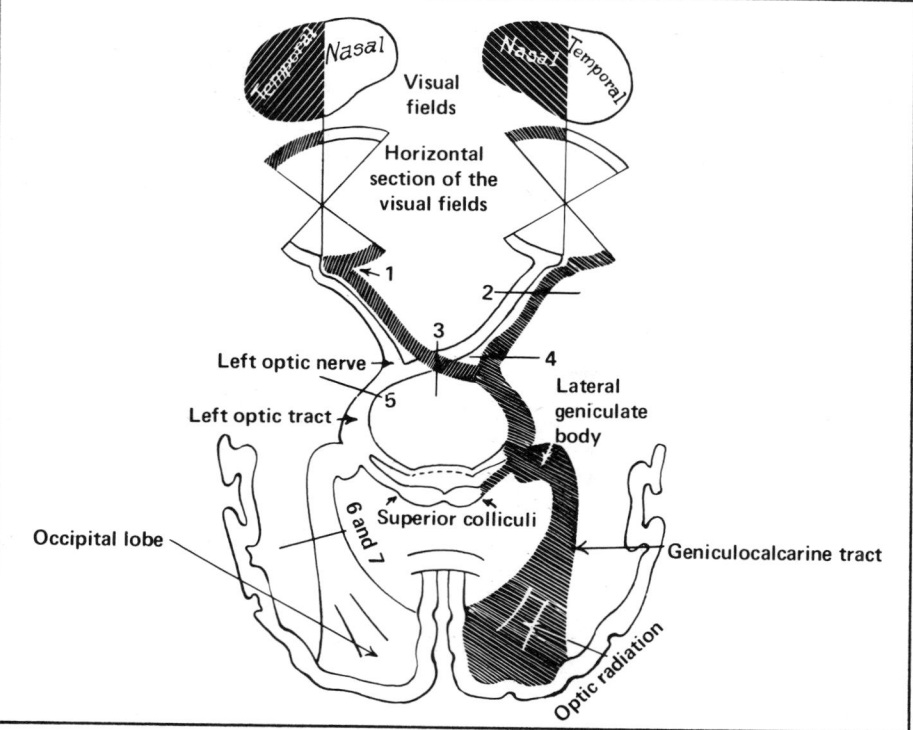

Figure 3–23. Visual field integrity. *(From Chusid, J. G. Correlative neuroanatomy and functional neurology (19th ed.). Los Altos, Calif.: Lange, 1985, p. 114, with permission.)*

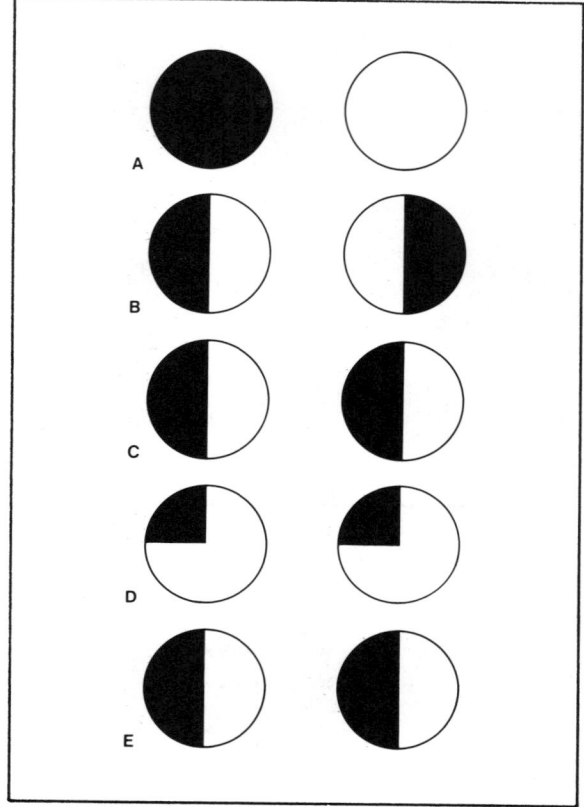

Figure 3–24. Five visual defects. **A.** Unilateral blindness. **B.** Bitemporal hemianopsia (optic chiasma). **C.** Left homonymous hemianopsia (right optic tract). **D.** Homonymous left upper quadrant defect (optic radiation, partial). **E.** Left homonymous hemianopsia (right optic radiation).

Assessment of Motor Activity

RATIONALE

The neurological component of motor activity involves the integration of a complex circuit of impulses. The impulse originates in the sensory peripheral nerves, is transmitted to the spinal cord, and ascends to the cerebral cortex for interpretation. The interpretation is made, an impulse descends from the precentral gyrus of the cerebral cortex to the brainstem. Here 80% of the fibers cross, descend into the spinal cord, and travel to the periphery to produce a response to the original impulse (Fig. 3–25).

PARAMETERS	FINDINGS	POSSIBLE ETIOLOGIES	DOCUMENTATION
	The methodology for assessing motor activity must be consistent and precise in order to monitor any subtle alterations. Early interventions may alleviate or reduce the potential for catastrophic neurological deficits. The patient is usually assessed supine in bed, assessing upper extremities initially and then lower extremities. Motor strength as well as movement are assessed in each limb, and symmetry is evaluated for discrepancies (Figs. 3–26 to 3–42).		Observations of limb movement and strength will be recorded q1h. Gradual or sudden decrease in movement or strength will be reported immediately.
1. Peripheral nervous system	1. Flaccid paralysis or weakness	1. Cervico-occipital neuralgia: Trauma, fractures, infection Phrenic neuralgia: Tumors, aortic aneurysms Brachial plexus lesion: Trauma, violent pulling of arms, fractures Tumors of neck, infections Sciatic nerve lesion: Herniated intervertebral disc	• Limbs $\dfrac{RA\mid LA}{RL\mid LL}$ • Movement Voluntary (V) On command (C) With stimulation (purposeful) (S) Withdraws (W) None (0) Decorticate (Decor) Decerebrate (Decer)
2. Central nervous system	2. Spastic paralysis or weakness	2. Neoplasms Infection Vascular lesions Toxic lesions Cerebral ischemia	• Strength + Strong − Weak 0 Absent *Example.* Patient with normal strength and moves all extremities voluntarily and to command: Limbs $\dfrac{\underset{VC}{+}\mid\underset{VC}{+}}{\underset{VC}{+}\mid\underset{VC}{+}}$

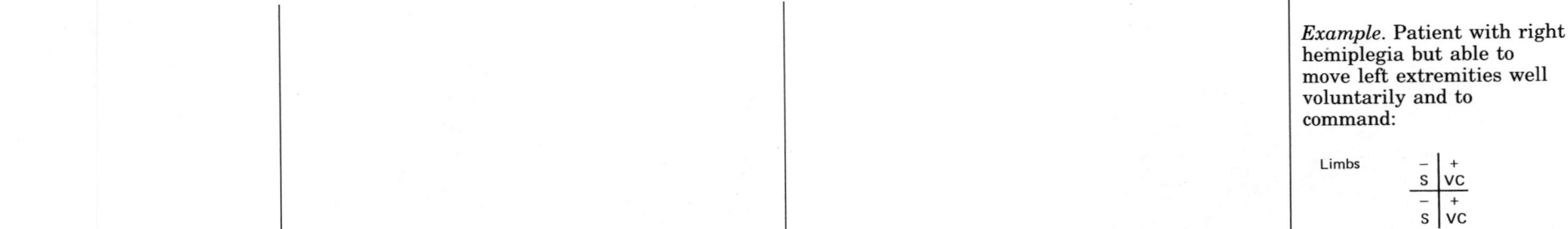

Example. Patient with right hemiplegia but able to move left extremities well voluntarily and to command:

Limbs

$$\frac{-}{S} \Big| \frac{+}{VC}$$
$$\frac{-}{S} \Big| \frac{+}{VC}$$

Example. Patient who is completely unresponsive.

Limbs

$$\frac{O}{O} \Big| \frac{O}{O}$$

Narrative documentation supports the symbolic recording by reflecting the response, level and nature of stimulus required to elicit the response, and whether the response was sustained or sporadic. The narrative note would also reflect any extenuating circumstance influencing a motor response: neuromuscular blockade, amputation, congenital defect.

POSSIBLE NURSING DIAGNOSES

- Injury, potential for
- Mobility, impaired: physical
- Self-care deficit (specify level: feeding, bathing–hygiene, dressing–grooming, toileting)

SPECIAL NOTE

Sensory Testing

Spinal cord and peripheral nerve injuries require evaluation of the patient's sensory perception and dermatome level. These observations would be used in conjunction with limb movement initially to establish a baseline and then continually to monitor progress. Limb movement is monitored in conjunction with the Glasgow coma scale to provide a more comprehensive assessment of the patient's neurological status.

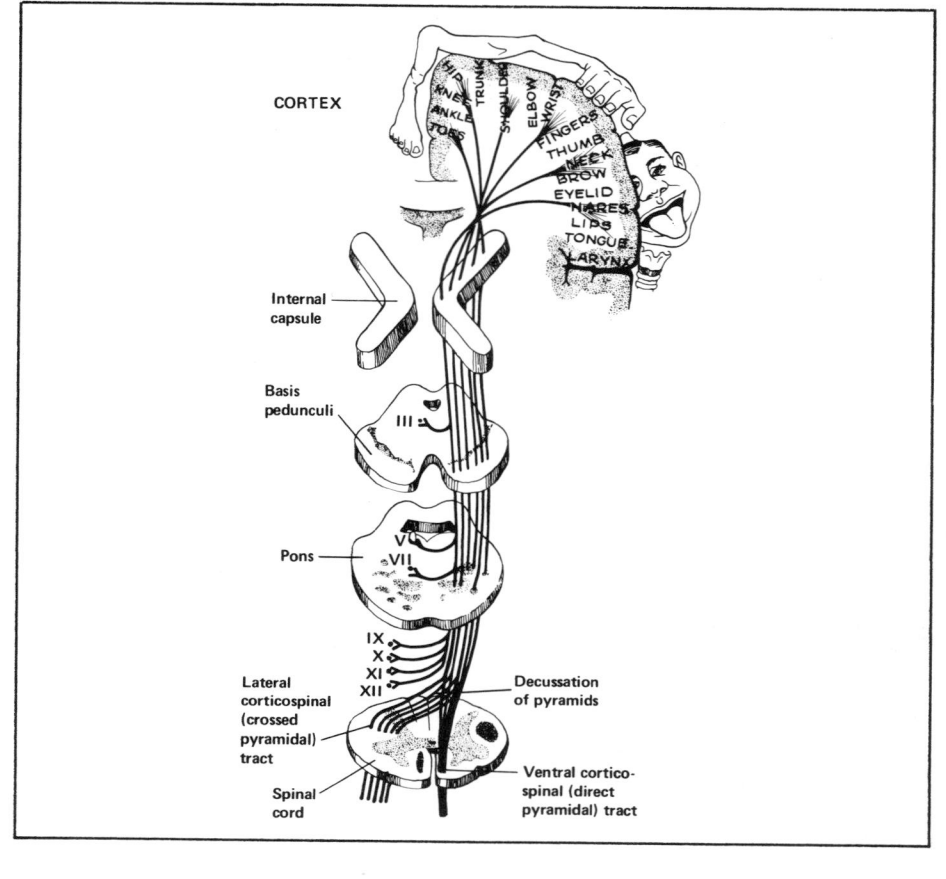

Figure 3–25. Motor pathway. *(From Chusid, J. G. Correlative neuroanatomy and functional neurology (19th ed.). Los Altos, Calif.: Lange, 1985, p. 191, with permission.)*

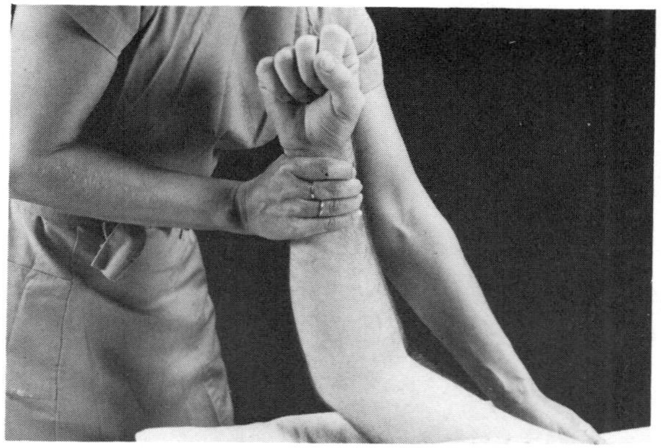

Figure 3–26. Triceps testing.

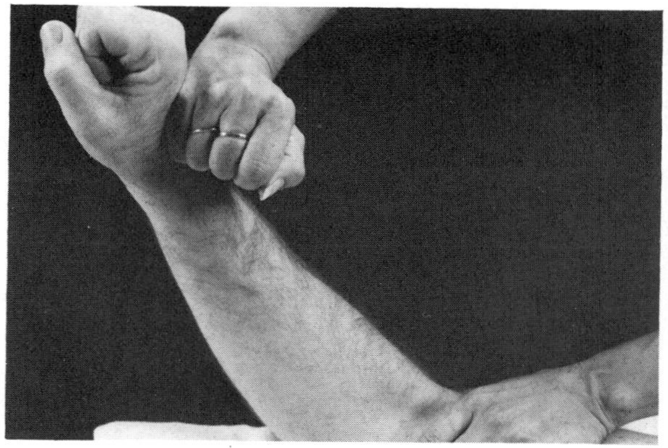

Figure 3–27. Wrist extensor testing.

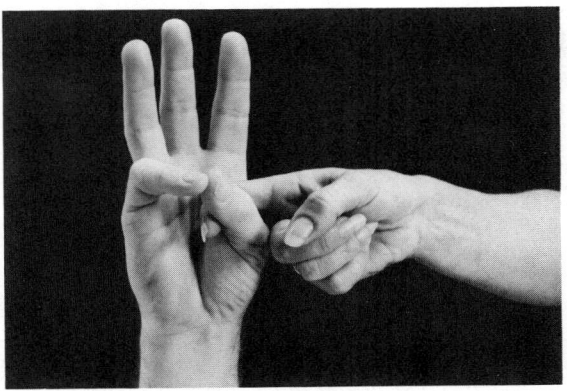

Figure 3–28. Opponens pollicis testing.

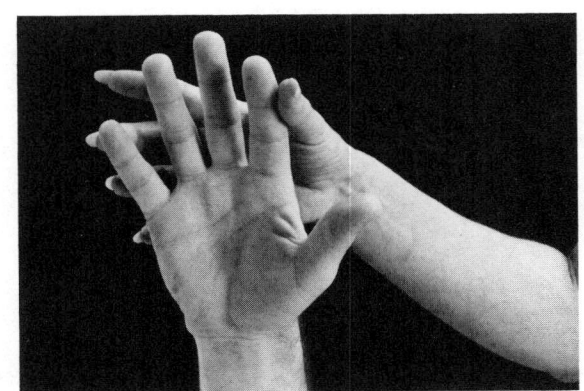

Figure 3–29. Dorsal interosseous testing.

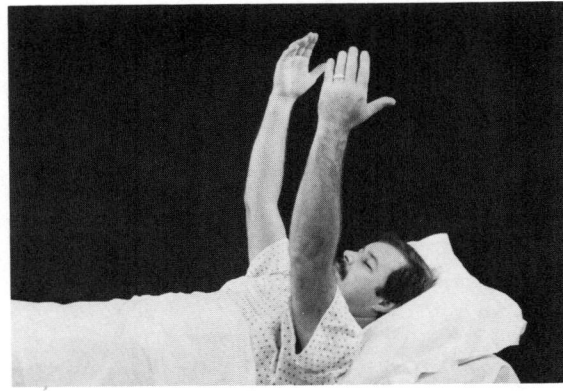

Figure 3–30. Residual hemiparesis testing (1).

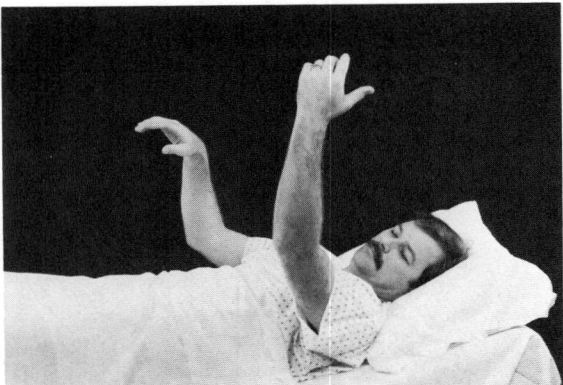

Figure 3–31. Residual hemiparesis testing (2).

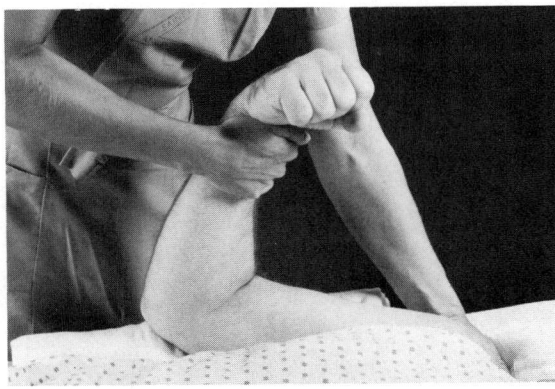

Figure 3–32. Biceps testing.

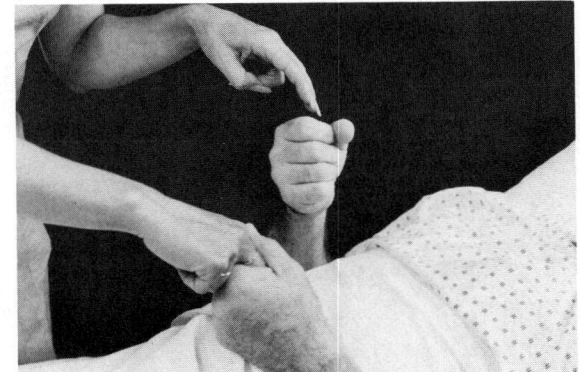

Figure 3–33. Hand grips.

(continued)

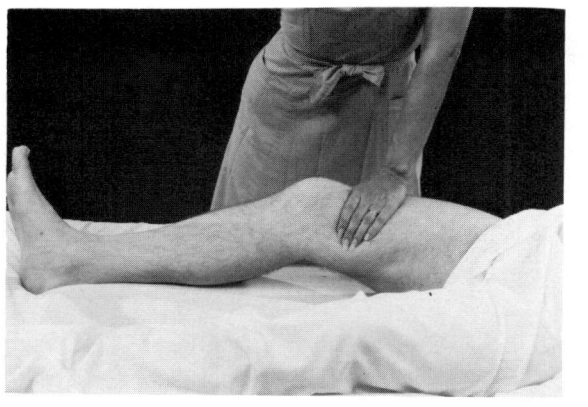

Figure 3–34. Flexor testing (L2,3).

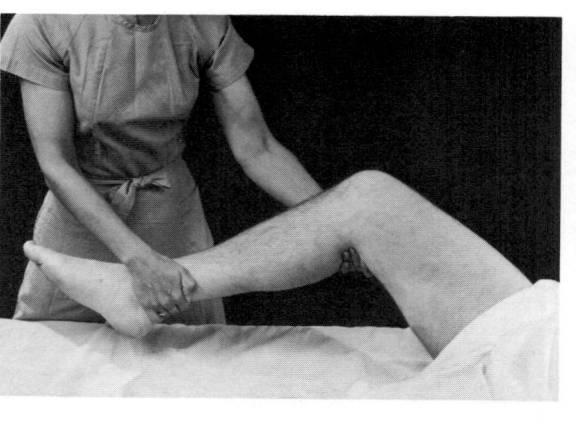

Figure 3–35. Flexor testing (L4,5; S1,2).

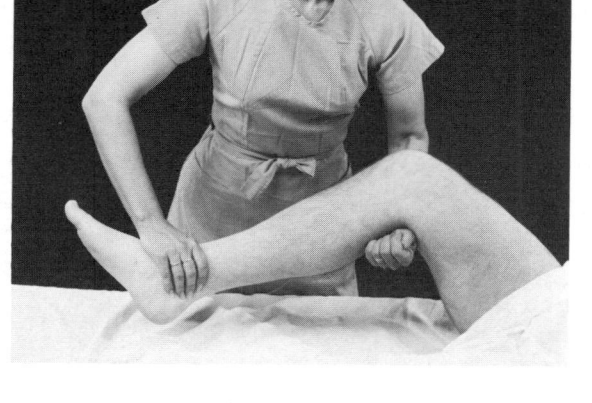

Figure 3–36. Extensor testing (L2,3,4).

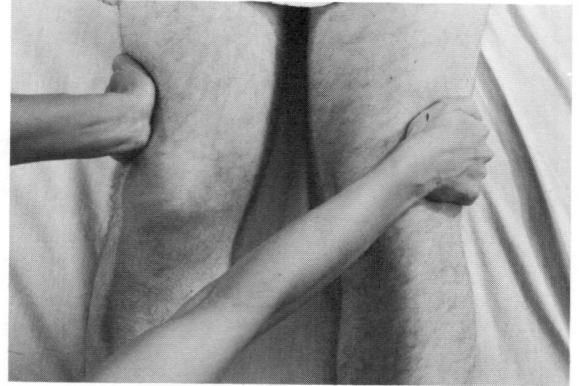

Figure 3–37. Abductor testing (L4,5; S1).

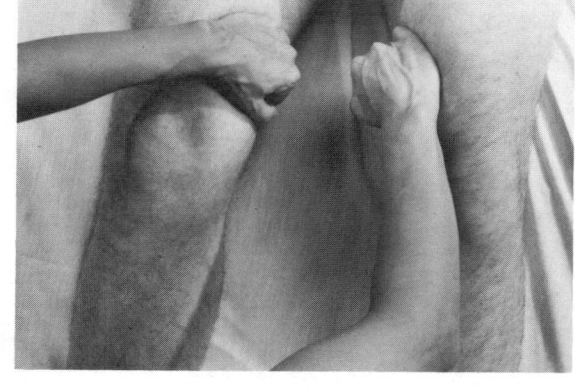

Figure 3–38. Adductor testing (L2,3,4).

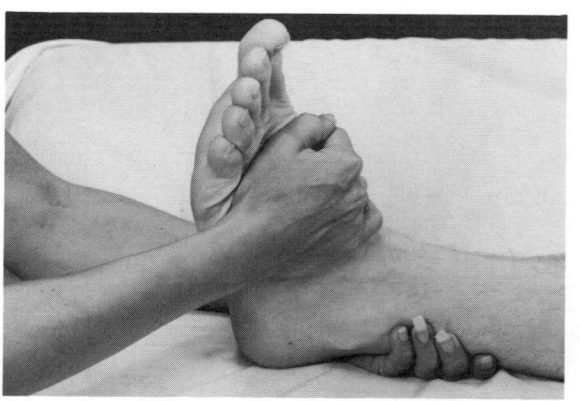

Figure 3–39. Dorsiflexion.

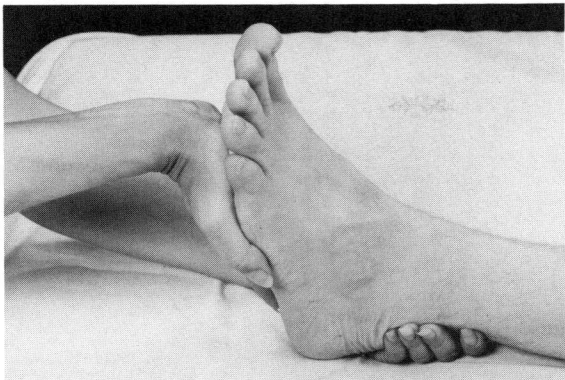

Figure 3–40. Plantar flexion.

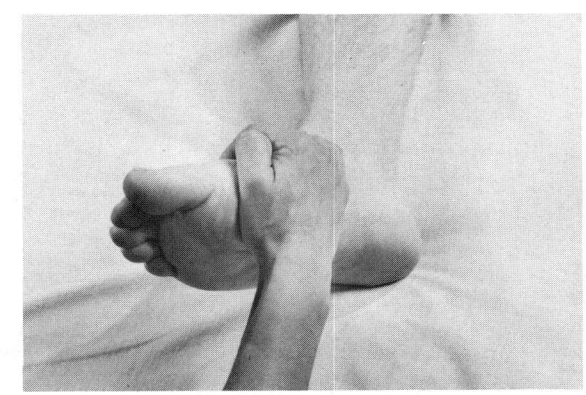

Figure 3–41. Inversion testing (sciatic nerve, L4,5).

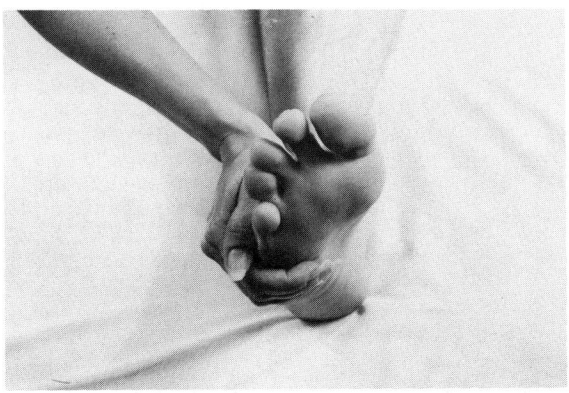

Figure 3–42. Eversion testing (sciatic nerve, L5; S1).

Assessment of Speech and Language

RATIONALE

Speech and language are extremely complex phenomena integrating numerous functions of the cortex: a circuitry of intake–transmission–integration–association–retrieval–output. The function of language involves several areas of the cerebral cortex including Broca's and Wernickes' areas. Dysfunctions can be divided into two groups: motor aphasia and sensory aphasia. A combination of both expressive and receptive aphasia is known as global aphasia.

PARAMETERS	FINDINGS	POSSIBLE ETIOLOGIES	DOCUMENTATION
1. Motor aphasia (expressive)	1. Speech is slow, poorly organized, with short sentence structure Single words used in place of sentences Difficulty naming objects (nouns) Able to comprehend written and spoken language	1. The motor center for speech is located on the cerebral cortex in the convolution adjacent to the motor strip in the dominant hemisphere (left side of brain in right-handed persons and right side of brain in left-handed persons). Broca's area (Brodman's area 44) functions as the memory bank for each spoken word. Superior to this is Brodman's area 9, the area responsible for writing ability	• Verbal response will be assessed q1h using the Glasgow coma scale • Findings are supported narratively and specifically address clarity and appropriateness of verbalizations • Any extenuating circumstances that would affect the quality of the response should be narratively indicated. This would include blindness, deafness, anatomic disorders of mouth and larynx, and congenital speech defects. Also note primary language used (if different) and level of literacy if known.
2. Sensory aphasia (receptive)	2. Unable to comprehend written and spoken language Learning not impaired May not be aware of dysfunction Use of wrong words or incomprehensible sounds Writing will exhibit proper grammatical construction but will be comprised of improper words	2. Sensory aphasia (word deafness) is a dysfunction in the temporal cortex in the posterior portion of the superior temporal gyrus (Brodman's area 22). Alexia (inability to understand printed words) is a dysfunction of the angular gyrus (Brodman's area 39). This combined aphasia, the inability to comprehend spoken and printed words, is known as Wernicke's aphasia (Fig. 3–43) Possible causative agents for disturbances in either expressive or sensory speech centers would be cortical in nature. This may be related to trauma, manipulation of the brain during surgery, cerebrovascular insufficiency (emboli, spasm), or invasive substances (tumor, blood, infection).	*Examples:* Motor aphasia, i.e., dysfunction with spoken word–printed word (expressive) • "Patient has difficulty naming specific objects" • "Patient uses incorrect words or phrases when expressing self but appears to understand

			and follow simple commands" • "Patient able to speak clearly and distinctly but unable to write name, numbers, sentences" Sensory aphasia, i.e., dysfunction with spoken word–printed word (receptive) • "Patient does not appear to understand spoken word and is unable to follow simple commands" • "Patient unable to read menu or newspaper" • "Patient's speech is proper in structure but uses wrong words or incomprehensible sounds." "Patient does not appear to be aware of this dysfunction" • "Patient uses correct sentence structure when writing but uses incomprehensible words or jargon"

POSSIBLE NURSING DIAGNOSES

- Communication, impaired: verbal
- Self-concept, disturbance in

SPECIAL NOTE

Speech and Language

Man is the only animal using its voice to express thoughts in words. Words are sets of symbols and sounds used alone and in combination to communicate. They are components of language, as are signs, gestures, body postures, and facial expressions. Consider the implications for a patient suddenly unable to use the spoken or printed word.

Exclusions

Aphasia and dysphasia both indicate a dysfunction of motor and sensory language as a result of a brain lesion in the primary speech centers. Excluded are language dysfunctions associated with psychiatric disease, dysfunction of the muscles necessary for the production of speech, and any alteration in the sense organs.

(continued)

Facilitating Communication

Frustration resulting from communication deficits for the patient, family, and staff can be reduced. Anticipate the patient's needs. Speak slowly, in normal volume, clearly, and distinctly. Use simple sentences. Ask only one question at a time and allow enough time for a response. Be patient. Experiment with alternate modes of communication, select the most beneficial, and use it consistently.

Alternatives

Alternate modes of communication available for the patient with a speech–language deficit (Fig. 3–44):
- Alphabet board
- Picture board
- Gestures
- Printed word
- Eye blinking

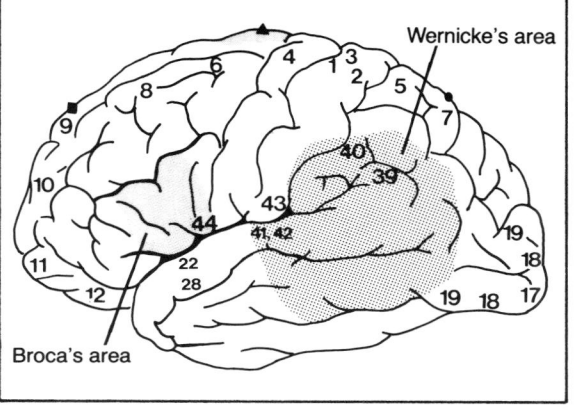

Figure 3–43. Lateral view of left hemisphere with Wernicke's and Broca's areas and selected Brodman's numbers superimposed. *(Adapted from* Core curriculum for neurosurgical nursing *(Vol. 1) (2nd ed.). Baltimore, Md.: American Association of Neuroscience Nurses, 1983, p. 37, and Chusid, J. G.* Correlative neuroanatomy and functional neurology *(19th ed.). Los Altos, Calif.: Lange, 1985, p. 247.)*

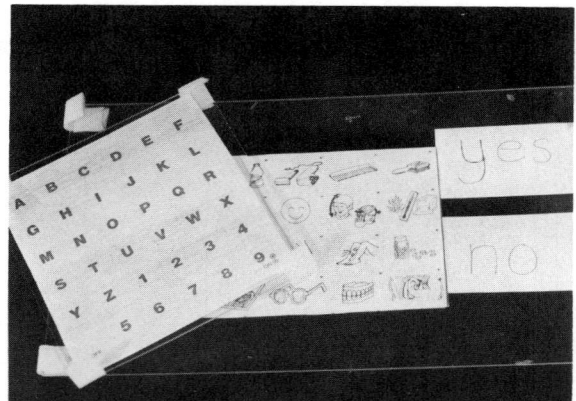

Figure 3–44. Various assist devices and available for the patient experiencing disordered speech and language.

Assessment of the Patient During a Generalized Seizure

RATIONALE   A seizure, a symptom of an irritative or destructive focus in the brain, results from an abnormal amount of electrical activity discharged in the cerebral cortex. The International Classification of Epileptic Seizures, as described by Gastant, is divided into two main categories: partial seizures and generalized seizures. Generalized seizures are discussed here because of the clinical impact on the patient and the importance of assessment by the critical care nurse.

PARAMETERS	FINDINGS	POSSIBLE ETIOLOGIES	DOCUMENTATION
1. Preictal phase	1. Subtle alterations in level of consciousness: Lethargy Subtle alterations in mental status: Confusion and disorientation Restlessness Preictal cry: Verbal response immediately prior to intraictal phase of a seizure Aura: Sensory manifestations experienced by the patient that may precede the onset of a seizure, such as bright, blinking lights	The electrical activity of the brain is an excitatory–inhibitory cycle. When a lesion is present, disruption of this cycle potentiates the excitatory phase, resulting in a seizure. The exact physiology is still not completely understood. The causes are multiple: trauma, infection, drugs, toxins, idiopathology, respiratory dysfunctions, metabolic disorders, cerebrovascular disorders.	Documentation of vital signs during seizure (if obtainable, respirations, pulse) and especially during the postictal phase, in conjunction with the Glasgow coma scale scoring in the postictal phase. Narrative documentation of:

2. Intraictal phase	2. Loss of consciousness
	Tonic–clonic motor activity
	Eye deviation: Direction of deviation usually dependent on type of seizure focus in the brain
	    Irritative lesion: Eyes deviate to opposite side of lesion
	    Destructive lesion: Eyes deviate toward side of lesion
	Pupillary response
	Incontinence of bladder or bowel
	Apnea
			• Time of onset and duration of seizure
			• Precipitating factors, i.e., trauma, infection, electrolyte imbalance, toxic drugs
			• Aura (if applicable): Sense involved, characteristics
			• Seizure activity: Describe completely, including body parts involved, sequence of activity, characteristics of movement
			• Pupil response
			• Incontinence

3. Postictal phase	3. Alteration in level of consciousness: Lethargy, stupor, hypersomnolence Alteration in mental status: Confusion, disorientation Residual neurologic deficit: Temporary paralysis–paresis (Todd's paralysis) Fatigue Headache Trauma sustained during intraictal phase, such as tongue biting Aspiration		• Respirations • Level of consciousness: Preictal, intraictal, and postictal phases • Postictal state: Physiological responses in addition to change in level of consciousness • Sequelae resulting from seizure: Injury, if any,

			such as tongue biting, bruising, aspiration • Notification of physician • Initiation of therapy and patient's response

POSSIBLE NURSING DIAGNOSES

- Level of consciousness, alteration in
- Airway clearance, ineffective
- Breathing patterns, ineffective
- Injury, potential for
- Mobility, impaired: physical

SPECIAL NOTE

Anticonvulsant Therapy

Patients on long-term diphenylhydantoin sodium (Dilantin) therapy may present with gingival hyperplasia. This finding should alert the critical care nurse to the probability of anticonvulsant therapy. Measures then can be taken to assure patient compliance to drug therapy and to provide seizure precautions (such as tongue blade, airway, and oral suction at the patient's bedside (Figs. 3–45 and 3–46).

Diphenylhydantoin sodium may be given by intravenous push but only in 0.9% saline (crystallization occurs in dextrose) and not at a rate to exceed 50 mg/min.

Safety

If patient is in process of having a generalized seizure, with clenched teeth, do *not* attempt to insert an oral airway or bite stick. Doing so may injure the patient or the nurse.

Diazepam (Valium) should be administered intravenously only if ventilatory support is immediately available.

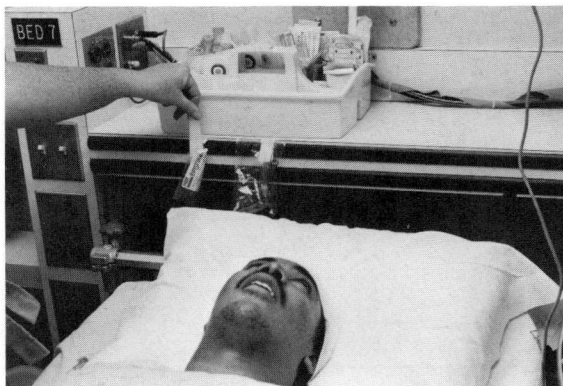

Figure 3–45. Proper insertion of a tongue blade can minimize tongue lacerations.

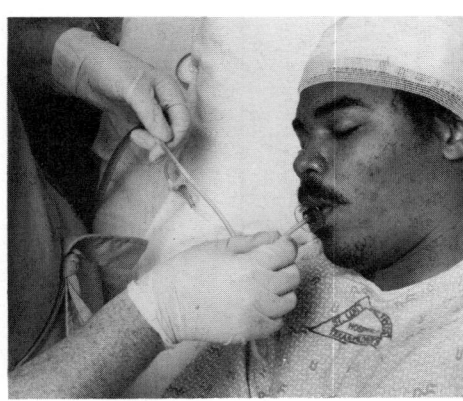

Figure 3–46. Maintain a patent airway by promptly suctioning the postictal patient.

Care of the Patient with Increased Intracranial Pressure

NURSING DIAGNOSIS	RATIONALE	DEFINING CHARACTERISTICS	EXPECTED OUTCOME
Injury, potential for	In accordance with the Monro–Kellie hypothesis, in the adult, increase in volume in any of the three components (blood, brain, cerebral spinal fluid) within the skull beyond the capacity of the compensatory mechanism will eventually elevate the intracranial pressure. This increase in the volume of the components and the subsequent rise in intracranial pressure can result from trauma, hydrocephalus, infection, tumors, metabolic disorders, or cerebrovascular anomalies. The medical regimen for treating IICP varies with each physician. Nursing interventions, however, are more standardized and are primarily directed toward preventing complications.	Manifestations of IICP may be initially mild if volume alterations within the skull develop slowly. The brain is compliant with respect to displacement, but devastating neurological dysfunction occurs precipitously when compliance limits are exceeded. Alteration in level of consciousness: decreased Motor function: deteriorated Pupil response: deteriorated Headache Vomiting Basic vital signs, alteration in 　Systolic BP increases with widening pulse pressure 　Pulse slows 　Breathing pattern deteriorates: Pathological breathing patterns associated with neurological dysfunction at the brainstem level	Neurological damage from uncontrolled IICP will be minimized.

NURSING INTERVENTIONS

All patients experiencing IICP, with or without monitoring device:

1. Vital signs every hour
2. Neurological vital signs with Glasgow coma scale q30min–1h
3. Intake and output hourly
4. Continuous ECG monitoring
5. Seizure precautions
   A. Airway and tongue blade at bedside
   B. Oral–nasal suction immediately available
   C. Side rails up and padded
6. Elevate head of bed to 30 degrees; prevent neck from flexion and maintain proper alignment. Venous drainage from the cranial vault via jugular veins is maintained and CBF will remain unimpaired
7. Maintain patent airway at all times
8. Mechanical ventilatory support available immediately
9. Minimize environmental stimuli
10. Avoid or minimize Valsalva maneuvers, such as coughing or straining at stool or with physical activity. The Valsalva maneuver causes the blood pressure to rise and venous drainage from the cranial vault to decrease, resulting in IICP
11. Administer pharmacological agents as appropriate; i.e., glucocorticoids, anticonvulsants, diuretics, hyperosmolar agents, barbiturates

Should a device be placed for intracranial pressure monitoring, additional interventions are indicated:

1. Obtain operative permit (as appropriate to institution policy)
2. Maintain sterile occlusive dressing
3. Inspect insertion site dressing hourly for any evidence of drainage. Record and report amount, color, time
4. Maintain a closed system with the intracranial pressure monitoring device (Fig. 3–47)
5. Intracranial monitoring system
   A. Maintain entire system free of air; readings will be accurate
   B. Recalibrate entire system q4h as appropriate to institution and manufacturer's recommendation (Fig. 3–48)
   C. Set scale of monitor at lowest possible, 0–25 mm Hg or 0–50 mm Hg, to provide adequate waveform definition (Fig. 3–49)
   D. Observe for fluctuations, pathological waveforms, or dampening. There are five identifiable wave forms:

   Normal:
   > The normal waveform is similar to the arterial waveform but smaller in amplitude. Normal ICP range is 4–15 mm Hg (Fig. 3–50)

   Abnormal:
   > The A wave or plateau wave is the most clinically significant (Fig. 3–51). It exhibits a range of 50–100 mm Hg. The waves occur randomly. Recurring or sustained A waves are an indication of cerebral decompensation, and the physician should be notified promptly
   > The B wave and C wave are indicative of changes in respiration and blood pressure and are not clinically significant (Figs. 3–52 and 3–53)
   > The dampened wave form may indicate a dysfunction of the ICP monitoring device. Prompt investigation of the dysfunction is essential

   E. Maintain transducer at the level of the ventricles, external landmarks being the outer canthus of the eye and the top of the ear (Fig. 3–54)
6. Calculate and record CPP and ICP hourly. CPP is that pressure needed to perfuse the brain, and the normal range is 80–90 mm Hg. It is calculated by subtracting the ICP from the mean arterial pressure (MAP).

$$CPP = MAP - ICP$$

   CBF is compromised if the CPP is below 60 mm Hg. Reduced CPP may result in irreversible brain damage or death
7. When an intraventricular catheter is used for monitoring ICP
   A. A ventricular drainage bag is used to collect CSF (Fig. 3–55)
   B. Note presence of fluid in tubing, fluctuation of fluid, color, clarity, and amount. Normally, cerebrospinal fluid should fluctuate with the heart rate and be clear and colorless. The amount will vary according to the level of the drainage system, size of the ventricles, and the ICP
   C. Drip chamber to CSF collection device should be level with the ventricles unless physician indicates otherwise, external landmarks being the outer canthus of the eye and the top of the ear

OUTCOME CRITERIA

All patients experiencing IICP, with or without monitoring device:

1. Blood pressure will be maintained between 10 and 15 mm Hg of baseline
   Pulse rate will be maintained between 10 measurements of baseline
   Temperature will be maintained below 100°F
2. Neurological status will remain stable or improve as evidenced by increase in Glasgow coma scale scores

(continued)

3. Urine output will be at least 30 ml per hour
4. Dysrhythmias will be identified and reported immediately. Therapy instituted as appropriate to minimize effects on the CBF and to maintain CPP
5. Complications related to seizure activity will be minimized or avoided
6. Intracranial venous drainage will not be compromised
7. Airway will remain unobstructed
8. Any ventilatory difficulties will be recognized and prevented or minimized
9. Exposure to loud noises, tactile stimulation will be minimal
10. Coughing, straining at stool will be minimized
11. Medications will be received appropriately and in a timely manner

Should a device be placed for ICP monitoring, additional outcome criteria are indicated:

1. Informed consent will be obtained prior to procedure
2. Dressing remains sterile and intact
3. Any CSF drainage from around the insertion site will be noted and corrected promptly. Accurate records of drainage will be maintained
4. Sterility of ICP monitoring device will be maintained
5. Intracranial monitoring system
   A. Waveform will be of an appropriate configuration
   B. Waveform will be accurate
   C. Waveform will be visible in size
   D. Any evidence of dysfunction or pathological condition will be promptly identified and measures instituted for correction
   E. Accurate recordings will be maintained
6. Indications of decreased CPP and increased ICP will be promptly identified and measures instituted for correction
7. When an intraventricular catheter is used for monitoring ICP
   A. CSF will be drained easily while maintaining sterility of the system
   B. Evidence of obstruction (fluid not fluctuating in tubing) or hemorrhaging (indicated by change in fluid color) will be identified and measures instituted for correction
   C. Integrity of the CNS ventricular system will be maintained; ventricular system collapse from the siphoning of CSF will be absent

DOCUMENTATION

All patients experiencing IICP, with or without monitoring device:

- Vital signs q1h. Sudden or gradual change will be noted and reported promptly
- Neurological vital signs with the Glasgow coma scale q30min–1hr. Sudden or gradual change will be immediately reported
- Intake and output recorded q1h
- ECG pattern will be noted q1h. Any dysrhythmia will be noted and reported immediately. A rhythm strip will be included in the nurse's notes at least q8h and when any dysrhythmias occur
- Documentation of administration, effect, and patient response to pharmacological agents

Should a device be placed for intracranial pressure monitoring, additional documentation is indicated:

- Note status and appearance of intracranial monitoring device, insertion site, and dressing. Record time, amount, and color of any drainage, and report immediately
- Note status of intracranial monitoring system; record and report any dysfunction immediately
     Note time recalibrated
     Note scale of monitor

Note changes in ICP or waveforms, precipitating factors, interventions (medical and nursing), and patient's response
Note level of transducer
- CPP and ICP every hour. Sudden or gradual change will be noted and reported immediately. Note precipitating factors interventions (medical and nursing) and patient's response
- Note and record when using an intraventricular catheter for monitoring ICP
  Presence of fluid in tubing
  Fluctuation of fluid in tubing
  Color, clarity, and amount of fluid in drainage collection device
  Level of drainage system in relation to CNS ventricles

SPECIAL NOTE

Monitoring Devices

There are three types of ICP monitoring devices; all monitor, but only one can drain.

Intraventricular catheter. Able to drain (Figs. 3–56, 3–57, and 3–58)
Subarachnoid screw or bolt (Figs. 3–59 and 3–60)
Epidural screw, bolt, or sensor (Figs. 3–61 and 3–62)

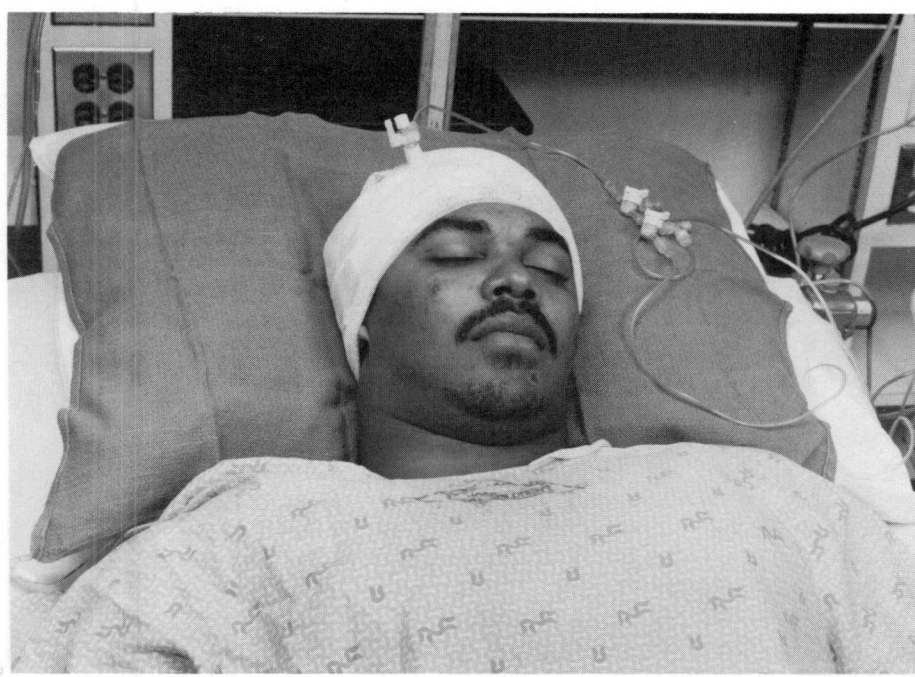

Figure 3–47. ICP monitoring systems should remain closed to reduce the risk of infection.

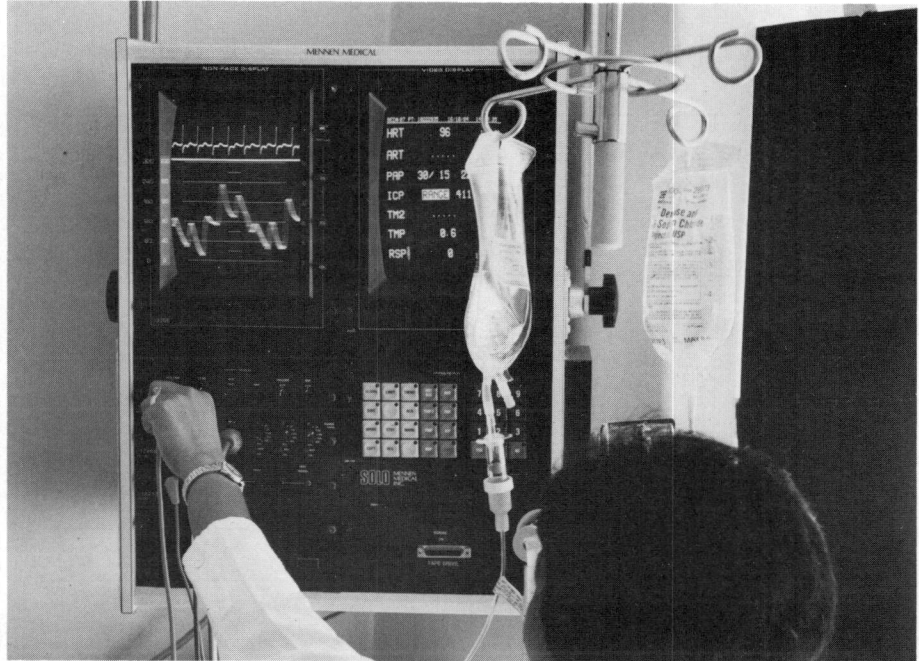

Figure 3–48. Proper calibration ensures accurate ICP measurement.

(continued)

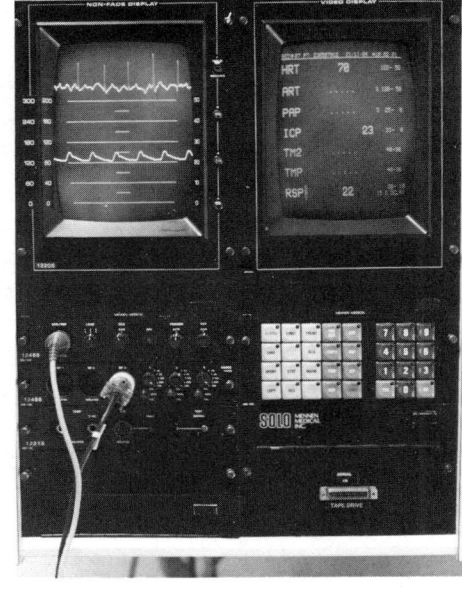

Figure 3–49. Waveform definition is enhanced with low scale monitor settings.

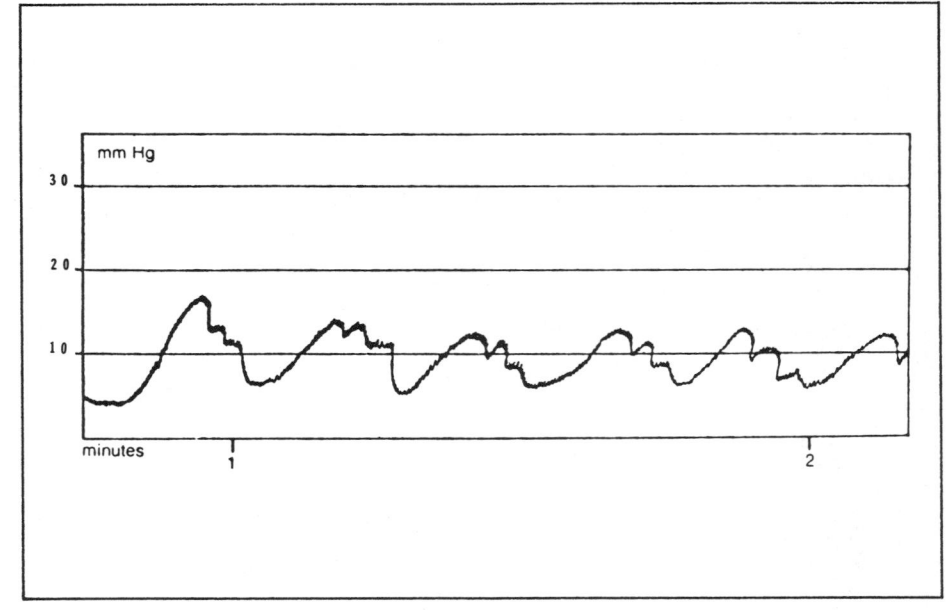

Figure 3–50. Normal ICP waveform. *(Figures 3–50 to 3–53 are from Nursing Photobook. Coping with neurologic disorders. Springhouse, Pa.: Springhouse, 1982, p. 87, with permission.)*

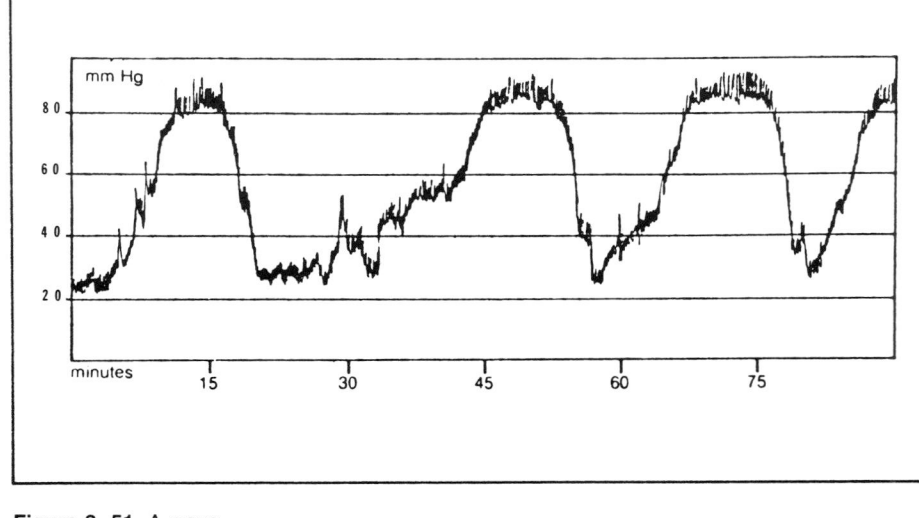

Figure 3–51. A wave.

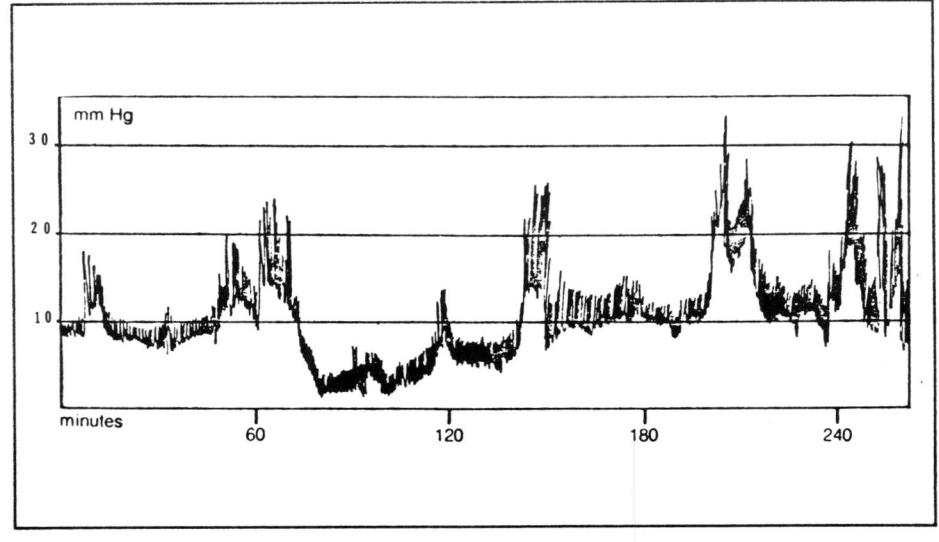

Figure 3–52. B wave.

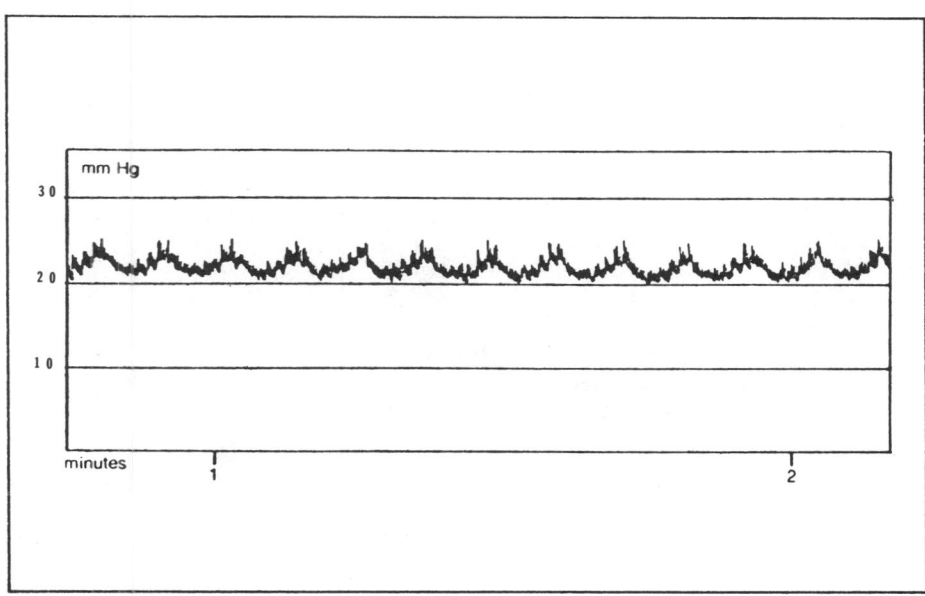

Figure 3–53. C wave.

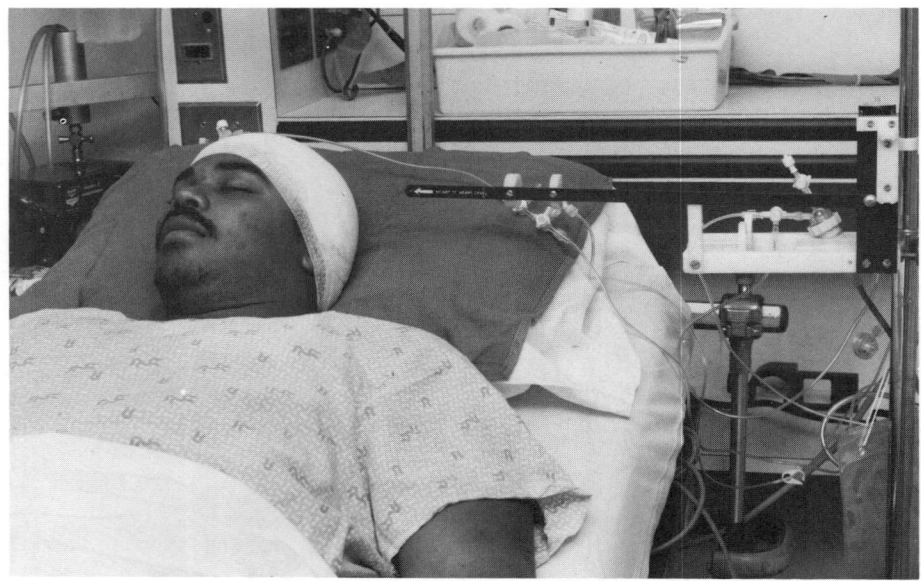

Figure 3–54. Transducer at level of lateral ventricle.

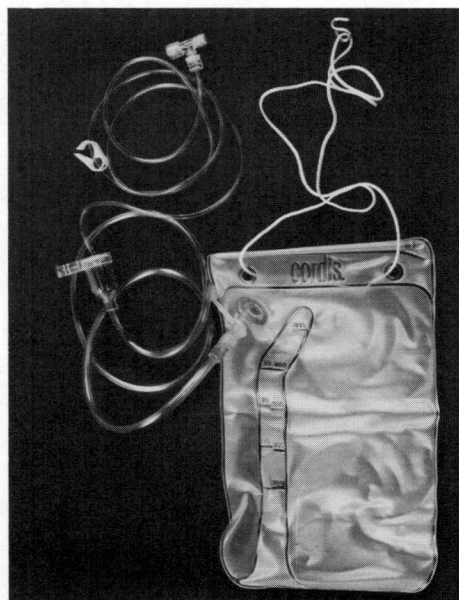

Figure 3–55. CSF collection bag. (Courtesy of Cordis Corporation, Miami, Fla.)

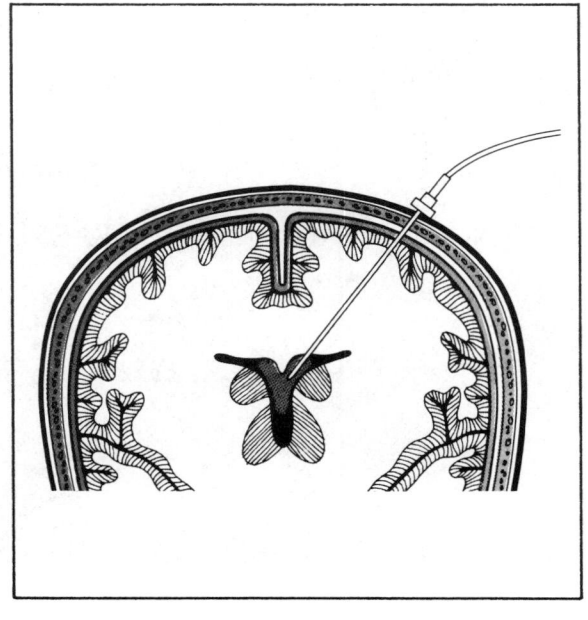

Figure 3–56. Intraventricular catheter placement. (From Nursing Photobook. Coping with neurologic disorders. Springhouse, Pa.: Springhouse, 1982, p. 82, with permission.)

(continued)

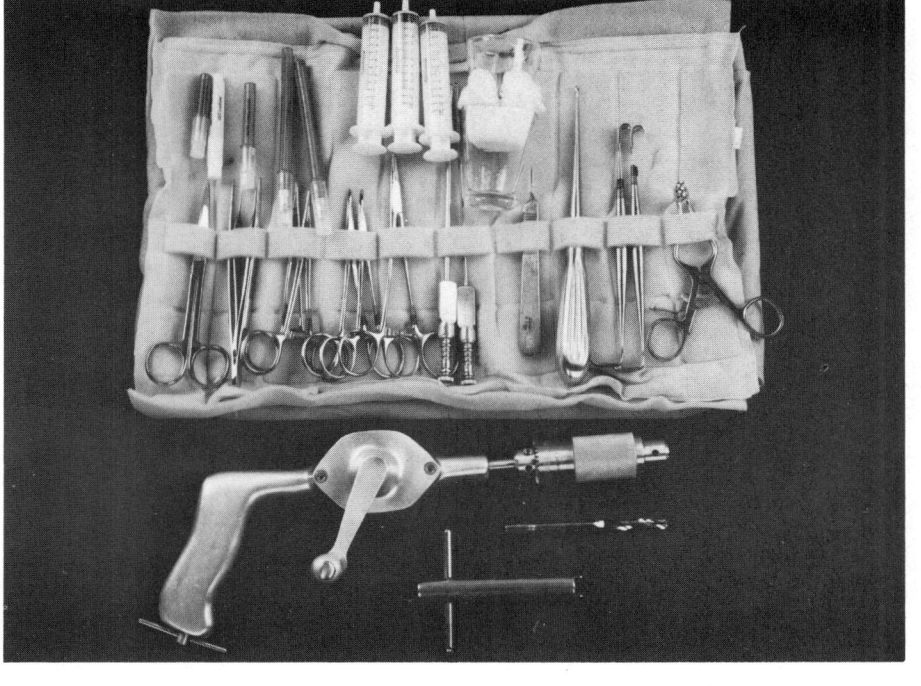

Figure 3–57. Ventriculostomy tray.

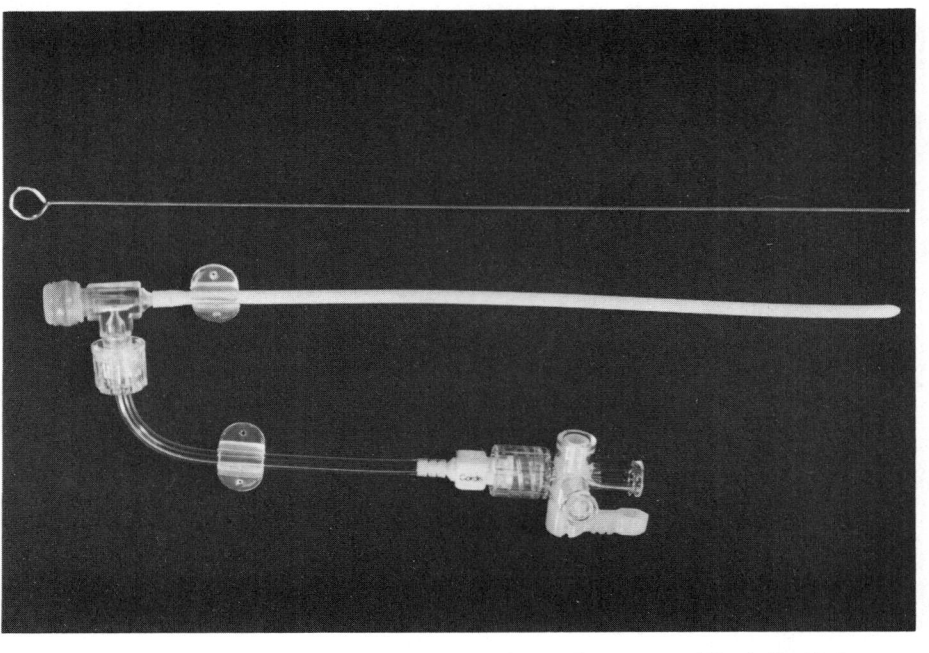

Figure 3–58. Intraventricular catheter. *(Courtesy of Cordis Corporation, Miami, Florida.)*

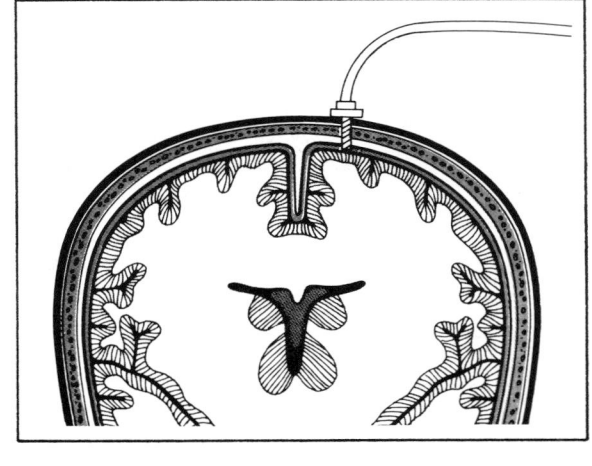

Figure 3–59. Subarachnoid screw placement. *(From Nursing Photobook. Coping with neurologic disorders. Springhouse, Pa.: Springhouse, 1982, p. 82, with permission.)*

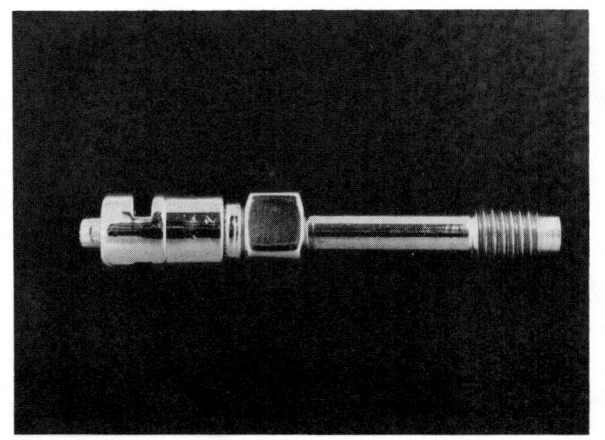

Figure 3–60. Subarachnoid screw.

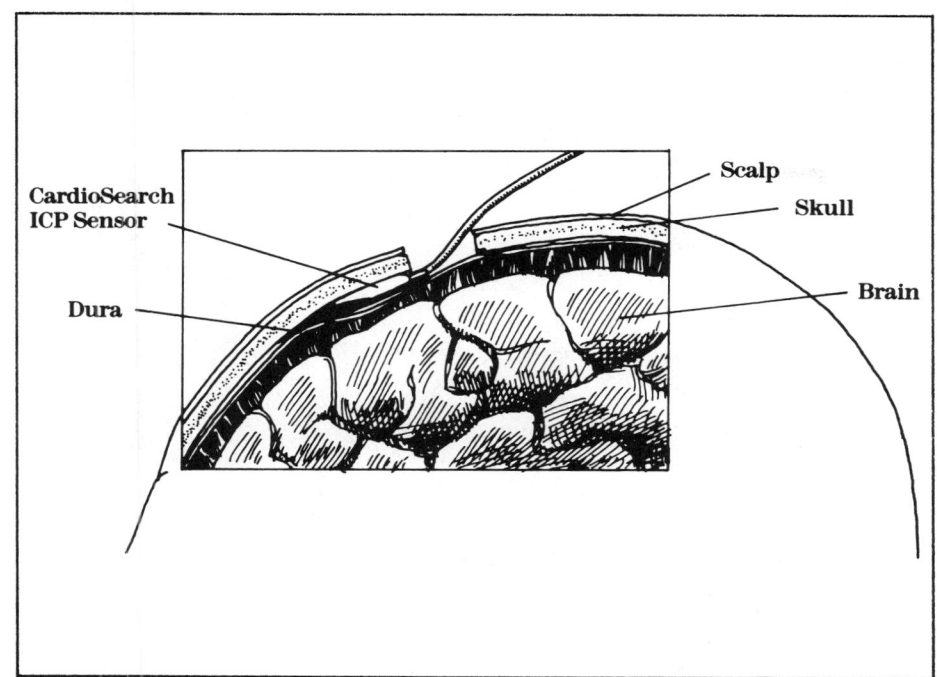

Figure 3–61. Epidural sensor placement. *(Courtesy of CardioSearch Inc., Tampa, Fla.)*

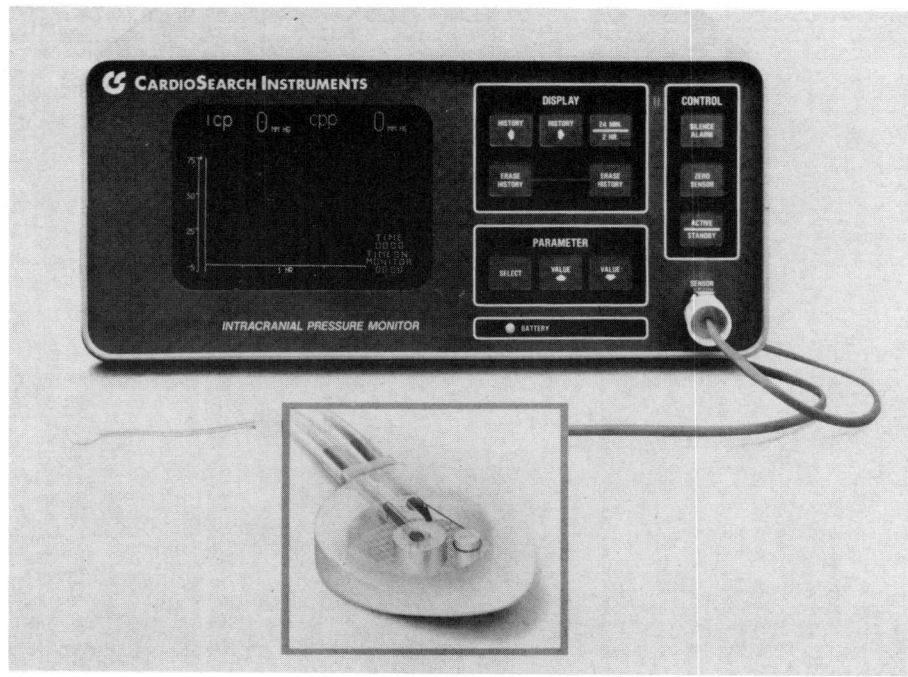

Figure 3–62. Epidural sensor. *(Courtesy of Cardiosearch Inc., Tampa, Fla.)*

Care of the Patient with Impaired Temperature Regulation Requiring Mechanical Intervention

NURSING DIAGNOSIS	RATIONALE	DEFINING CHARACTERISTICS	EXPECTED OUTCOME
Injury, potential for	Man is homeothermic and is able to maintain a constant temperature as a result of various nervous system interactions, chemical, metabolic, and physical in nature. The hypothalamus is the brain's center for temperature control. Many patients with neurological disorders experience extreme fluctuations in body temperature, which can interfere with cerebral metabolism causing stupor, coma, delirium, and seizures.	Body temperature below 96°F (35.5°C) Body temperature above 101°F (38.3°C) Neurological impairment of temperature regulatory mechanism refractory to all interventions except the hypothermia–hyperthermia blanket	No complications associated with use of the hypothermia–hyperthermia blanket will occur

NURSING INTERVENTIONS

1. Obtain physician's order: Use of the hypothermia machine is an intense method of treatment, and most institutions require a physician's order for its use
2. Review procedure with patient and family: Directions for use of the blanket are usually supplied with machine and in nursing procedure manuals
3. Cover the blanket with a thin sheet prior to placement on or under the patient: Allows for conduction and protects skin from direct contact
4. Prepare skin and bony prominences: Apply oil-based lotion to provide lubrication without potentiating effects of blanket; wrap heels and elbows with cotton socks and gauze to minimize potential for frostbite (Fig. 3–63)
5. Insert rectal probe for automatic temperature readings: Tape securely; turn machine to automatic cool–heat
6. Monitor temperature q1h to validate probe readings
7. Monitor vital signs q1h
8. Observe for evidence of effectiveness, adverse effects, and patient's response
9. Reposition patient q1h

OUTCOME CRITERIA

1. Patient's temperature will be above 96°F (35.5°C) and below 101°F (38.3°C)
2. Patient will exhibit no untoward sequelae from mechanical intervention for temperature control: frostbite, shivering, burns

DOCUMENTATION

- Temperature q1h. Sudden elevation will be noted and reported immediately
- Placement of patient on hypothermia blanket. This reflects physician's order, patient–family teaching, physical preparation of patient prior to initiating therapy

- Evidence of effectiveness, adverse effects, and patient's response
- Discontinuation of therapy

Shivering

Shivering is counterproductive during treatment for hyperpyrexia. It is the body's mechanism for rewarming and may indicate treatment is too aggressive.

Frostbite

Frostbite is evidenced by redness of skin that is cold to the touch. With severe frostbite, the skin is white. Rewarming should be gradual.

Determination of Brain Death

Most states have established guidelines for determining brain death including serial EEGs. For the EEG reading to be valid, a patient must be normothermic. This is very important in the age of organ harvest. The hypothermia blanket may be used to gradually rewarm those patients who otherwise lack the neurological control.

Drift

Core temperature is more reflective of the patient's actual temperature and may be more helpful in controlling temperature drift. This phenomenon occurs after therapy is stopped, but temperature continues to fall another 1 or 2 degrees before stabilizing.

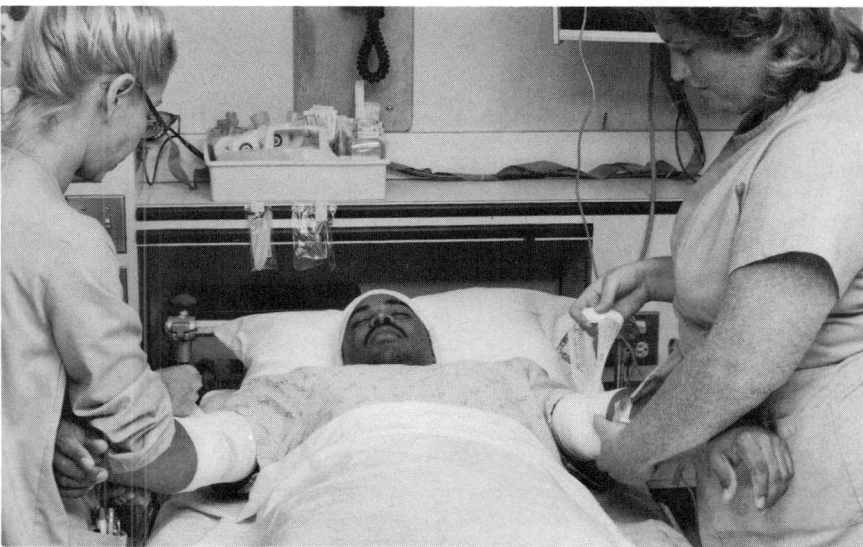

Figure 3–63. Application of protective padding.

Care of the Patient Requiring Cervical Stabilization by Skeletal Traction

NURSING DIAGNOSIS	RATIONALE	DEFINING CHARACTERISTICS	EXPECTED OUTCOME
Injury, potential for	Cervical spine injury whether due to trauma, surgery, degenerative disease, or infection may require skeletal traction for cervical stabilization. The dangers of instability and resulting cord damage outweigh the ease of using soft or hard cervical collars for stabilization. Proper nursing care and assessment can be instrumental in preserving what little function is spared, making rehabilitation quicker and easier. Subluxation and some spinal cord injuries are potentially reversible.	History of cervical spinal cord injury Displacement or fracture of cervical vertebrae confirmed by radiological examination Motor–sensory deficits Posterior ligament rupture Abnormal alignment of vertebral column Instability of vertebrae and spinal cord	No complications associated with use of skeletal traction for cervical stabilization will occur.

NURSING INTERVENTIONS

Preinsertion

1. Obtain permit as per institution policy
2. Explain procedure to patient and family
3. Assist physician with insertion of skeletal traction device, as appropriate

Postinsertion

1. Vital signs hourly
2. Motor assessment hourly
3. Monitor ventilatory status: the cervical vertebrae house the nerves controlling ventilation, the muscles used for respiration, and the diaphragm
   A. Tidal volume q4h
   B. Vital capacity q4h
   C. Incentive spirometer q2h
4. Sensory assessment q1h
5. Intake and output q1h
6. Continuous ECG monitoring
7. Reposition patient hourly; side-back-side (log roll) unless contraindicated
8. Care for and maintain cervical traction
   A. Two varieties of tongs and a halo brace are available for skeletal traction and stabilization:
      a. Tongs: Gardner–Wells, Crutchfield (Figs. 3–64 and 3–65) The concept of the two types of tongs is basically the same. They differ with respect to pin placement and angle of pin entry. The tongs are stabilized to the skull table by two pins. Weights are then suspended from the tongs by a rope and

pulley to provide the traction. Confinement to bed with this type of traction prevents flexibility in activity

    b. Halo (Figs. 3–66 and 3–67) The halo is stabilized to the skull table by four pins. Traction may be applied by one of two methods: by weights suspended by a rope and pulley or by stabilizing bars attached to a hard plastic, lined, vest-type jacket. When the halo is stabilized with the bars and jacket, the patient is no longer confined to the bed

B. Care of cervical traction has two specific components

    a. Skin care

        Pin site care to be performed q8h; usually consists of observation and cleaning

        Observe pressure areas under the halo jacket, particularly the shoulders and scapulas

    b. Maintaining traction

        Rope suspended properly; knot away from pulley (Figs. 3–68 and 3–69)

        Weights hang freely away from the bed and are suspended off the floor

OUTCOME CRITERIA

Preinsertion

1. Permission for procedure will be obtained
2. Patient–family will express understanding of the procedure for cervical stabilization by skeletal traction
3. Placement of cervical traction completed without extending or compromising the neurological dysfunction; proper alignment accomplished

Postinsertion

1. Blood pressure will be maintained between 10 and 15 mm Hg of baseline
   Pulse rate will be maintained between 10 measurements of baseline
   Temperature will be maintained below 100°F
2. Motor response will remain stable or improve as evidenced by an increase in the Glasgow coma scale score and as indicated by limb movement on the critical care flowsheet
3. Ventilatory status
   A. Tidal volume will be maintained between 2 and 4 ml per pound of body weight
   B. Vital capacity will remain three times tidal volume
   C. Lung dysfunction will be minimized or improved, as demonstrated by increased levels achieved on the incentive spirometer
4. Sensory response will remain stable or improve, as evidenced by response noted in narrative note on the critical care flowsheet
5. Urine output will be at least 30 ml per hour
6. Dysrhythmias will be promptly identified and treated to maintain cerebral perfusion pressure
7. Skin integrity and body alignment will be maintained while in bed
8. Vertebral alignment will be attained as documented by radiologic examination
9. Pin sites will heal promptly and remain free of infection
10. Suspension apparatus will be unobstructed

DOCUMENTATION

Preinsertion

- Permit obtained
- Patient–family verbalizes understanding of the use of skeletal traction for cervical stabilization
- Radiological examination completed following insertion of traction device

(continued)

Postinsertion

- Vital signs q1h. Changes will be noted and reported promptly
- Motor assessment q1h. Changes will be noted and reported promptly
- Ventilatory status. Changes will be reported promptly
    Tidal volume q4h
    Vital capacity q4h
    Ventilatory support and treatment: Note frequency and patient response
- Sensory assessment q1h. Changes will be noted and reported promptly
- Intake and output q1h. Decrease in output will be noted and reported promptly
- ECG rhythm and with rhythm strip at least q8h. Note and report dysrhythmias immediately
- Activity and positioning of patient
    Frequency
    Skin integrity
    Position (side-back-side)
- Status of traction
    Traction device
        Tongs: Type, pin site status
        Halo: Presence of jacket, pin site status
    Weights
        Poundage used: Note all changes in weights and patient's response
        Status of rope and pulley

SPECIAL NOTE

Transport

These patients should be transported only with a physician in attendance, as it may become necessary to alter the traction in some fashion, e.g., to transfer from bed to x-ray table or operating room table or to fit into an elevator should it be necessary in transportation. The physician needs to assume the responsibility for maintaining proper cervical traction once the skeletal traction is altered.

Closed Reduction

Some cervical spine injuries involving subluxation (facets of the vertebrae involved become overlapped and occasionally locked) are reduced mechanically by progressive addition of weights to the skeletal traction until the desired alignment is achieved. The physician is the one who adds the weights. Each change in weights is followed with an x-ray film. Serial cervical spine films are the most accurate means of determining correct alignment and stabilization of a cervical injury. Tomograms are a more definitive diagnostic means for determining the extent of a cervical injury. They may indicate if skeletal traction has been sufficient to stabilize the cervical injury or if surgical intervention is warranted.

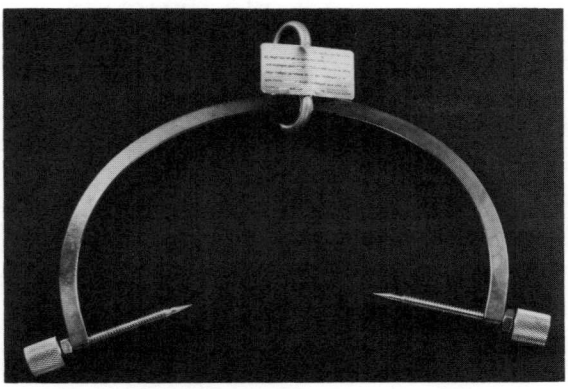

Figure 3–64. Gardner–Wells tongs.

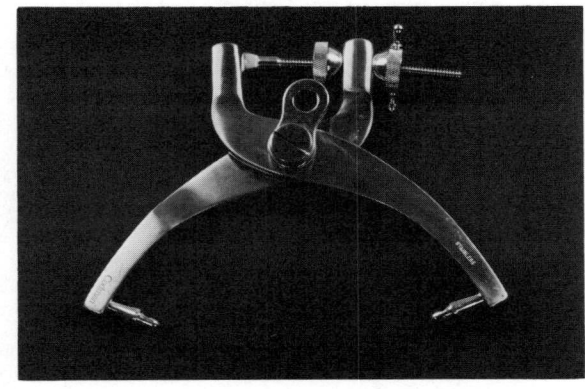

Figure 3–65. Crutchfield tongs.

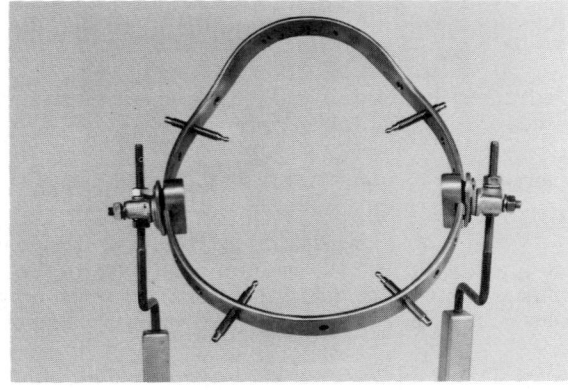

Figure 3–66. Halo brace for skeletal traction.

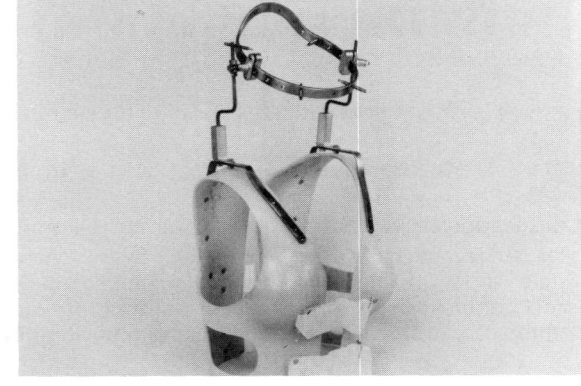

Figure 3–67. Halo brace and Minerva jacket with stabilizing bars.

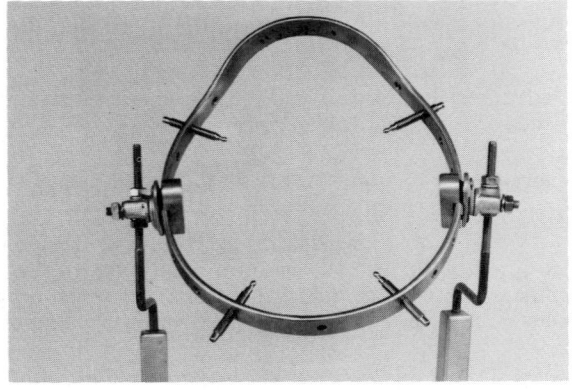

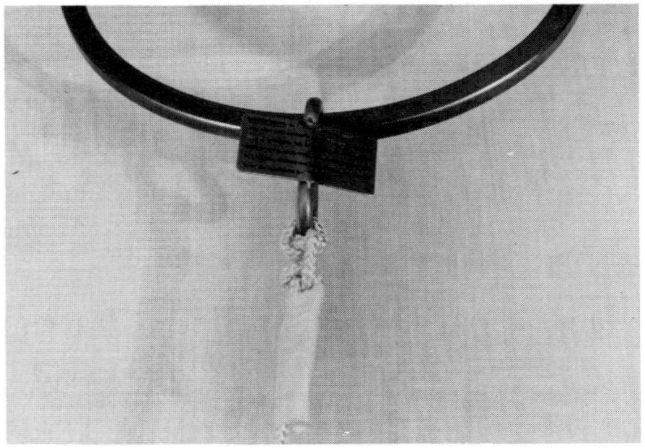

Figure 3–68. Wrap knot ends with tape to prevent slippage.

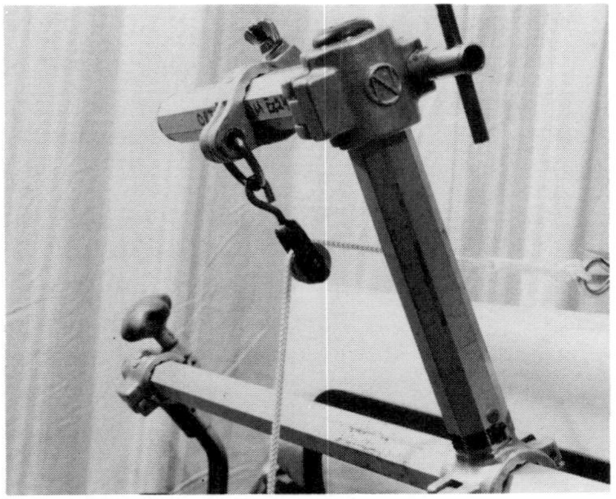

Figure 3–69. Maintain adequate distance between the knot and the pulley.

Glossary

Accommodation: Adjustment of the lens for distant vision by relaxation of the ciliary muscles.

Anisocoria: A condition in which the two pupils are not of equal size. May be benign (congenital) or pathological.

Aphasia: Impaired or absent communication by speech, writing, or signs, due to dysfunction of brain centers in the dominant hemisphere.

Motor aphasia: Any of the varieties of aphasia in which the power of expression by writing, speaking, or signs is lost.

Sensory aphasia: Loss of the ability to comprehend written or spoken words.

Autonomic dysreflexia: In subacute spinal cord injury, diffuse, uncontrolled sympathetic discharge of neuronal impulses below the level of the spinal cord lesion.

Autoregulation: Tendency of the blood flow to an organ or part to remain at or return to the same level despite changes in the pressure in the artery that conveys blood to it.

Baroreceptors: Sensory nerve ending in the wall of the atria of the heart, vena cava, aortic arch, and carotid sinus, sensitive to stretching of the wall resulting from increased pressure from within and functioning as the elicitation point of central reflex mechanisms that tend to reduce that pressure.

Central nervous system: Brain and spinal cord inclusive.

Cerebral ischemia: Local anemia in the cerebrum due to mechanical obstruction of the blood supply.

Cerebral perfusion pressure: A measure of compliance of intracranial pressure and cerebral blood flow, calculated as mean arterial pressure minus the intracranial pressure.

$$CPP = MAP - ICP$$

Craniosynostosis: Premature ossification of the skull and obliteration of the sutures.

Dysarthria: Disturbance of articulation due to emotional stress or to paralysis, incoordination, or spasticity of the muscles used for speaking.

Extraocular movements: Movement of eye in any and all fields of gaze.

Glasgow coma scale: Standard tool for evaluating the level of consciousness as defined by eye opening, verbal response, and motor response.

Homeothermic: Warm-blooded

Hydrocephalus: A condition marked by an excessive accumulation of fluid dilating the cerebral ventricles.

Hyperthermia. Hyperpyrexia, therapeutically or pathologically induced.

Hypothermia: Reduction of total body temperature, therapeutically or pathologically induced.

Intracranial pressure: Pressure exerted within the skull by its components: blood, brain, cerebrospinal fluid.

Neurofibromatosis: Von Recklinghausen disease; multiple neurofibromas; small, discrete, pigmented skin lesions (café au lait spots) that develop in infancy or early childhood followed by development of multiple slow-growing neurofibromas, usually subcutaneous, along the course of any peripheral nerve.

Nystagmus: Ocular ataxia, rhythmic oscillation of the eyeballs, may be horizontal, vertical, or rotary.

Ophthalmoplegia: Paralysis of cranial nerves III, IV, and VI separately or in combination.

Piloerection: Erection of hair due to action of arrectores pilobrum muscles; goosebumps.

Reticular activating system: The cellular and fibrous plexus in the brainstem producing impulses resulting in cortical arousal and contributing to conscious awareness.

Seizure: Disturbance of cerebral function due to excessive neuronal discharge. A generalized seizure is characterized by loss of consciousness with alternating tonic spasms and clonic jerking of the body.

Bibliography

Allan, D. Assessing levels of consciousness: Glascow coma scale. *Nursing* (Oxford), 1984, *14,* 668–669.

American Association of Neuroscience Nurses. Park Ridge, Ill.: American Association of Neuroscience Nurses, 1983. *Core curriculum for neurosurgical nursing* (2nd ed.).

Blacker, H. Starting the neurologic exam. *Patient Care,* 1983, *17,* 75–84.

Blacker, H. Evaluating sensory and motor systems. *Patient Care,* 1983, *17,* 121–136.

Fisher, J. Assessment of pupil and eye responses and their significance. *Journal of Emergency Nursing,* 1982, *8*(4), 211–212.

Hickey, J. *The clinical practice of neurological and neurosurgical nursing.* Philadelphia: Lippincott, 1981.

Hickey, M. Nursing diagnosis in the critical care unit. *Dimensions of Critical Care Nursing,* 1984, *3*(2), 91–96.

Johnson, L. If your patient has increased intracranial pressure, your goal should be: No surprises. *Nursing 83,* 1983, *13,* 58–63.

Jones, C., & Cayard, C. Care of ICP monitoring devices: A nursing responsibility. *Journal of Neurosurgical Nursing,* 1982, *14,* 255–260.

Jones, S. The use and misuse of hypothermia blankets. *RN,* 1984, *47,* 55.

March, K. Look into my eyes. *Journal of Neurosurgical Nursing,* 1983, *15,* 213–221.

Nikas, J. *The critically ill neurosurgical patient.* New York: Churchill Livingstone, 1982.

Smith, S. Continuous intracranial pressure monitoring: Implications and applications for critical care. *Critical Care Nurse,* 1983, *3,* 42–51.

Teasdale, G., & Jennett, B. The description of "conscious level": A case for the Glasgow coma scale. *Scottish Medical Journal,* 1982, *27*(1), 79.

Walleck, C. A. A neurologic assessment procedure that won't make you nervous. *Nursing* (Horsham), 1982, *12,* 50–58.

Youmans, J. Developmental and acquired anomalies, vascular disease. In *Neurological Surgery* (Vol. III). Philadelphia: Saunders, 1982.

Youmans, J. Trauma, benign spine lesions. In *Neurological surgery* (Vol. IV). Philadelphia: Saunders, 1982.

4

RENAL SYSTEM

Adrianne Ward Cosby

Assessment of the Pertinent Renal History

RATIONALE

Knowledge of patient history is one of the most important aspects of caring for a patient at risk for developing, or already exhibiting, renal disease. Based on information obtained by the nurse, specific treatment may be instituted that will be instrumental in reversing or halting the progression of renal pathology. Data obtained from the history may give the only etiological clues that relate to the current clinical presentation. The nurse must be able to determine historically important facts, to identify the patient at risk, and to select and prioritize the data that will affect the patient most seriously during his or her hospitalization.

PARAMETERS	FINDINGS	IMPLICATIONS FOR NURSING CARE

1. Family history	1. X-linked traits (single gene disorder or defective gene on X chromosome)
	    Alport's syndrome (hereditary nephritis with deafness)
	    Fabry's disease (angiokeratoma)
	    Nephrogenic diabetes insipidus
	  Autosomal dominant traits
	    Polycystic renal disease
	    Renal tubular acidosis
	    Renal glycosuria
	  Autosomal recessive traits
	    Congenital nephrosis
	    Medullary cystic disease (particularly when combined with familial history of calculi)
	    Medullary sponge kidney
		1. Awareness of family history is important because many renal disorders have definite genetic transmission as autosomal dominant and recessive traits. In addition, many common disorders, such as diabetes and essential hypertension appear to have a strong familial predisposition. However, actual disease names may not be known by the patient. Familial histories of "stones," "bleeding into urine," "uremic poisoning," or "kidney failure" may be the only information available to the patient and the nurse

2. Past health history	2. Systemic lupus erythematosus
	  Diabetes mellitus
	  Amyloidosis
	  Scleroderma
	  Other states
	    Hypertension
	    Streptococcal infections
	    Gout
		2. It is important to recognize that certain previously diagnosed conditions have implications for the renal system. Patients with scleroderma or lupus erythematosus (because of the nephrosclerotic changes related to their primary disease) almost always have some concomitant degree of renal impairment that can develop into failure if not treated properly. In addition, many relatively innocuous conditions, such as streptococcal infections, may lead to renal complications, specifically poststreptococcal glomerulonephritis. A history of chronic urinary tract infection or unexplained hematuria should alert the nurse to the possibility of potential renal impairment

3. Patient profile	3. Medication therapy
	    Antibiotics (cephalosporins, tetracyclines)
	    Analgesics (especially phenacetin compounds)
	    Chemotherapeutic agents
		3. Lifestyle may present several biohazards for the renal system. Seemingly therapeutic antibiotic administration can have a profoundly detrimental effect on the kidneys, as can many other commonly prescribed medications (e.g., nonsteroidal anti-inflammatory agents). Exposure to nephrotoxins in activities of daily living or working also may predispose the patient to renal insult. Information on the precise nature of employment, hobbies, and so on must be obtained

4. Present problem	(platinum complexes, methotrexate)
	Toxin exposure
	   Chemicals (ethylene glycol, paraquat)
	   Heavy metals (lead, mercury)
	4. Decreased renal perfusion (prerenal or intrarenal causes)
	   Edema
	   Polyuria
	   Oliguria
	   Urine color change
	Intrarenal or postrenal damage (frequently obstructive)
	   Renal colic pain
	   Nocturia
	   Dysuria
		4. Unless the patient has a previously documented renal problem, few symptoms in the history may be available to suggest renal disease. Because of the kidneys' loss of urine-concentrating ability in early failure or insufficiency, change in urinary volume is probably the most commonly seen alteration. Symptoms *suggestive* of urologic dysfunction must be closely examined (e.g., true frequency vs polyuria)

5. Review of systems	**5. A.** Renal
	
	B. Cardiovascular
	
	C. Pulmonary
	D. Central nervous system
		5. A. Fluid volume, alteration in: excess
		   Tissue perfusion, alteration in: renal
		B. Fluid volume, alteration in: excess
		   Fluid volume, deficit, actual
		C. Gas exchange, impaired
		D. Level of consciousness, alteration in: decreased

Assessment of Renal Function

RATIONALE

The kidney has six major functions: elimination of metabolic waste products, regulation of fluid volume, regulation of electrolytes, assistance in maintenance of acid-base balance, regulation of blood pressure, and erythropoietin production. Since all of these functions can be impaired to varying degrees in renal pathology, the critical care nurse must develop expertise in recognizing clinical manifestations characteristic of pathological dysfunction.

PARAMETERS	FINDINGS	POSSIBLE ETIOLOGIES	DOCUMENTATION
1. Fluid balance	1. Normal urine output: 1500 cc/day (exclusive of insensitive losses); amounts and frequency of voidings vary **A.** Anuria: Less than 50 cc/24 hours; essentially no urine output **B.** Oliguria: Less than 30 cc/hour or 400 cc in 24 hours	1. **A.** Usually a result of complete renal failure. If lasting beyond 24 hours, it is suggestive of • Cessation of renal blood flow; glomerular filtration ceases. Etiologies are 　Trauma 　Bilateral renal artery embolization 　Profound shock with peripheral vasoconstriction • Obstruction of urinary flow. Etiologies are 　Bilateral ureteral obstruction (carcinoma, trauma, calculi) 　Urethral obstruction (calculi, carcinoma) • Widespread renal parenchymal damage, including the glomerulus, tubules, and interstitium. Etiologies may include 　Cortical necrosis: Destruction of the entire renal cortex 　Glomerulonephritis: Inflammatory and necrotic changes of the glomerulus **B.** A urine volume insufficient to excrete the metabolic end products, even at maximal concentration. Etiologies may be • Prerenal in origin, suggestive of decreased blood volume for glomerular filtration, seen in 　Volume depletion (hypovolemia) 　Impaired cardiac function (shock states) • Postrenal in origin, suggestive of obstruction of urinary flow, such as 　Benign prostatic hypertrophy 　Calculi 　Carcinoma 　Hematoma	1. Urine output and overall volume status q1h. Trends toward declining volumes (either gradual or sudden) will be reported immediately. Sudden oliguria in conjunction with clinical signs of volume depletion constitute a situation that must be corrected immediately. Sudden polyuria may precipitate electrolyte or fluid shifts and will also be reported immediately.

		• Intrarenal lesions may be responsible for widespread tubular alterations and disruption of the glomerular basement membrane, as in
		    Acute tubular necrosis (ATN)
		    Acute cortical necrosis
		    Acute glomerulonephritis	

	C. Polyuria: More than 1500 cc/24 hours (must be differentiated from frequency, in which volumes urinated are smaller but daily volume still totals approximately 1500 cc)	**C.** Suggests diminished tubular reabsorption. Etiologies include • Increased volume (either intravenous or psychogenic water intake) • Decreased vasopressin, as in diabetes insipidus • Tubular defect, such as analgesic nephropathy or polycystic renal disease • Iatrogenic causes, such as diuretics	

2. Electrolyte balance	**2.** Normal electrolyte balance
	  A. Normal serum potassium: 3.5–5.0 mEq/L
	      Hyperkalemia: Above 5.0 mEq/L
		2. A. Indicative of either glomerular damage with decreased glomerular filtrate or tubular disorders affecting distal tubule excretion. Etiologic factors are
		• Renal failure, with decreased glomerular filtration rate (GFR)
		• Tissue breakdown (potassium released in large quantities as the major intracellular cation)
		• Severe hypoxia (lack of tissue oxygen preventing potassium entering the cells)
		• Acidosis (pH and bicarbonate affecting potassium exchange; cellular absorption of H+ to compensate for acidosis, with shift of potassium to extracellular space)
			2. Laboratory data will be scrutinized carefully for changes. ECG abnormalities (e.g., peaked T-waves due to hyperkalemia) indicative of abnormal laboratory values constitute life-threatening situations that must be confirmed by laboratory data and treated immediately

	B. Normal serum calcium: 8.7–10.7 mg/dl Hypocalcemia: Below 8.7 mg/dl	**B.** Indicative of decreased renal tubular threshold for calcium secretion or reabsorption, such as in renal hypercalciuria. Serum calcium may also occur in decreased levels due to • Renal disease of any etiology (probable cause: lack of vitamin D-promoted intestinal reabsorption) • Acidosis, either metabolic or renal tubular (calcium is lost from bones in an acid environment)	
	C. Normal serum phosphorus: 2.5–4.5 mg/dl Hyperphosphatemia: Above 4.5 mg/dl	**C.** Hyperphosphatemia: Characterized by inability to excrete increasing loads. • Renal disease, indicative of decreased glomerular filtration and decreased tubular excretion	

(continued)

PARAMETERS	FINDINGS	POSSIBLE ETIOLOGIES	DOCUMENTATION
3. Acid-base balance	3. Normal acid-base values Plasma pH normal 7.35–7.45 HCO_3 normal 22–26 mEq/L **A.** Simple metabolic acidosis Plasma pH below 7.35 HCO_3 below 22 mEq/L Pco_2 below 36 (compensatory change) **B.** Simple metabolic alkalosis Plasma pH above 7.45 HCO_3 above 26 mEq/L Pco_2 above 46 (compensatory change)	• Lymphoproliferative disorders with increased destruction of malignant cells • Lactic acidosis, ischemia, increased phosphate levels 3. **A.** Metabolic acidosis: Suggests a tubular defect, blocking hydrogen ion transport and ammonia excretion. Diabetic ketoacidosis, lactic acidosis, starvation states, or excessive bicarbonate loss that cannot be fully compensated also play a role in acidosis formation **B.** Metabolic alkalosis: Suggests renal tubular chloride loss or tubular retention of bicarbonate in conjunction with hypokalemia. Excessive gastrointestinal loss of acids from vomiting contributes to alkalosis	3. In observing laboratory data and clinical symptomatology of acid-base disturbance, the potential for sudden changes in the clinical picture or electrolyte abnormalities will be recognized and reported immediately
4. Systemic blood pressure regulation	4. Normal blood pressure varies by age, sex, mental status, position of patient, and equipment or operator **A.** Age under 50: Abnormal above 140/90 mm Hg **B.** Age over 50: Abnormal above 150/95 mm Hg	4. Hypertension: Renal disorders are the most frequently encountered cause of secondary (nonessential) hypertension. The basic mechanism involves decreased tissue perfusion under increased pressure. Factors contributing are cardiac contractility (affected by decreased venous return, poor venous filling, decreased circulating blood volume) and problems with vascular resistance (influenced by vessel tone, lumen, and blood viscosity). The most frequently seen etiologic factors are • Renovascular hypertension: Caused by atherosclerotic occlusion of the renal arteries, with decreased GFR • Primary renal diseases: In which widespread destruction of the glomerulus and microvasculature also decreases GFR. Increasing vascular resistance leads to hypertension, with subsequent reflex bradycardia and decreased cardiac output potentiating the cycle • Other disease states: Primarily exhibiting hypertension mediated by hormonal abnormalities rather than prerenal or intrarenal vascular problems, e.g., aldosteronism with increased aldosterone secretion and decreased plasma renin action and pheochromocytoma with increased catecholamine production	4. Blood pressure will be monitored q1h, more often in hypertensive emergencies (diastolic 120 or above). Hypertensive emergencies predispose the patient to hypertensive encephalopathy, seizures, and intracerebral hemorrhage. Blood pressure changes will be reported immediately

5. Secretion of erythropoietin	5. Normal hemoglobin
	  A. Male: 14–18 g/dl
	    Abnormal: Below 14 g/dl
	  B. Female: 12–16 g/dl
	    Abnormal: Below 12 g/dl
	  Normal hematocrit
	  A. Male: 41–51%
	    Abnormal: Below 41%
	  B. Female: 37–47%
	    Abnormal: Below 37%
		5. Anemia: The kidney is responsible for production of the glycoprotein, erythropoietin, which stimulates red blood cell production. The widespread damage to the renal parenchyma that occurs in renal disorders of any origin is responsible for anemia from two etiologic standpoints
		• Decreased erythropoietin production as a product of declining renal function
		• Decreased cell survival of the circulating red blood cells due to the toxic environment present in renal failure, resulting from systemic acidosis and elevated levels of metabolic wastes
		
		Other contributing factors are
		
		• The presence of anemia, which may increase plasma flow to the glomerulus, but no increase in cellular flow since fewer cells exist. This produces decreased glomerular filtration, which contributes to renal failure and further potentiates anemia
		• Tendency toward gastrointestinal bleeding, mediated by the toxic effects of renal failure on the gastric mucosa, thus increasing loss via the gastrointestinal system
		Note: Abnormally high hemoglobin and hematocrit levels may occasionally be seen if fluid loss or imbalance has led to hemoconcentration
			5. The laboratory data diagnostic of anemia will be followed, and *critically* low levels will be noted (hemoglobin below 8 g/dl, hematocrit below 25%). These must be reported and treated immediately, particularly if occurring in conjunction with gastrointestinal loss, since the anemia may potentiate renal failure via cardiac decompensation

6. Excretion of metabolic waste products	6. Normal waste product levels (normal ratio of BUN:creatinine—10:1)
	  A. Blood urea nitrogen: Normal 8–24 mg/dl
	  B. Serum creatinine: Normal 0.5–1.5 mg/dl
	  BUN above 50 mg/dl and creatinine normal at 1.0 mg/dl
	  BUN above 75 mg/dl and creatinine increased to 2.0 mg/dl
	  BUN above 100 mg/dl and creatinine above 4.0 mg/dl
		6. Elevated waste product levels: Both urea nitrogen and creatinine are indices of GFR and, consequently, renal function.
		  A. BUN above 50 mg/dl and creatinine normal at 1.0 mg/dl may be indicative of severe volume depletion, hemorrhage, or high protein intake.
		  B. BUN above 75 mg/dl and creatinine increased to 2.0 mg/dl is indicative of definite decline in glomerular filtration, as may be seen in prerenal azotemia. If not treated, may progress
		  C. BUN above 100 mg/dl and creatinine above 4.0 mg/dl is indicative of frank renal failure, with decompensation throughout the
			6. Blood urea nitrogen and creatinine levels will be noted and upward trends reported immediately. The higher the levels seen, the greater is the degree of probable failure and, thus, the greater potential for life-threatening electrolyte, acid-base, and fluid disturbances. High levels may indicate lack of response to conservative methods and need for

(continued)

PARAMETERS	FINDINGS	POSSIBLE ETIOLOGIES	DOCUMENTATION
		glomerulus due to ischemic–necrotic changes. *Note:* The 10:1 ratio is normally maintained if the pathology is of renal origin. A normal creatinine in the presence of a rising BUN may indicate nonrenal causes.	more aggressive interventions

POSSIBLE NURSING DIAGNOSES

- Fluid volume deficit, potential
- Fluid volume, alteration in: excess
- Cardiac output, alteration in: decreased
- Tissue perfusion, alteration in: renal
- Gas exchange, impaired

SPECIAL NOTE

Symptomatology

The nurse must be aware that, although these clinical manifestations of renal system malfunction are extensive, they are only a few of the clinical symptoms that may occur. Renal dysfunction affects virtually every other major body system, all of which may exhibit minor to life-threatening symptomatology. Laboratory and clinical data must be viewed within the overall picture of major system alterations resulting from as well as contributing to renal malfunction.

Assessment of Pertinent Laboratory Data

RATIONALE Due to the multiplicity and complexity of kidney functions, potential impairment may be reflected by a number of laboratory tests. Attention to the data provided, in addition to observations of symptomatology, will assist critical care nurses in developing clinical impressions and estimating the degree of dysfunction.

PARAMETERS	FINDINGS	POSSIBLE ETIOLOGIES	DOCUMENTATION
1. Blood urea nitrogen	1. Blood urea is a product of protein metabolism and is primarily filtered in the glomerulus Normal range: 8–24 mg/dl	1. Above 25 mg/dl: Indicative of impairment Blood urea nitrogen above 100 mg/dl: Indicative of such a high level of metabolic waste product retention that the patient is at risk for seizures and metabolic encephalopathy Serum urea levels are always elevated in renal disease; it is a fair measurement of GFR and urine flow rate. Factors attributed to increased levels are • High dietary protein intake • Catabolic state • Current fluid volume status • Renal impairment of any etiology	• Laboratory results outside normal range: correlating laboratory findings with hydration status and central nervous system—peripheral neuromuscular status • Urine volume changes, with either associated volume disorders indicating decreased GFR or normal volume status indicative of possible interstitial or tubular dysfunction This documentation will be made q2h or more often, depending on clinical presentation. • Communication of laboratory results to appropriate personnel
2. Serum creatinine	2. Serum creatinine is a more sophisticated index of true renal function (less affected by external factors than BUN). It exists in a 1:10 ratio with BUN but is not influenced by as many factors, since it is filtered freely Normal range: 0.5–1.5 mg/dl	2. Above 1.5 mg/dl: Indicative of impairment As with blood urea nitrogen, a creatinine elevation above 10 mg/dl is indicative of risk for seizures Increased levels are a direct result of intrarenal pathology and, as such, make creatinine level a reliable indicator of acute and, more specifically, chronic decline in function. A normal serum creatinine level combined with an elevated BUN suggests intact tubular function and probable • Hypovolemia • Decreased renal perfusion • Hypercatabolism	
3. Serum complement	3. Complement C3 and C4 are part of the complement system activated in immune complex reactions Normal range: 55–130 mg/dl for Complement C3 Normal range: 20–40 mg/dl for Complement C4	3. Abnormal: Below 55 mg/dl for Complement C3 Abnormal: Below 20 mg/dl for Complement C4 Decreased serum levels of C3 and C4 indicate deposition of this substance on the glomerular basement membrane, with resulting inflammatory changes. Etiologies include • Poststreptococcal acute glomerulonephritis • Lupus nephritis	

4. Bence–Jones protein	**4.** Urine positive for Bence–Jones protein	**4.** Bence–Jones protein is specifically diagnostic of multiple myeloma. The abnormal protein collects in the tubules and, in states of dehydration, is indicative of tubular damage. The protein may be found occasionally in the urine of patients with macroglobulinemia
5. Quantitative creatinine clearance	**5.** Quantitative creatinine clearance is a urine examination in which creatinine, because of its constant rate of excretion by the kidney and close parallel to urine flow, is used as an index of glomerular filtration rate (GFR) Normal range: Male, creatinine clearance of 110–140 ml/min; female, 95–125 ml/min	**5.** Abnormal: Male, below 110 ml/min; female, below 95 ml/min A low clearance rate is indicative of decreased renal function due to decreased GFR
6. Glomerular filtration rate	**6.** GFR, using a specific substance that is well filtered by the glomerulus and not reabsorbed by the tubules, is an examination frequently performed to observe the ability of the kidney to remove substances from the blood. Insulin is the substance most frequently used in testing Normal range: Male, 88–174 ml/min; female, 87–147 ml/min	**6.** Abnormal: Male, below 88 ml/min; female, below 87 ml/min A decreased GFR obtained using insulin clearance is indicative of decreased glomerular flow-filtration rate
7. Gram stain and culture of urine	**7. A.** Gram stain of urine demonstrates the number of bacteria present, as well as the quality of the specimen **B.** Culture of urine demonstrates numbers and types of organisms present in the urine	**7. A.** A value of greater than one bacterial cell per field is indicative of significant numbers of bacterial organisms and, therefore, urinary tract infection of any location **B.** Greater than 10^5 organisms/ml is indicative of high bacterial count rather than contamination and probable urinary infection. Types of organisms are usually considered to be either contaminants, such as *Escherichia coli* or *Staphylococcus epidermidiis,* or true urinary bacteria related to infection, such as *Pseudomonas aeruginosa*
8. Urinalysis	**8. A.** Any deviation from yellow straw in color	**8. A.** Any deviation from yellow straw color is considered abnormal; altered color is indicative of secretion of abnormal material • White: Pus, phosphate crystals, seen in urinary tract infection, any source, hyperphosphatemic states • Red or red–brown: Hemoglobin, myoglobin; Hematuria of any cause (infection, burns, trauma, vascular derangement, muscle injury or extreme exercise (Fig. 4–1)) • Red–purple: Porphyria

(continued)

PARAMETERS	FINDINGS	POSSIBLE ETIOLOGIES	DOCUMENTATION
	B. Any deviation from clear in clarity	• Green: *Pseudomonas* (Urinary infection) • Orange–brown: Bile (Hepatic dysfunction) **B.** Turbidity is indicated by any deviation from clear and is indicative of abnormal substances or debris. The substances detected are likely to be • Crystals: Indicate concentration in the tubules of such substances as uric acid • Red cells: Indicate either an inflammatory response of the tubules, such as pyelonephritis, or trauma or inflammatory response elsewhere in the urinary tract • White cells: Indicative of inflammatory response of the tubules or urinary tract • Casts: Indicative of intrarenal problems (decreased flow allows the abnormal material to form casts) • Hyaline casts: Decreased nephron flow combined with increased protein levels; caused by any renal pathology, febrile states, and congestive heart failure • Waxy casts: Decreased nephron flow combined with tubular epithelial cells; indicative of parenchymal damage; seen in glomerulonephritis • Granular casts: Decreased nephron flow and cellular debris; caused by renal damage of any etiology • Red cell casts: Decreased flow and microvascular damage to the glomerules; caused by glomerulonephritis, collagen diseases, malignant hypertension, acute tubular necrosis • White cell casts: Decreased flow and large numbers of white cells; indicative of a major inflammatory process and leukocyte entrapment by the tubules; caused by pyelonephritis, glomerulonephritis, interstitial nephritis • Broad casts: Indicative of decreased flow and damage to multiple nephrons (formed in collecting ducts); may be composed of any elements; always seen in renal failure	

C. Below 1.001 specific gravity

C. An index of urine concentration in renal medulla and loop
- Below 1.001: Suggests fluid overload, post-obstructive diuresis or the diuretic phase of acute renal failure (ARF)
- Above 1.030: Suggests volume depletion, hemoconcentration

D. Above 7.0 pH

D. A reflection of urine acidity or alkalinity. A low urine pH would indicate laboratory error, may possibly be seen in urinary tract infections. Alkaline urine (pH greater than 7.0) indicates abnormal tubular acid loss (renal tubular acidosis) or uncompensated alkali loads, such as urinary tract infection by urea-splitting organisms, alkalosis

E. Presence of protein greater than 10 mg%

E. Indicative of glomerular capillary or tubular damage. One of the hallmark signs of renal disease, such as Fanconi's syndrome, tubulo-interstitial disorders, heavy metal toxicity. May also be mediated to some degree by hypercatabolism (fever, strenuous exercise)

F. Presence of glucose

F. Indicative of glomerular or tubular abnormalities, such as sclerosis and altered permeability. Seen in diabetes mellitus when renal glucose threshold is exceeded and in renal glycosuria

G. Presence of occult blood

G. Indicative of intrarenal (glomerular, capillary, or tubular) dysfunction or postrenal damage
May be associated with betadine contamination or menstrual blood in females

H. Presence of ketones

H. Associated with lypolysis or altered basement membrane permeability. Etiological factors include diabetic ketoacidosis, some dietary regimens, maple syrup urine disease

I. Presence of bilirubin

I. Indicative of an increased level of conjugated bilirubin (unconjugated bilirubin is not excreted by the kidney); glomerular filtration reflects elevated levels in hepatic disorders

9. Urine sodium

9. Normal range: 40–220 mEq/L in 24 hour specimen or 20–40 mEq in random specimen

9. Abnormal: Below 20 mEq; above 40 mEq

10. Urine osmolality

10. Normal range: 350–400 mOsm/kg

10. Abnormal: Below 350 mOsm/kg; above 400 mOsm/kg
Indicative of loss of renal ability to conserve

(continued)

PARAMETERS	FINDINGS	POSSIBLE ETIOLOGIES	DOCUMENTATION
		sodium and concentrate urine. High urine osmolality values (greater than 400 mOsm) combined with low urine sodium values (below 20 mEq) indicate possible prerenal causes or acute glomerulonephritis. Low osmolality values (below 350 mOsm) combined with high sodium values (above 40 mEq) indicate possible obstruction or acute tubular necrosis.	

POSSIBLE NURSING DIAGNOSES

- Fluid volume, alteration in: excess
- Fluid volume, deficit, actual
- Tissue perfusion, alteration in: renal

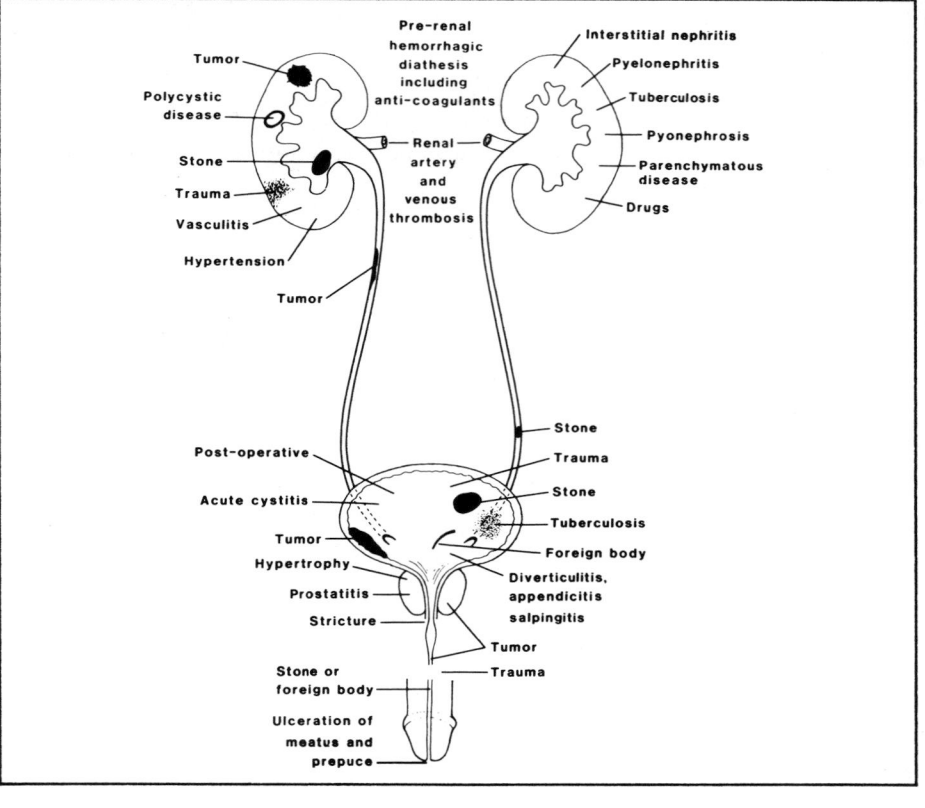

Figure 4–1. Common etiologic sites of hematuria. *(From Earle, D. Manual of clinical nephrology. Philadelphia: Saunders, 1982, p. 90, with permission.)*

Assessment of Fluid and Electrolyte Status

RATIONALE

Fluid and electrolyte disturbances are among the most frequently seen and least understood manifestations of renal pathology. To understand the important role of renal regulation of fluids and electrolytes, nurses must be aware that all cellular metabolic processes are regulated or facilitated by body water and cellular ions and cations. They must comprehend normal serum constituents and distribution, as well as regulation, in order to understand disturbances in volume, composition, distribution, and their sequelae. Observation, assessment, and appropriate reporting of these disturbances will frequently prevent or lessen life-threatening complications.

PARAMETERS	FINDINGS	POSSIBLE ETIOLOGIES	DOCUMENTATION
1. Dehydration	1. Dehydration (volume depletion). Abnormal combined loss of water and sodium chloride without reduction in intracellular water and electrolytes. Reabsorption of salt and water occurs unless GFR falls to extremely low levels as volume depletion progresses. Dry mucous membranes Decreased skin turgor Lethargy Postural hypotension Decreased insensible loss, i.e., perspiration and tearing Hyperventilation Decreased urine volume and increased specific gravity	1. Symptoms arise from decreased cardiac output (decreased plasma volume), and decreased intercellular space of subcutaneous tissue, and cerebral tissue Blood loss Plasma loss (burns) Vomiting Diarrhea Fistula drainage Diuretics Severe gastroenteritis Nasogastric suction	*Note:* These observations will be recorded at least q2h or more often depending on clinical presentation. • Urine volume changes (either increase or decrease), especially dramatic changes • Change in fluid status, evidence of either volume depletion or volume excess • Change in electrolyte status, particularly abnormal values. Observe and report *immediately* any electrolyte abnormalities that place the patient at risk for life-threatening arrhythmias (e.g., potassium less than 3.0 mEq/L or above 6.0 mEq/L) • Any clinical condition that places the patient at risk for sudden associated electrolyte abnormalities (e.g., gastrointestinal bleeding or blood sequestration in the intestine, the breakdown of which places the patient at risk for sudden hyperkalemia)
2. Overhydration	2. Overhydration (volume excess). Extracellular fluid volume excess with expanded interstitial cell volume Edema Dyspnea Normal skin turgor Rales Jugular venous distention Hypertension Increased urine volume and decreased specific gravity	2. Edema occurs because of decreased plasma colloid oncotic pressure, increased permeability of the capillary wall, and obstruction of regional lymphatic flow. All symptomatology is related to increased intravascular load that cannot adequately be excreted by kidneys Congestive heart failure Nephrotic syndrome Cushing's syndrome	
3. Hypokalemia	3. Hypokalemia (serum potassium below 3.5 mEq/L). Potassium is normally excreted by the kidneys (filtered by the glomeruli) and by the gastrointestinal tract (excreted in stool)	3. Hypokalemia may result from inadequate dietary intake, temporary cellular shift (alkalosis), extrarenal loss (sweating, gastrointestinal loss), or intrarenal potassium loss. Symptomatology is related to the effect of potassium de-	

ECG manifestations
Depressed ST segment
Flattened or inverted T-wave (Fig. 4–2)
Prolonged PR interval
Sinus bradycardia
First and second degree block
Atrial flutter
Paroxysmal atrial tachycardia
Atrioventricular dissociation
Ventricular fibrillation
U-waves
Ventricular tachycardia
Premature atrial and ventricular beats
Anorexia
Muscle weakness
Lethargy
Confusion
Predisposition to digitalis toxicity

pletion on cardiac muscle, skeletal muscle, and gastric mucosa
Inadequate intake (iatrogenic)
Gastrointestinal loss
Diuretics (high-flow urine output state)
Diabetic ketoacidosis
Postobstructive diuresis (high-flow urine output state)
Leukemia
Antibiotics

4. Hyperkalemia

4. Hyperkalemia (serum potassium greater than 5.0 mEq/L). Seen in ARF or CRF when GFR decreases to below 10 ml/min. The kidneys are unable to excrete the continually increasing load, especially if tissue breakdown is evident
ECG manifestations
Increased rate
Peaked T-waves (Fig. 4–3)
Widened QRS complex
Atrial arrest
Cardiac standstill and ventricular fibrillation
Sinus and atrioventricular blocks
Weakness
Flaccid paralysis

4. Symptomatology is produced by the effects of high potassium levels on cardiac and skeletal muscles
Acidosis
Use of beta-blockers
Digitalis overdose
Hypercatabolism
Addison's disease
Drugs (e.g., spironolactone)
Blood administration

5. Hypocalcemia

5. Hypocalcemia (serum calcium below 8.7 mg/dl). Calcium, after absorption, is either deposited in bone or excreted by the kidneys. Renal excretion is mediated by serum calcium levels and parathyroid horomone levels
ECG manifestations
Tachyarrhythmias
Prolonged QT interval (after correction for age, sex, heart rate) (Fig. 4–4)
Prolonged ST segment
Tetany (Chvostek's and Trousseau's signs)
Muscle cramps
Convulsions

5. Symptomatology relates to the effects of serum calcium levels on neuromuscular irritability and excitability of the cardiac cellular membrane
Hypoalbuminemia
Decreased parathyroid activity (whether idiopathic or surgically acquired)
Hypomagnesemia
Acute pancreatitis
Osteoblastic metastases
Nephrotic syndrome
Disturbances in vitamin D metabolism

(continued)

PARAMETERS	FINDINGS	POSSIBLE ETIOLOGIES	DOCUMENTATION
6. Hypercalcemia	**6.** Hypercalcemia (serum calcium above 10.7 mg/dl). Facilitated by increased gastrointestinal absorption and increased bone resorption 　ECG manifestations 　　Decreased rate 　　Shortened QT interval (after correction for age, sex, heart rate) (Fig. 4–5) 　　Shortened ST segment 　Muscle weakness 　Obtundation–coma	**6.** Symptomatology again relates to the effect of calcium in regulating cardiac stability and cellular excitability, and neuromuscular excitability. 　Hyperparathyroidism 　Malignancies 　Granulomatous diseases (e.g., sarcoidosis) 　Recovery from ARF (diuretic phase)	
7. Hyponatremia	**7.** Hyponatremia (serum sodium below 135 mEq/L). Sodium is selectively reabsorbed or excreted in the tubules and is mediated by a number of mechanisms for concentration or dilution of water load 　Anorexia and nausea 　Weakness 　Orthostatic syncope 　Circulatory collapse	**7.** In *hypertonic hyponatremia,* serum sodium is decreased, but plasma osmolality is increased, probably because of such substances as glucose or urea. In *isotonic hyponatremia,* serum sodium is decreased and plasma osmolality is normal, suggesting the presence of elevated protein or lipid levels. *Hypotonic hyponatremia* shows decreases in both serum sodium and osmolality levels. In *decreased sodium and osmolality,* the extracellular volume must be elevated. If *extracellular volume is low,* etiological factors to be considered are hemorrhage, gastrointestinal loss, diuretics, and adrenal failure. If *extracellular volume is normal,* etiologies to be considered are renal failure, syndrome of inappropriate antidiuretic hormone (SIADH), and water intoxication. If *extracellular volume is increased,* one must suspect such etiologies as congestive heart failure (CHF), liver failure, or renal failure	
8. Hypernatremia	**8.** Hypernatremia (serum sodium above 148 mEq/L) 　Edema 　Pulmonary congestion	**8.** Cause is partially mediated by extracellular volume Increased extracellular volume with increased serum sodium. • Iatrogenic • Primary aldosteronism Normal extracellular volume with increased serum sodium • Hypercapnea • Excessive diaphoresis • Nephrogenic diabetes insipidus Decreased extracellular volume with elevated serum sodium • Gastrointestinal loss	

9. Hypophosphatemia	**9.** Hypophosphatemia (serum phosphorus less than 2.5 mg/dl). Normally selectively reabsorbed by the glomerulus and, questionably, the tubules (influenced by parathyroid hormone and vitamin D)
	    Weakness
	    Respiratory failure
	    Cardiomyopathy
	    Obtundation
	    Coma
	    Seizures
	    Osteomalacia
		• Diuresis
		• Renal failure
		9. Gastrointestinal
		  • Inadequate intake
		  • Antacid therapy
		  • Diarrhea
		Renal
		  • Hyperparathyroidism
		  • Glycosuria
		  • Diuretics
		  • Fanconi's syndrome
		Other
		  • Insulin administration
		  • Acute respiratory alkalosis
		  • Catecholamine administration

10. Hyperphosphatemia	**10.** Hyperphosphatemia (serum phosphorus above 4.5 mg/dl)
	    Tetany
	    Hypotension
	    Cardiac arrest
		10. May be transient or chronic depending on renal excretion capabilities
		Decreased GFR
		Decreased tubular reabsorption
		  • Hypoparathyroidism
		  • Acromegaly
		  • Thyrotoxicosis
		Sudden extracellular phosphate shift
		  • Cytotoxic drugs
		  • Rhabdomyolysis
		  • Laxative abuse
		  • Phosphate enemas

11. Hypomagnesemia	**11.** Hypomagnesemia (serum magnesium less than 1.7 mg/dl). Magnesium is filtered in the glomerulus and the loop, dependent upon percentage of renal function still existing. This is mediated to some degree by parathyroid hormone
	    Coarse tremors
	    Hypertension
		11. Symptoms are related to the effect on cardiac and skeletal muscle
		Gastrointestinal
		  • Malabsorptive insufficiency
		  • Pancreatic insufficiency
		  • Alcoholism
		Renal
		  • Hypercalcemia
		  • Hyperaldosteronism
		  • Acute tubular necrosis (diuretic phase)
		  • Diuretic therapy
		  • Glycosuria
		  • Hyperthyroidism

12. Hypermagnesemia	**12.** Hypermagnesemia (serum magnesium above 2.8 mg/dl). Dependent upon GFR
	    ECG manifestations
	      Prolonged PR interval
	      Broadened QRS complex
	      Elevated T-waves
		12. Symptoms related to effect on central nervous system and cardiac system
		    Eclampsia
		    Adrenal insufficiency
		    Acute renal insufficiency
		    Magnesium-containing antacids

(continued)

PARAMETERS	FINDINGS	POSSIBLE ETIOLOGIES	DOCUMENTATION
	Muscle weakness Paralysis Confusion Hypotension		

POSSIBLE NURSING DIAGNOSES

- Fluid volume, alteration in: excess
- Fluid volume, deficit, actual
- Fluid volume, deficit, potential
- Tissue perfusion, alteration in: renal

SPECIAL NOTE

Dehydration

The nurse should be aware of the difference between pure dehydration and volume depletion. Pure dehydration refers to the evenly distributed loss of water in the body and is usually seen only in the syndrome of diabetes insipidus (neurogenic or nephrogenic) and in patients with lack of access to water (due to either immobility or illness). Volume depletion refers primarily to loss in the extracellular fluid of both water and solutes and is used as the basis for discussion because of the frequency with which it is seen.

Volume Excess

For the purposes of this assessment skill, volume excess with the features of expanded extracellular and intracellular volume is discussed because of the frequency with which it is encountered in clinical practice. Hypotonic excess characterized by pathological water ingestion is observed less frequently.

Third Spacing

In assessing fluid balance, the nurse must be aware of the third-space syndrome, a sudden and massive fluid shift into a potential space mediated by decreased plasma proteins, increased capillary permeability, or lymphatic blockage. This syndrome is frequently encountered after major surgery (particularly retroperitoneal), infections (peritonitis), trauma, burns, or liver disease, with rapid development of ascites. The fluid may be localized in a specific area or widely diffused. Remobilization of the fluid usually occurs approximately 1 week postinsult and at that time presents a threat related to rapid reexpansion of intravascular volume.

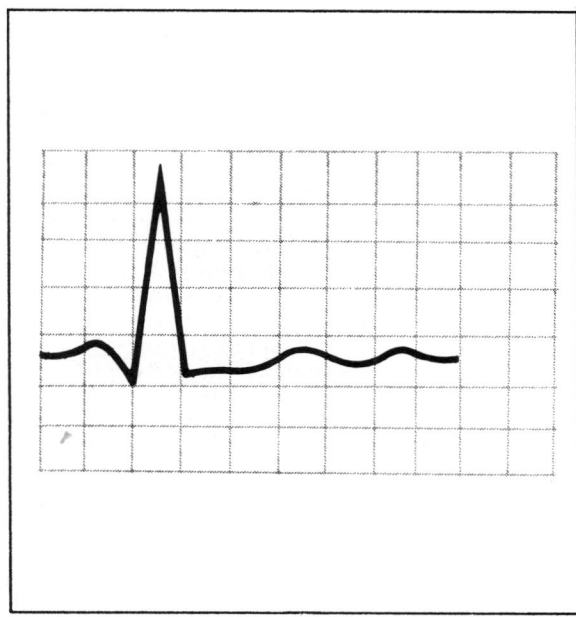

Figure 4–2. ECG changes characteristic of hypokalemia.

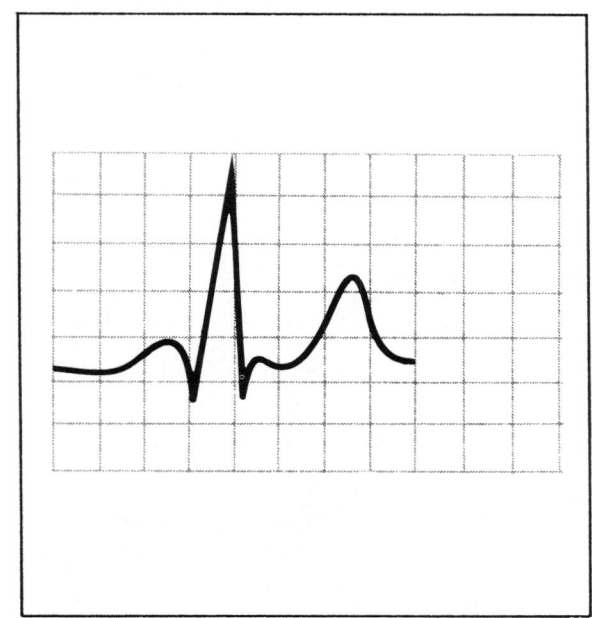

Figure 4–3. ECG changes characteristic of hyperkalemia.

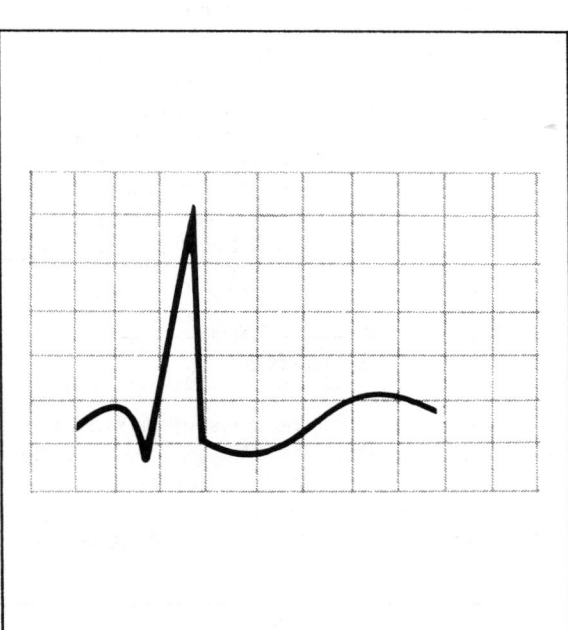

Figure 4–4. ECG changes characteristic of hypocalcemia.

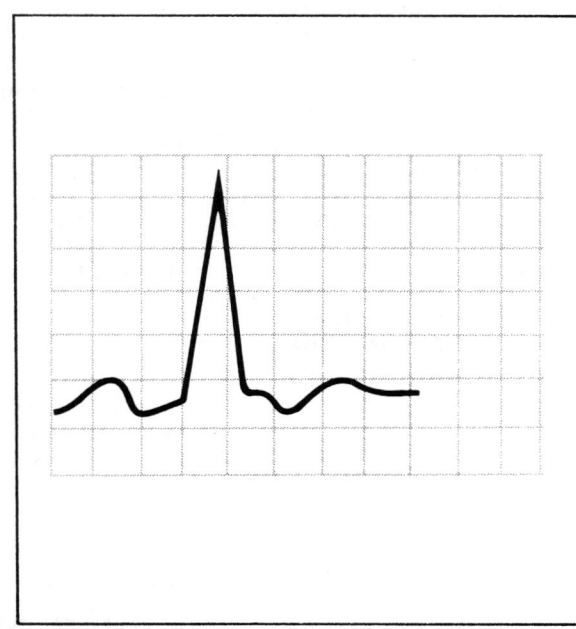

Figure 4–5. ECG changes characteristic of hypercalcemia.

Assessment of Acid-Base Balance

RATIONALE

Body acidity or alkalinity expressed as pH, or hydrogen concentration, is regulated in three ways: by the blood buffers, by the respiratory system, and by the renal system. The kidneys are responsible for maintenance of balance via excretion of acids and reabsorption of bicarbonate. When renal malfunction occurs, however, the buffer system and lungs are frequently incapable of compensating adequately. For the purpose of this assessment skill, emphasis is on *metabolic* abnormalities primarily mediated by the renal system.

PARAMETERS	FINDINGS	POSSIBLE ETIOLOGIES	DOCUMENTATION
1. Metabolic acidosis: A reduction in bicarbonate concentration and increase in hydrogen ion concentration	1. • Laboratory data Plasma pH below 7.35 P_{CO_2} normal (36–46 mm Hg) HCO_3 below 22 mEq/L *Compensatory change* P_{CO_2} below 36 mm Hg • Physical findings Neurological: Altered mental status, confusion, somnolence, coma Gastrointestinal: Nausea, vomiting Respiratory: Hyperventilation, Kussmaul respirations	1. • Bicarbonate loss (carbonic anhydrase inhibition) via reaction with systemic acid environment; lactic acidosis in diabetic ketoacidosis, renal disease, starvation Excessive bicarbonate loss from the gastrointestinal tract, pancreatic drainage, diarrhea, or ureterosigmoidostomy Bicarbonate loss from the kidney, carbonic anhydrase inhibitors (acetazolamide, benzolamide) • Retention of fixed acids (acids other than in form of CO_2, derived from sulfur- and phosphorus-containing proteins) seen in renal failure with decreased ammonium ion excretion due to decreased functioning mass Acid ingestion: Salicylates, ethylene glycol, methanol, or lysine or arginine hydrochloride	• Disorientation, stupor, decrease in responsiveness • Muscle fasciculations, convulsions • Loss of appetite, emesis • Impaired gastrointestinal motility • Change in respiratory rate, rapid and deep respirations • Shallow respirations These should be documented q2h and more often if changes occur. • Laboratory data: Notation of observation and reporting of arterial blood gases will be made each time blood gases are drawn, especially 20–30 minutes after treatment is initiated or altered
2. Metabolic alkalosis: An increase in bicarbonate concentration and a reduction in hydrogen ion concentration	2. • Laboratory data Plasma pH above 7.45 P_{CO_2} normal (36–46 mm Hg) HCO_3 above 26 mEq/L *Compensatory change* P_{CO_2} above 46 mm Hg • Physical findings Neuromuscular: Muscle cramps, tetany, seizures Gastrointestinal: Gastric retention, ileus Respiratory: Hypoventilation, hypoxia	2. • Acid loss: Vomiting, nasogastric suction or chloride-losing diarrhea Iatrogenic acid loss, mediated by the renal system in diuretic and mineralocorticoid administration Hypokalemia associated with renal acid loss • Bicarbonate gain, rapid bicarbonate administration, hypovolemia, posthypercapneic states	

POSSIBLE NURSING DIAGNOSES

• Gas exchange, impaired
• Tissue perfusion, alteration in: pulmonary
• Tissue perfusion, alteration in: renal

Assessment of Altered Urine Volume

RATIONALE

Although a serious and life-threatening clinical entity, acute renal failure (ARF) has a prognosis such that, if properly treated, 50–60% of patients may regain normal renal function. A variable percentage of the remaining 40% will go on to develop chronic renal insufficiency or failure. Since renal failure, regardless of etiological process, is the most common type of renal dysfunction that the nurse in a critical care area will observe, it is vital to immediately and accurately assess impending renal failure or its stages in order to treat and diminish possible sequelae. The most easily assessed alteration is urine volume.

PARAMETERS	FINDINGS	POSSIBLE ETIOLOGIES	DOCUMENTATION
1. Onset phase	1. Onset phase: Period of time in which the kidney has sustained, or is continuing to sustain, renal insult, with failure of compensatory mechanisms • Urine volume: Decreases to less than 25% of normal • Time span: Hours to days, possibly weeks (lasts from precipitating event to beginning of oliguria–anuria) Indicative of • Renal blood flow: Decreases to less than 30% of normal • Filtration clearances: Decrease to less than 15% of normal	Since renal failure of different etiologies will be managed differently and response depends on the specificity of treatment, it is important for the nurse to understand the causative factors that will influence treatment. 　　ARF may be logically categorized into three groups, according to etiology (Fig. 4–6) 　　*Prerenal failure:* Caused by decreased renal blood flow or drop in systemic pressure; most frequently due to hypotension or hypovolemia. Renal hypoperfusion or vasoconstriction occurs; tubular reabsorption of sodium, water, and urea occurs. Examples of causative conditions are	Since the critical care nurse has no practical method for measuring renal blood flow or filtration clearance at the bedside, the best and most noted index of decreasing renal function is the urine volume. Flowsheet comments, *in addition to notification of physician,* will reflect urinary output in the following phases
2. Oliguric–anuric phase	2. Oliguric–anuric phase: Period of time in which renal decompensation is complete and uremia ensues • Urine volume: Decreased to less than 10% of normal • Time span: Lasts 1–2 weeks Indicative of • Renal blood flow: Decreased to less than 30% of normal • Filtration clearances: Decreased to less than 15% of normal	• Volume depletion: Actual loss of extracellular fluid volume, whether from excessive diuresis, gastrointestinal loss, hemorrhage or third-space loss, with intracellular or intracompartment entrapment of fluid • Decreased cardiac output: General circulatory insufficiency that results in hypotension, due to pericardial tamponade, cardiogenic shock, or severe CHF • Peripheral vasodilatation: Leading to hypotension, either from sepsis or antihypertensive drugs • Renal artery stenosis–occlusion: Decreasing renal blood flow and glomerular filtration	• Onset: A gradual decrease from 60–70 cc/hr, allowing for variables such as intravenous infusion rate and possible diuretic administration, to less than 30 cc/hr • Oliguric–anuric: Approximately 10 cc/hr or less • Early diuretic: An increase to approximately 100 cc/hr or more • Late diuretic: A possible increase of more than 200 cc/hr
3. Early diuretic phase	3. Early diuretic phase: Period of time in which cellular renewal occurs; urine volume increases due to the inability of these cells to concentrate urine • Urine volume: Steadily increases to 100% or more of normal • Time span: Lasts 1–2 weeks	Prerenal failure usually responds to prompt treatment of the underlying etiology. If not, it progresses rapidly to intrarenal failure. 　　*Intrarenal failure:* Pathological physiological or structural changes at specific sites within the	• Recovery: A stabilization at approximately 60–70 cc/hr with a return to normal renal volume of 1500 cc/24 hr

4. Late diuretic phase	Indicative of • Renal blood flow: Increases to greater than 25% of normal • Filtration clearances: Still decreased to less than 15% of normal; BUN and creatinine levels become stationary **4.** Late diuretic phase: Period of time in which cellular renewal continues, with reestablishment of tubular function • Urine volume: Increases to greater than 100% of normal • Time span: Variable Indicative of • Renal blood flow: Increases to greater than 40% of normal • Filtration clearances: Increases to greater than 40% of normal	kidney itself, resulting in impaired function. The sites include • Tubular: Characterized by obstruction of the tubules by cells, casts, or ischemic edema and arteriolar vasoconstriction; reabsorption and secretion capabilities are impaired. Tubular site damage is most often characterized by acute tubular necrosis (ATN) (the most common cause of intrarenal failure). Etiologies include ischemia (e.g., prolongation of prerenal causes), exogenous toxins (e.g., contrast media reactions, antibiotics, heavy metal exposure), or endogenous toxins (e.g., transfusion reactions, hyperuricemia, multiple myeloma, rhabdomyolysis)
5. Convalescent phase	**5.** Convalescent phase: Period of time in which glomerular function returns to normal. Depending on a multitude of factors (e.g., age, etiological process), values may not revert to absolute normal. However, function is adequate to maintain bodily homeostasis • Urine volume: Approximately 100% of normal • Time span: Lasts 4–6 months Indicative of • Renal blood flow: Approximately 100% of normal • Filtration clearances: Approximately 100% of normal	• Vascular: Characterized by inflammation, scarring, or occlusion of the renal micro- and macrovasculature with resulting decrease in glomerular function. Etiologies include vasculitis (e.g., polyarteritis nodosa or Wegener's granulomatosis), arterial occlusion or thrombotic states (e.g., postpartum renal failure or thrombocytopenia purpura, which lead to necrosis of the renal cortex), and malignant hypertension, regardless of etiology, causing fibrosis and necrosis of the arterioles • Glomerular site: Characterized by an alteration in the glomerular apparatus usually to the capillary mesangial cells, with deposition of complement and other debris on the glomerular basement membrane. This pathological change alters the glomerular membrane's permeability and thus decreases glomerular filtration. Etiologies include primary glomerulonephritis, in which the renal pathology occurs alone (e.g., membranoproliferative glomerulonephritis), or secondary glomerulonephritis associated with systemic diseases (e.g., subacute bacterial endocarditis, systemic lupus erythematosus, or Goodpasture's syndrome) • Interstitial: Characterized by edema and infiltration of the renal interstitium by inflammatory cells, leading to tubular atrophy, microvascular changes, and glomerular pathology. Actual mechanism is unclear, but the

(continued)

PARAMETERS	FINDINGS	POSSIBLE ETIOLOGIES	DOCUMENTATION
		etiological factor appears to be a possible hypersensitivity reaction to drugs, such as allopurinol, antibiotics, diuretics, nonsteroidal anti-inflammatory agents, and phenytoin • Papillary: Characterized by severe inflammatory or vascular alterations of the papilla, with fibrosis and scarring of renal arterioles. Etiologies include pyelonephritis associated with urinary infections, diabetes mellitus, and analgesic abuse Intrarenal failure, owing to the multitude of etiological entities and the profound morphological changes taking place, is not as easily treated as prerenal failure, and is apt to produce more serious sequelae *Postrenal failure:* Generally a result of obstruction of urine flow from the kidney. Bilateral obstruction is, of course, the more severe and results in hydroureter and hydronephrosis. The retained urine causes edematous changes of the renal parenchyma, with loss of concentrating ability, loss of tubular function with loss of acid-secreting ability, and pathological changes in the glomeruli with decreased GFR. Examples of causal factors are • Urethral obstruction: Such as strictures or valve malfunction • Bladder neck obstruction: Due to benign prostatic hypertrophy, prostatic or bladder carcinoma, or autonomic neuropathy • Ureteral obstruction: Either outside the ureters from trauma or masses or inside the ureters from calculi or clots Postrenal failure is more easily treated than intrarenal failure and usually more easily reversible, depending upon the degree and length of obstruction, location of lesion, and presence or absence of infection. The postobstructive diuresis that occurs after relief of obstruction must be observed closely, since sodium and water can be lost in large quantities as tubular function attempts to return to normal	

POSSIBLE NURSING DIAGNOSES

• Fluid volume, alteration in: excess
• Fluid volume, deficit, potential
• Tissue perfusion, alteration in: renal

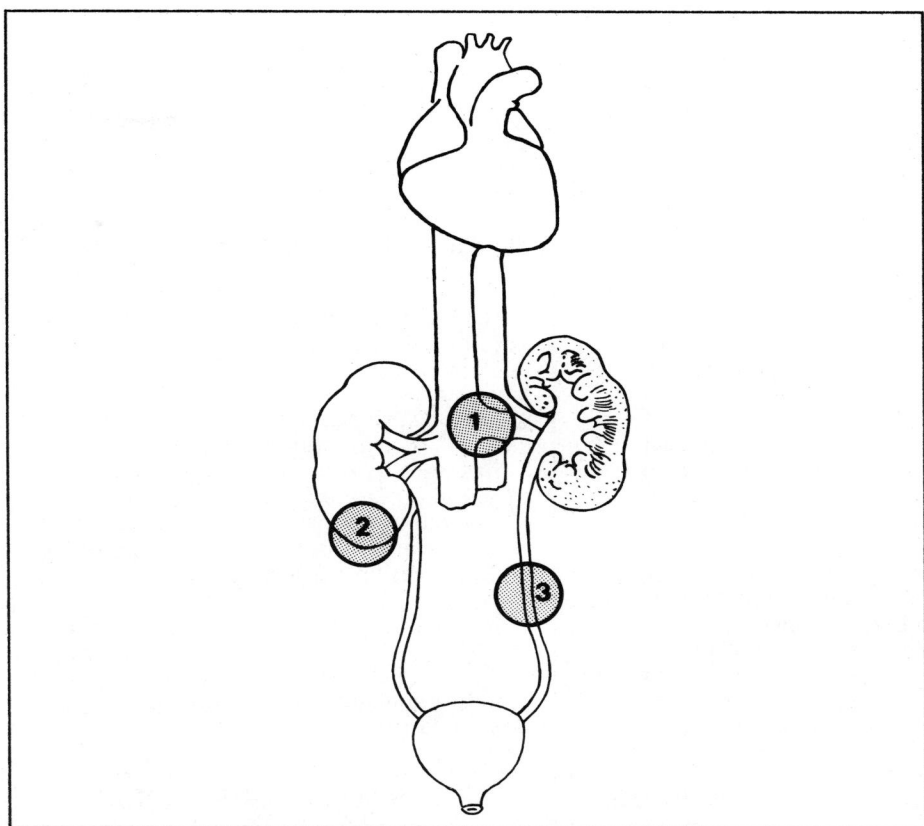

Figure 4–6. Etiologic sites of acute renal failure: prerenal (**1**), intrarenal (**2**), and postrenal (**3**).

Assessment of the Renal Failure Patient Requiring Hemodialysis

RATIONALE STATEMENT

Hemodialysis is the removal of nitrogenous waste products and fluid from the blood by a machine, using a semipermeable membrane for filtration (Fig. 4–7). It is the treatment of choice for the uremic symptoms of acute renal failure (ARF). It is the chief therapeutic modality for selected drug overdose, patient maintenance in chronic renal failure (CRF) or while awaiting transplantation. Although hemodialysis will alleviate the life-threatening sequelae of uremia, this is only accomplished on a short-term basis. Hemodialysis will not return the patient to a completely normal physiological state. Complications may arise from the procedure itself, as well as from exacerbation of symptoms of the underlying disease process. Although a patient being dialyzed (whether for ARF or CRF) in the critical care area will be attended by a hemodialysis nurse specially trained in procedural treatment and intervention, the critical care nurse still retains responsibility for patient assessment pre- and postdialysis as well as for appropriate intervention.

PARAMETERS	FINDINGS	POSSIBLE ETIOLOGIES	DOCUMENTATION
1. Procedural A. Blood loss	1. A. Detection of more than 0.45 ml/min of blood in effluent fluid line by a blood leak sensor, confirmed by Hemostix test of dialysate bath. Physical symptoms: Weakness, increased heart rate, decreased blood pressure	1. A. Related to filter (Fig. 4–8) rupture, or systemic continuous heparin infusion rather than regional heparinization	1. A. Increased heart rate Decreased blood pressure Weakness Type of blood loss, estimated blood loss
B. Dialysis disequilibrium	B. Headache, impaired concentration, restlessness, confusion, twitching, jerking, generalized seizure	B. Poorly understood; it is speculated that a too rapid fluid shift leads to difficulty in urea transfer across blood–brain barrier (i.e., urea more easily removed from blood than from cerebral tissue, with fluid shift to brain resulting in cerebral edema)	B. Headache, impaired concentration, restlessness, confusion, muscle twitching, asynchronous limb jerking, seizures
C. Hypotension	C. Systolic blood pressure decrease of 40 mm Hg or more from baseline	C. At beginning of dialysis, probably related to inadequate circulatory blood volume (occurs more frequently in women) with rapid volume shift; late in dialysis, probably related to excessive ultrafiltration combined with increased speed of filtration in high-performance dialyzer (too rapid fluid shift). Very frequently seen in patients with cardiac decompensation, due to inability to tolerate rapid fluid–electrolyte shifts; administration of antihypertensive medication before dialysis	C. Systolic blood pressure decreased 40 mm Hg under baseline
D. Cardiac dysrhythmia	D. ECG evidence of atrial flutter, atrial fibrillation	D. Frequently due to underlying heart disease, rapid volume and electrolyte shifts, es-	D. Cardiac dysrhythmias

E. Air embolus	**E.** Detection by air bubble detector of air in line. Symptoms: Elevated heart rate, decreased blood pressure, restlessness, shortness of breath	pecially if serum potassium is rapidly decreased in digitalized patients **E.** Usually technical misadventure, inflow of air around needles due to suction from blood pump or foaming of blood	**E.** Anxiety, coughing, shortness of breath, chest pain

2. Uremic
  A. Anemia
	2. A. Weakness, blood pressure decrease, pulse increase
	  Hemoglobin: Male, below 14 g/dl; female, below 12 g/dl
	  Hematocrit: Male, below 41%; female, below 37%
		2. A. In ARF patients, related to decreased erythropoietin secretion and decreased red blood cell survival. Aggravated by blood loss in dialysis, frequent blood collection for laboratory determinations, and uremic effects on gastric mucosa, with possible steroid administration potentiating gastrointestinal hemorrhage (Fig. 4–9)	**2. A.** Hemoglobin and hematocrit determinations

B. Dialysis dementia	**B.** Speech disturbances, mutism, gait apraxia, slow wave EEG abnormalities, seizures, psychosis	**B.** Mechanism poorly understood; possibly related to aluminum toxicity	**B.** Speech disturbances, mental confusion
C. Hypertensive crisis	**C.** Systolic blood pressure increased 40 mm Hg over baseline, encephalopathy, papilledema, cardiovascular decompensation	**C.** Generally related to widespread vascular changes in the kidney due to renal pathology; may be seen after dialysis as a by-product of increased cardiac output with removal of fluid volume excess; also seen as a result of insufficient ultrafiltration in hemodialysis	**C.** Systolic blood pressure elevations of 40 mm Hg over baseline
D. Hyperkalemia	**D.** Serum potassium increased to 6.0 mEq/L or above, associated ECG abnormalities	**D.** The primary electrolyte disturbance seen in renal disease and the most emergent in terms of life-threatening arrhythmias. In and of itself, it is an index of need to hemodialyze, is seen occasionally in inadequate dialysis, or very frequently is caused by patient's dietary indiscretions. It is important to note that any etiology of red cell lysis (e.g., transfusion mismatch or severe upper gastrointestinal bleeding that allows blood to remain in the intestinal tract) will cause precipitous potassium increases	**D.** Serum potassium determinations
E. Septicemia	**E.** White blood cell count increased above 10 mm³, elevated temperature, hypotension, elevated heart rate	**E.** Lymphocyte depression is present in ARF and CRF. Acidosis and hyperosmolar states constitute an environment conducive to bacterial growth. Other contributing factors are immunosuppressant medications used in treatment of underlying renal disease, decreased protein dietary intake, severe pruritis resulting in scratching with secondary skin infections, and frequent instrumentation	**E.** White blood cell determinations, elevated temperature, elevated heart rate, hypotension

(continued)

PARAMETERS	FINDINGS	POSSIBLE ETIOLOGIES	DOCUMENTATION
F. Secondary hyperparathyroidism	**F.** Serum phosphorus increased above 4.5 mg/dl, associated ECG abnormalities	**F.** Decreasing renal function leads to phosphate retention and decreased serum calcium, which stimulates parathyroid hormone levels and increases phosphate excretion. Complete renal failure precludes phosphate excretion, even in the face of high parathyroid hormone levels; decreased calcium intestinal absorption and inability of the kidney to metabolize parathyroid hormone also mediate development	**F.** Serum phosphorus determinations, ECG abnormalities
G. Accelerated arteriosclerotic cardiovascular disease (ASCVD)	**G.** Chest pain, ECG showing ST depression, fatigue	**G.** Accelerated in CRF patients secondary to hypertension and elevated triglyceride levels (impaired breakdown in end stage renal disease)	**G.** Chest pain, ECG abnormalities, nausea, weakness
H. Pericarditis	**H.** Atypical chest pain, pericardial friction rub	**H.** Unknown etiology (suspected unidentified uremic toxin), usually an indication of need for dialysis; may be exacerbated by the renal failure patient's susceptibility to viral organisms and poor anticoagulation control during dialysis	**H.** Atypical chest pain, pericardial rub
I. Hepatitis	**I.** Jaundice, Hb_sAg positive, IgG antibody positive	**I.** Probably viral in origin, either A, B, or non A–non B. Facilitated by diminished immune response, frequent blood transfusions, dialysis environment induced	**I.** Jaundice, increasing abdominal girth, Hb_sAG and IgG determinations
J. Fluid overload	**J.** Increase of weight of over 3 pounds since last dialysis, S_3, shortness of breath, rales, jugular venous distention (JVD)	**J.** Related to renal inability to excrete sodium and water. Considered to be one of the primary indicators of need for dialysis if symptomatic. Also influenced by dietary indiscretion, possible inadequate dialysis	**J.** Weight determinations, rales, S_3, JVD, shortness of breath
K. Ileus	**K.** Absent bowel sounds, nausea, vomiting, anorexia, abdominal distention	**K.** Results from decreased fluid intake, altered dietary regimen, and use of phosphate-binding antacids	**K.** Absent bowel sounds, nausea, vomiting, anorexia, distention

POSSIBLE NURSING DIAGNOSES

- Airway clearance, ineffective
- Cardiac output, alteration in: decreased
- Breathing pattern, ineffective
- Fluid volume, alteration in: excess
- Gas exchange, impaired
- Tissue perfusion, alteration in

SPECIAL NOTE

Complications

The nurse should be aware that the parameters presented are only some, and certainly not all, of the complications involved in renal failure. These complications may prove to be the most likely to be seen in the intensive care area. From the patient's viewpoint, however, other complications may be equally or even more distressing, such as extreme pruritis or peripheral neuropathy. In individualizing a care plan, the nurse must keep in mind that problems of a life-threatening nature and those more mundane may coexist. To that end, the nurse may be able to utilize multiple nursing diagnoses.

Medications

The nurse must be aware of the fact that many drugs are dialyzable. Some drugs, therefore, should be administered after dialysis. Additionally, the nurse should expect that since the kidneys excrete many medications, many classes of pharmacological agents will be ordered in much reduced dosages. One exception to this may be antihypertensive medications which may be ordered in increased dosages.

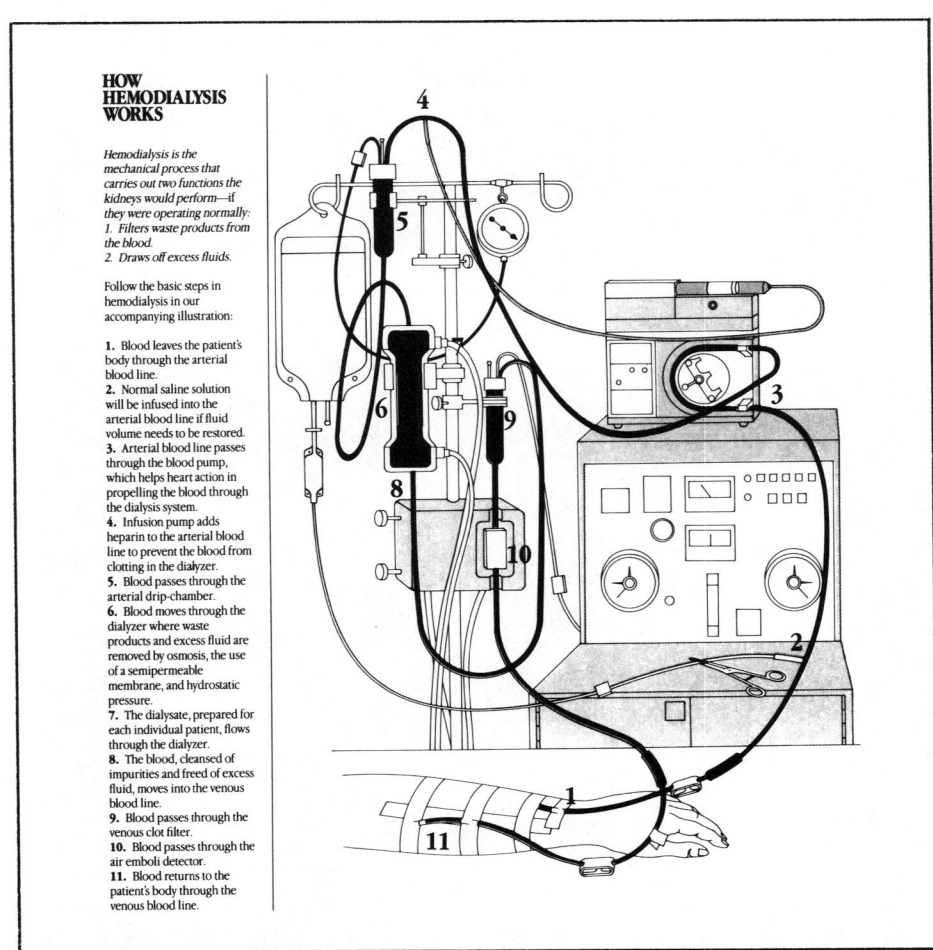

HOW HEMODIALYSIS WORKS

Hemodialysis is the mechanical process that carries out two functions the kidneys would perform—if they were operating normally:
1. Filters waste products from the blood.
2. Draws off excess fluids.

Follow the basic steps in hemodialysis in our accompanying illustration:

1. Blood leaves the patient's body through the arterial blood line.
2. Normal saline solution will be infused into the arterial blood line if fluid volume needs to be restored.
3. Arterial blood line passes through the blood pump, which helps heart action in propelling the blood through the dialysis system.
4. Infusion pump adds heparin to the arterial blood line to prevent the blood from clotting in the dialyzer.
5. Blood passes through the arterial drip-chamber.
6. Blood moves through the dialyzer where waste products and excess fluid are removed by osmosis, the use of a semipermeable membrane, and hydrostatic pressure.
7. The dialysate, prepared for each individual patient, flows through the dialyzer.
8. The blood, cleansed of impurities and freed of excess fluid, moves into the venous blood line.
9. Blood passes through the venous clot filter.
10. Blood passes through the air emboli detector.
11. Blood returns to the patient's body through the venous blood line.

Figure 4–7. Basic hemodialysis schematic. *(From Reed, S. B. Giving more than dialysis. Nursing 82, 1982, 12(4), 59, copyright 1982, Springhouse Corporation, with permission.)*

(continued)

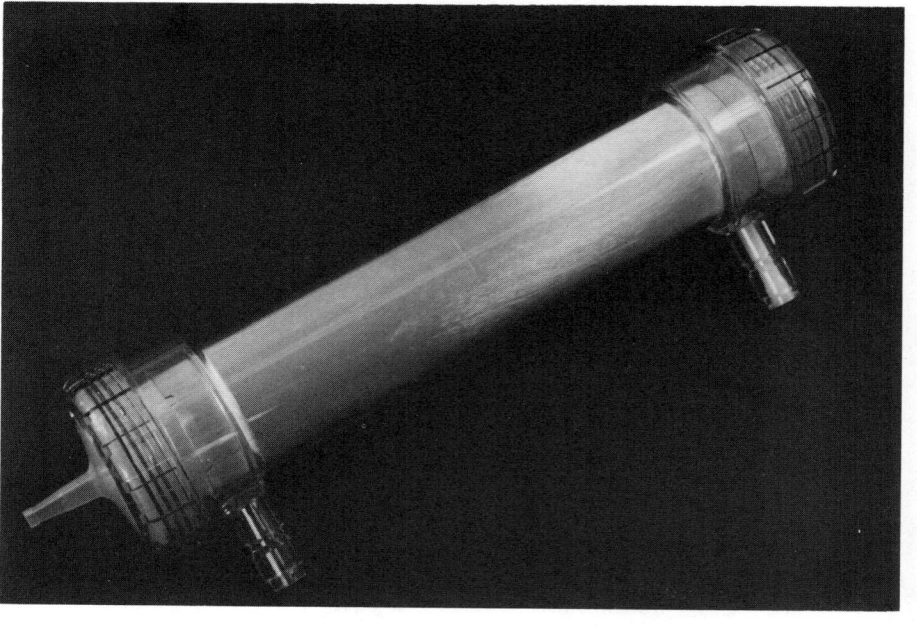

Figure 4–8. An example of a typical hemodialysis filter.

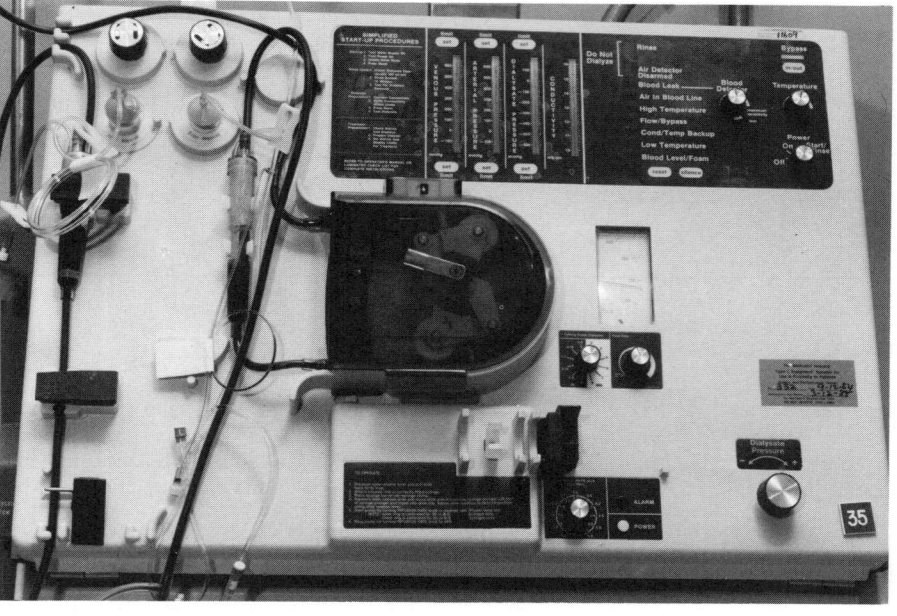

Figure 4–9. One of many hemodialysis machines in current use.

Care of the Patient with a Hemodialysis Access Site

NURSING DIAGNOSIS	RATIONALE	DEFINING CHARACTERISTICS	EXPECTED OUTCOME

Injury, potential for	Access to the circulation and thus attachment to the hemodialysis machine are usually accomplished by surgical insertion of an external cannula (Fig. 4–10) or an internal graft (bovine or autologous) or surgical creation of an arteriovenous fistula (Fig. 4–11). The nurse must recognize and instruct other staff that the vascular access is the patient's lifeline to the hemodialysis machine. Close observation must be made to prevent injury to the access, with resultant need for surgical revision and an extended hospital stay	1. Clotting
		  Absent bruit
		  Absent thrill (palpable buzzing sensation over fistula–graft)
		  Cold, clammy, pulseless, cyanotic access hand or leg
		  Separation of serum in cannula (clear areas)
		2. Infection
		  Temperature elevation
		  Erythema of access arm or leg
		  Increased edema of access arm or leg
		  Purulent drainage
		    Cannula insertion site
		    Needle puncture site on fistula–graft
		  Increased WBC (greater than 10,000)
		  Pain in extremity (increased with movement)
		3. Mechanical injury (tip dislodged in cannula or loss of anastomosis in fistula/graft)
		4. Sudden hematoma formation (drastic in size), internal
		5. Arterial bleed with resulting complications of shock, external
			No injury will occur at the hemodialysis access site or limb

NURSING INTERVENTIONS

General

1. Place sign over head of bed, "No B/P or venipunctures in (R/L) (arm/leg)"
2. Blood from access site must be drawn by RN familiar with the technique (if acceptable according to hospital policy)
3. Discourage patient from sleeping or lying in a position that exerts pressure on the access extremity
4. Discourage tight clothing, identification bands, tape over extremity
5. Instruct patient to report any signs or symptoms, such as numbness, tingling, or pain, to the nursing staff
6. Report any change in vascular access site immediately to appropriate personnel
7. Elevate access extremity if edema occurs postoperatively
8. As soon as is feasible, begin patient teaching regarding care of the access.

Specific: Cannula

1. Ensure that cannula is loosely wrapped in Kerlex; avoid any constriction or tangling of lines
2. Ensure that two cannula clamps are present, clipped at all times to the outside of the Kerlex. (If T-tube is in place, the two clamps should be on the T-tube)
3. *Unwrap* Kerlex to visibly inspect insertion site once per shift. Never cut Kerlex to remove it. Observe for presence of drainage at insertion site. Culture if purulent
4. Auscultate at connection of arterial and venous lines for bruit q2h
5. Observe for clotting q2h; check for serum separation (areas of clear serum and blue-black clot)
6. Check color, warmth, capillary filling, and pulses in the hand or leg distal to the access when auscultating q2h
7. Cleansing of the cannulated area is not recommended during routine inspection. Site care will be performed during dialysis. If necessary because of drainage, it should be done gently using hydrogen peroxide

Specific: Fistula–Graft

1. Auscultate at fistula–graft site for bruit q4h
2. Palpate fistula–graft for palpable thrill (buzz usually felt over AV anastomosis in fistula or near venous insertion in graft)
3. Observe surgical insertion site every shift for signs and symptoms of infection. Culture any purulent drainage noted
4. Check color, warmth, and capillary filling in hand or leg distal to fistula–graft when auscultating q4h
5. Discourage patient from picking at scabbed areas (previous dialysis needle insertion sites)
6. Area may be cleansed gently with hydrogen peroxide daily

OUTCOME CRITERIA

General

1. The access extremity will not be used for blood pressure determination or venipuncture
2. Blood drawing from access site will occur without procedural errors
3. No pressure will be placed on the access extremity during sleep
4. The access site will remain free of external constriction
5. The patient will immediately report any noted change in the access extremity
6. The complications occurring in vascular access will be treated promptly
7. Edema in access extremity will be minimized
8. Patient will state (or demonstrate) procedure for care of the access site

Specific: Cannula

1. No unnecessary exposure of surgical site or tangling of cannula lines will occur
2. Clamps necessary for control of emergent hemorrhage will be available
3. No site drainage will be present; if detected it will be cultured promptly
4. Bruit will be detected
5. Cannula will remain free of clotting
6. Complications of arterial steal in the access extremity will be minimized or prevented
7. No injury will occur to the cannula during cleaning procedure

Specific: Fistula–Graft

1. Bruit will be detected
2. Thrill will be detected (if present initially)
3. Anastomosis site will be drainage free; if present, it will be cultured promptly

(continued)

4. Circulatory complications of arterial steal in the access extremity will be minimized or prevented
5. Secondary infections from previous needle insertion will be prevented
6. No injury will occur to the fistula–graft during cleaning procedure

DOCUMENTATION

General

- Presence of precaution sign with date and time placed
- Date and time blood drawn with patency of access noted following procedure
- Notation of patient's sleeping position, with reference to position of access extremity
- Lack of constrictive devices over access extremity
- Any abnormality noted by patient
- Any abnormality noted by nurse
- Observation of access extremity edema
- Patient teaching; evidence of learning

Specific: Cannula

- Kerlex placement over access extremity
- Two clamps present on outside of Kerlex or on T-tube
  (if absent, interventions taken)
- Status of insertion site, including presence of drainage
- Presence of bruit
- Patency of cannula lines by inspection
- Access extremity condition and any abnormalities or changes noted
- Cleansing of insertion site if necessary, solution used, and redressing

Specific: Fistula–Graft

- Presence of bruit
- Presence of palpable thrill
- Status of surgical site, including culture of any drainage
- Status of access extremity
- Patient's verbalization of understanding of teaching
- Cleansing procedure, with solution used

Note: Any abnormalities documented will include notification of physician, interventions taken, and patient response to therapy.

SPECIAL NOTE

Arterial Steal

An arterial steal syndrome may develop in fistula or graft, particularly in the arm. If the radial artery is not tied off distal to the anastomosis, poor arterial flow may shunt blood from the fingers to the anastomosis. Signs and symptoms of decreased arterial flow in the hand will occur, despite the fact that the fistula–graft is still patent. This must be reported immediately to facilitate surgical correction if necessary.

Access Maturation

An internal access (fistula–graft) will take 4–6 weeks to mature for use. During this time, when the extremity may be edematous and painful for the patient, extra care in moving should be taken. Edema will prevent the thrill from being palpated; the bruit must be auscultated.

Blood Sampling

Routine blood drawing from the access is *not* recommended except during dialysis. However, if blood drawing from the access site (outside dialysis) is acceptable practice, the following procedure should be used.

1. Cannula
   A. Unclamp T-tube
   B. Cleanse end cap with germicidal solution
   C. Withdraw 3–4 cc of blood to discard
   D. Cleanse cap again and withdraw amount of blood needed
   E. Cleanse cap and irrigate T-tube with low-dose heparinized saline (5 cc)
   F. Reclamp T-tube
2. Fistula–Graft
   A. Cleanse area well with germicidal solution
   B. Insert needle (smallest gauge possible) of syringe into graft (or vein of fistula—do not insert at fistula anastomosis site)
   C. Withdraw blood needed
   D. Hold pressure to prevent arterial bleed for 5–10 minutes
   E. Place Band-Aid over site
   F. Do not draw blood from immature fistula–grafts (less than 6 weeks old)

Special Considerations

In patients with coagulopathies, especially disseminated intravascular coagulopathy (DIC), the cannula should be inspected q1h and the graft or fistula q2h.

Patients with already superficially infected fistulas–grafts are at great risk for arterial bleed if infection necroses through vessel walls or suture lines. Observe closely.

Aneurysm of graft (occasionally fistula) may occur. Observe closely for rupture and arterial bleed. Apply direct pressure.

Clotting can readily occur if arterial flow is decreased secondary to hypotensive episodes. Vascular access must be observed closely during and after these occurrences and changes reported immediately.

Temporary Circulatory Access

Many institutions now use the subclavian insertion site for temporary circulatory access for dialysis. Blood drawing and site care (outside dialysis) should be indicated and performed according to institutional policy (Fig. 4–12).

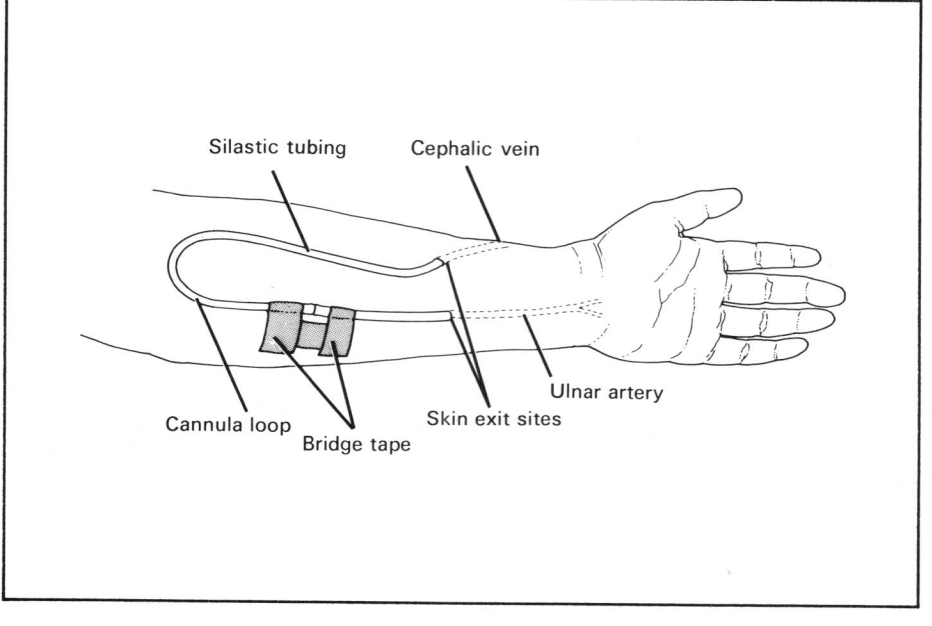

Figure 4–10. An external arteriovenous cannula in the arm is used for temporary access. *(From Hirsch, J., & Hannock, L. (Eds.). Mosby's manual of clinical nursing procedures. St. Louis, Mo.: Mosby, 1981, p. 115, with permission.)*

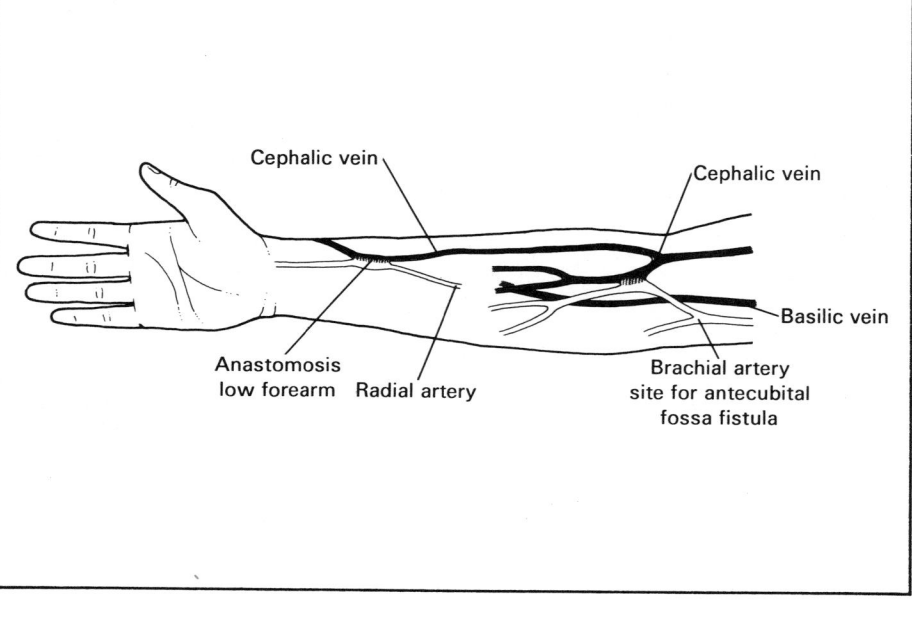

Figure 4–11. An internal arteriovenous fistula in the arm is used for chronic access. *(From Hirsch, J., and Hannock, L. (Eds.). Mosby's manual of clinical nursing procedures. St. Louis, Mo.: Mosby, 1981, p. 118, with permission.)*

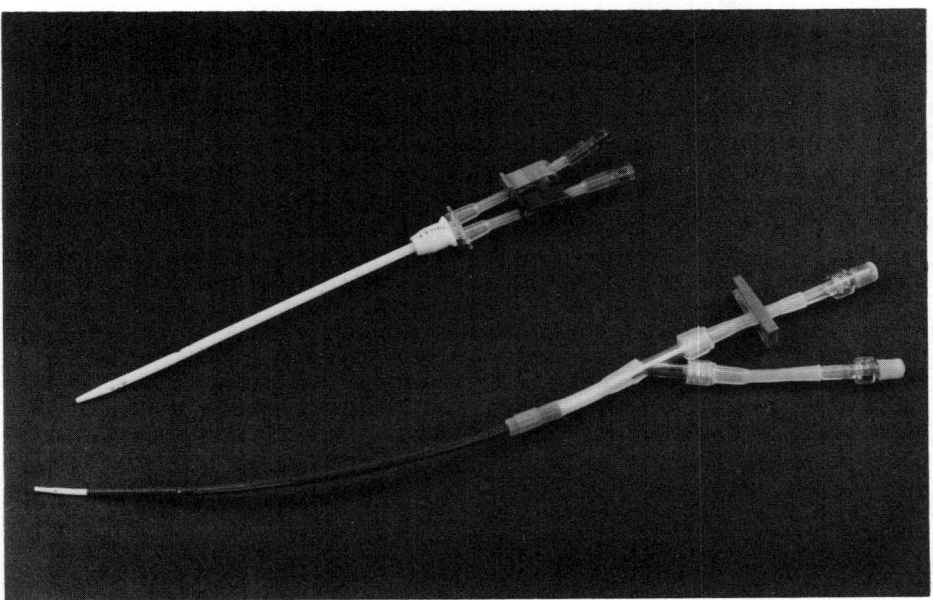

Figure 4–12. Shiley catheters (commonly used for acute access).

Care of the Patient Requiring Peritoneal Dialysis

NURSING DIAGNOSIS	RATIONALE	DEFINING CHARACTERISTICS	EXPECTED OUTCOME

Fluid volume, alteration in: excess	Peritoneal dialysis has been long established as a viable treatment methodology for both ARF and CRF. It differs from hemodialysis in that, during peritoneal dialysis, the patient's own peritoneum is used as the semipermeable membrane to filter out fluid and solutes (Fig. 4–13). Peritoneal dialysis is not as efficient a technique but has advantages in that it is better tolerated by patients unable to tolerate rapid fluid and electrolyte shifts. It also differs from hemodialysis in that manual performance of peritoneal dialysis can be safely delivered by nursing staff in the ICU without the months of training required for hemodialysis. It is important for the critical care nurse to understand procedural principles and techniques in order to perform this skill	Marked azotemia (BUN more than 100, creatinine above 5.0)
		Marked hyperkalemia (potassium 6.0 mEq/L or above)
		Marked metabolic acidosis
		Uremic symptoms
		  Gastrointestinal: anorexia, nausea and vomiting
		  Central nervous system: Changes in mental status, confusion
		  Cardiovascular: Pericarditis, CHF, pulmonary congestion
			• Body fluid and electrolyte balance will be restored to acceptable levels.
			• Serum BUN and potassium levels will be reduced
			• Fluid load will be reduced as ordered

NURSING INTERVENTIONS

General: Intermittent Peritoneal Dialysis

1. After insertion of peritoneal catheter (usually inserted in the operating room), check vital signs and weight, and gather equipment
   Skin preparation tray
   Masks and gloves
   Prewarmed dialysate solution (to decrease discomfort and increase peritoneal vasodilation)
   Medication additives (e.g., potassium in digitalized patients to decrease rapid changes in serum potassium; heparin to decrease fibrin deposition inside peritoneal catheter; antibiotics either prophylactically or for patients with peritonitis)
   Peritoneal dialysis administration tubing and collection bag
   Dialysis flow sheet
2. Bag, tubing, and drainage apparatus are set up, purged, and placed at bedside
3. Skin preparation is accomplished using aseptic technique
   Nurse performs handwashing technique using germicidal solution
   Patient and nurse don masks
   Dressing over peritoneal catheter is removed; site is inspected
   Catheter is scrubbed (nurse uses sterile gloves) with germicidal solution from tip to insertion site for 5 minutes
   Catheter is covered with sterile towel and held off abdomen
   Abdomen is scrubbed with germicidal solution for 5 minutes, starting at insertion site and working outward
   Abdomen is draped

Catheter cap is removed; tip of catheter is scrubbed for 5 minutes

Tubing is connected to catheter; catheter is redressed using aseptic technique

4. The nurse begins instillation of dialysate, with infusion time, dwell time, and outflow times specified by order. Total exchange time should approximate 1 hour (e.g., infusion time, 10 minutes; dwell time, 30 minutes; outflow time, 20 minutes)

Specific

1. Record vital signs q1h.
2. Record central venous pressure (CVP) q1h
3. Continuous ECG monitoring
4. Record weight determination q12h
5. Record intake and output q1h
6. Record BUN, electrolyte, and creatinine levels q6h
7. Record hemoglobin and hematocrit q24h
8. The lungs will be assessed q2h by auscultation
9. The abdomen will be assessed q4h by auscultation and palpation
10. The first dialysate exchange will be sent for culture, then cultured daily

OUTCOME CRITERIA

1. Temperature will remain below 100°F. Pulse will remain within 10 measurements of baseline. Respirations will remain between 5 and 7 measurements of baseline
   Blood pressure will remain between 20 and 30 mm Hg of baseline
2. CVP will remain between 4 and 10 mm Hg
3. Cardiac dysrhythmias will be promptly detected and interventions initiated
4. Weight will decrease 1–2 pounds q24h (if therapeutically indicated)
5. Urine output will remain at least 30 cc/hr (if patient not anuric)
6. Directional trends (specifically, hyperkalemia, hyperosmolar state) will be promptly identified and appropriate personnel notified
7. Directional trends (specifically blood loss) will be promptly identified and appropriate personnel notified
8. Complications associated with impaired respiratory status will be avoided
9. Complications suggestive of intestinal dysfunction or trauma will be avoided
10. Dialysate cultures will remain free of bacterial growth
11. Complications associated with mechanical failure, trauma, or infection will be avoided

DOCUMENTATION

Document the following in addition to actual peritoneal dialysis procedure administration on specialized flow sheet (Fig. 4–14):

- Vital signs q1h
- CVP ready q1h
- Presence of any ECG abnormalities (will be represented by rhythm strip); otherwise rhythm strip q8h
- Weight determination q12h (especially noting weight gain)
- Intake and output q1h
- Serial BUN, creatinine, glucose, and electrolyte determinations q6h, and results of other laboratory work
- Hemoglobin and hematocrit determinations q24h
- Bilateral breath sounds q2h

(continued)

- Abdominal assessment q4h
- Color and consistency of dialysate exchanges; notation of specimens sent for culture

Note: Documentation will include any abnormalities noted, notification of physician, interventions taken, and patient response to therapy.

SPECIAL NOTE

Dialysate Characteristics

The nurse should be aware of the characteristics of dialysate outflow:
Clear pale yellow: Normal
Cloudy: Infection, peritonitis
Brown: Bowel perforation
Amber: Bladder perforation
Blood tinged: Common for first through fourth exchanges; if it continues, may indicate abdominal bleeding or coagulopathy

IPD

Intermittent peritoneal dialysis (IPD) is essentially manual performance of peritoneal dialysis via permanent indwelling catheter. This is frequently the type of peritoneal dialysis performed in a hospital setting and is usually performed for 36–48 hours at a time.

CAPD

Continuous ambulatory peritoneal dialysis (CAPD) is performed by the patient at home via indwelling catheter 24 hours a day. Exchanges are performed by the patient, timed to his or her convenience. Equilibrium time is generally longer than with IPD.

CCPD

Continuous cycling peritoneal dialysis (CCPD) is usually performed at night. It exchanges 6–8 L over 9–10 hours via an automatic cycler machine. Can be performed by the patient or the nurse (Fig. 4–15).

Dextrose Solutions

Dextrose concentration in dialysate solution will be ordered by the physician. A solution of 1.5% is most commonly used, and 2.5% is also available. A solution with a concentration of 4.25% dextrose is also available and is used for rapid fluid removal. Patients receiving this concentration should be observed carefully for signs of excessive or too rapid fluid depletion.

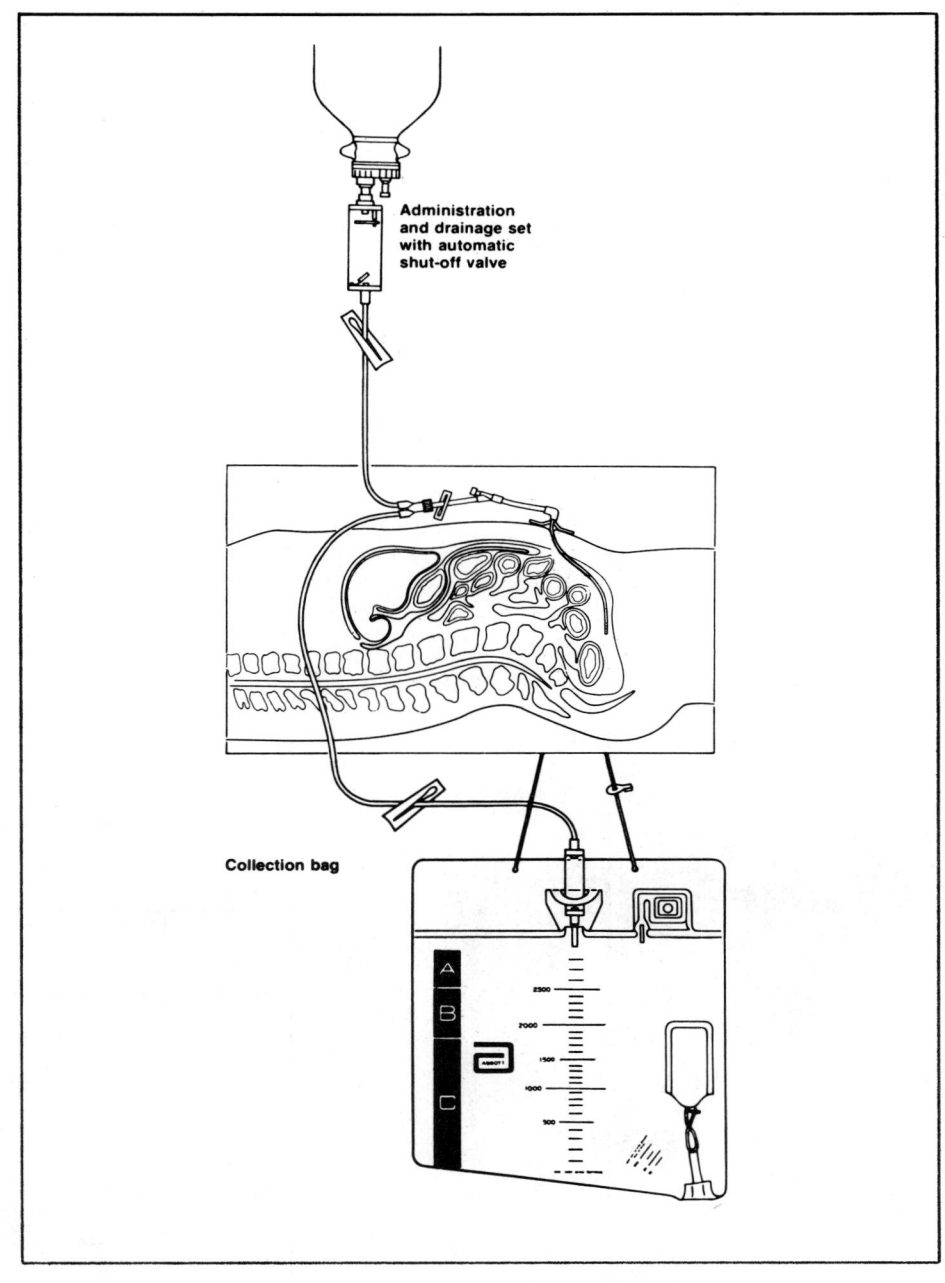

Administration and drainage set with automatic shut-off valve

Collection bag

Figure 4–13. Basic peritoneal dialysis schematic. *(From Richard, C. Nursing implications in prevention of complications in peritoneal dialysis.* Heart & Lung, *1975, 4(6), 891, with permission.)*

(continued)

PERITONEAL DIALYSIS FLOWSHEET

DATE	EXCHANGE NUMBER	DIALYSATE	OTHER ADDITIVES	SOLUTION IN			SOLUTION OUT			** DIFF.	** BALANCE
				Start	Finish	Volume	Start	Finish	Volume		

**
+   refers to fluid retained by the patient
−   refers to fluid lost by the patient

Figure 4–14. An example of a peritoneal dialysis flowsheet.

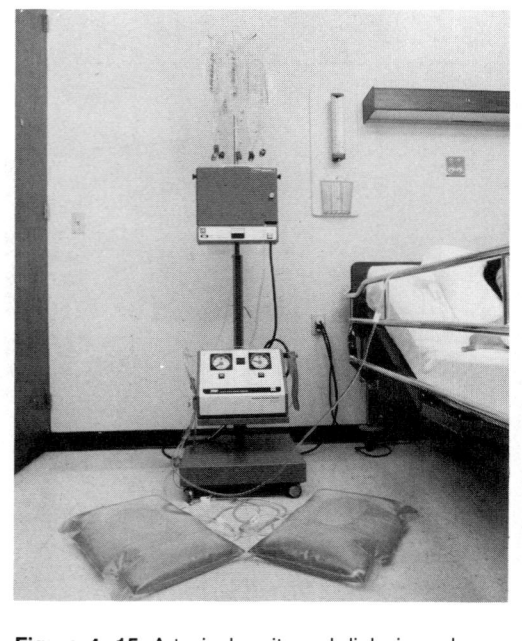

Figure 4–15. A typical peritoneal dialysis cycler.

Care of the Patient with a Peritoneal Dialysis Catheter

NURSING DIAGNOSIS	RATIONALE	DEFINING CHARACTERISTICS	EXPECTED OUTCOME
Injury, potential for	The peritoneal dialysis catheter is the patient's lifeline to peritoneal dialysis treatment. Although the ICU patient may be receiving peritoneal dialysis via a cycler, thus freeing the nurse of the obligation of performing the actual procedure, the nurse is still responsible for observation of the peritoneal catheter and potential symptomatology (on and off dialysis) that may indicate peritonitis or associated problems (Fig. 4–16)	Sudden, severe abdominal pain, tenderness, rigidity of abdominal wall Stool or flatus passed into peritoneal outflow Temperature elevation over 100°F Blood passed through catheter into peritoneal outflow Decreased or absent bowel sounds (obstruction) Poor outflow Increased leakage from insertion site Nausea, vomiting	No injury will occur at the peritoneal dialysis access site

NURSING INTERVENTIONS

1. Maintain strict asepsis in handling peritoneal catheter
2. Encourage patient to keep hands away from abdominal dressing
3. Observe dialysate outflow for color, consistency, quantity
4. Observe peritoneal catheter for presence of tissue and possible fibrin formation
5. Monitor vital signs q4h, after dialysis, especially temperature
6. Make sure catheter is capped when off dialysis
7. Maintain sterile dressing over catheter when off dialysis
8. Report any abdominal pain or rigidity
9. Observe for drainage at insertion site (if dressing removed) and report

OUTCOME CRITERIA

1. No breaks in sterile technique will occur during catheter manipulation
2. Patient will verbalize understanding of necessity of maintaining sterile dressing
3. Complications associated with mechanical trauma or infection will be avoided
4. Complications of catheter occlusion will be avoided
5. Temperature will remain below 100°F
6. Integrity of the closed system (postdialysis) will be maintained
7. Complications associated with infected insertion site will be avoided
8. Complications of peritonitis will be minimized or eliminated
9. Complications associated with technical misplacement or catheter dislodgement will be minimized

DOCUMENTATION

- Reason for catheter manipulation, with notation of maintenance of aseptic technique
- Initiation of patient teaching regarding catheter, patient response, lack of understanding or knowledge deficit (specify)
- Dialysate outflow characteristics
- Peritoneal catheter status

- Vital signs q4h
- Presence or absence of cap
- Presence or absence of sterile dressing, including intact state and drainage noted
- Any complaints of abdominal pain or change in abdominal assessment
- Presence or absence of drainage at insertion site

Note: Any abnormalities noted will include notification of physician, intervention taken, and patient response to therapy

SPECIAL NOTE

Poor Outflow

The patient may be on IPD or CCPD. CCPD patients must be observed constantly for poor outflow, as catheter problems may lead to pooling in the abdomen with resulting diaphragmatic elevation and respiratory distress.

Peritonitis

The importance of sterile technique in handling the peritoneal catheter *cannot* be overemphasized. Each successive episode of peritonitis causes more scarring of the peritoneum and decreases the potential efficiency of dialysis.

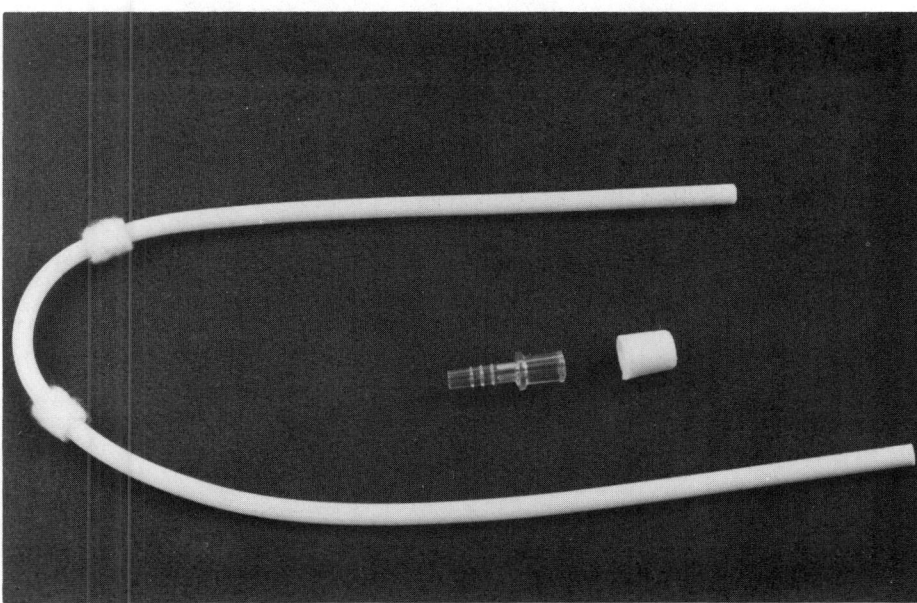

Figure 4–16. A permanent peritoneal dialysis catheter (Tenckhoff).

Care of the Patient Requiring Hemofiltration

NURSING DIAGNOSIS	RATIONALE	DEFINING CHARACTERISTICS	EXPECTED OUTCOME

Fluid volume, alteration in: excess	Hemofiltration has been recognized as an alternative treatment methodology for patients with renal dysfunction. It has proved valuable, particularly with reference to hemodialysis patients unable to tolerate rapid fluid shifts and with peritoneal dialysis patients following retroperitoneal surgery. Most recently, the indications for hemofiltration have been expanded to include any patient with multiple organ failure and fluid–electrolyte disturbances. The technique allows for continuous removal of small amounts of fluid and electrolytes by using the patient's arterial pressure gradient to propel blood through a capillary hemofilter similar to those filters used in hemodialysis. Thus, drastic volume and electrolyte shifts are avoided, while filtration of toxins occurs (Fig. 4–17)	General
		  Congestive heart failure refractory to diuretic therapy; parenteral nutrition administrations to patients requiring volume restriction
		  Hyperkalemia
		  Azotemia
		Specific
		  Pulmonary edema, ARDS
		  Refractory hypernatremia
		  Poisoning
		  Drug intoxication
			No hypotensive crisis or electrolyte abnormalities will occur while on hemofiltration

NURSING INTERVENTIONS

General

1. Blood lines and hemofilter are rinsed and filled with heparinized saline and albumin solution (Fig. 4–18).
2. The nurse assists the physician in cannulation of the femoral artery and vein
3. Blood flow is opened to capillary hemofilter
4. Heparin is infused (via pump) into arterial blood line
5. Measuring container for ultrafiltrate is positioned as low as possible at bedside to exert negative pressure (40 cm water). Clamps are opened
6. Ultrafiltrate should be inspected for signs of RBCs, indicating rupture of a fiber and need to replace unit
7. Ultrafiltrate flow rate will be observed for sudden decrease, may signify clotting within the circuit

Specific

1. Vital signs will be taken q15min (for 1 hour) during initiation of treatment, then q1h
2. Intake and output will be measured q1h
3. Continuous ECG monitoring
4. BUN and electrolyte determinations q6h
5. Weight recorded pretreatment and daily thereafter
6. The uncovered femoral access sites will be observed q2h. (Site care will be performed according to policy of institution)
7. Blood lines and hemofilter will be observed for clotting q2h
8. CBC determinations will be done daily
9. Clotting studies (prothrombin, partial thromboplastin time) will be performed q6h
10. Ultrafiltrate will be tested with Hemostix q4h
11. Uninterrupted heparin infusion will be maintained q1h

OUTCOME CRITERIA

1. Temperature will remain below 100°F. Pulse will remain between 10 measurements of baseline
   Blood pressure will remain between 10 and 15 mm Hg of baseline
   Respirations will remain between 5 and 7 measurements of baseline
2. Output will remain at least 30 cc/hr (if patient is not anuric)
3. Cardiac dysrhythmias will be promptly noted and interventions initiated
4. Electrolyte imbalance, specifically hyperkalemia or hypernatremia, will be promptly identified. Physician will be notified
5. Weight will decrease ± not more than 1 pound q24h
6. Complications associated with vascular trauma, infection, or catheter malalignment will be minimized or eliminated
7. Complications associated with technical misadvanture will be minimized
8. WBC count elevations, hemoglobin and hematocrit decrease will be promptly identified and physician notified
9. Laboratory values indicating lack of appropriate anticoagulation will be promptly identified and physician notified
10. Complications associated with ruptured hemofilter will be minimized or eliminated
11. Complications of over or under anticoagulation will be minimized or eliminated

DOCUMENTATION

- Vital signs q15 min during initiation of procedure, then q1h
- Intake and output q1h
- Any ECG dysrhythmias (will be represented by a rhythm strip); otherwise rhythm strip q8h
- BUN and electrolyte levels drawn, with results
- Daily weight (include weight preprocedure)
- Status of femoral access site, including site care if performed
- Patency of hemofilter and blood lines q2h
- CBC determinations drawn, with results
- Clotting studies drawn, with results
- Hemostix testing ultrafiltrate, with results
- Continuous heparin infusion (including amount, rate, and patency of lines and connections q1h)

   Note: Any notation of abnormality will include notification of physician, interventions taken, and patient response to therapy.

SPECIAL NOTE

Nomenclature

As the use of this technique increases, synonymous terms have been associated with continuous arteriovenous hemofiltration; a few are diafiltration, ultrafiltration, continuous flow filtration, and slow continuous hemofiltration. These terms may vary slightly in their meanings.

Coagulopathies

Because of the necessity of continuous heparin infusion, hemofiltration may be contraindicated in patients with coagulopathies or in those at severe risk for internal hemorrhage.

Air Embolus

Because of lack of an air-bubble detector in the system, all lines must be completely free of air, and observation and prevention of air embolus is a priority.

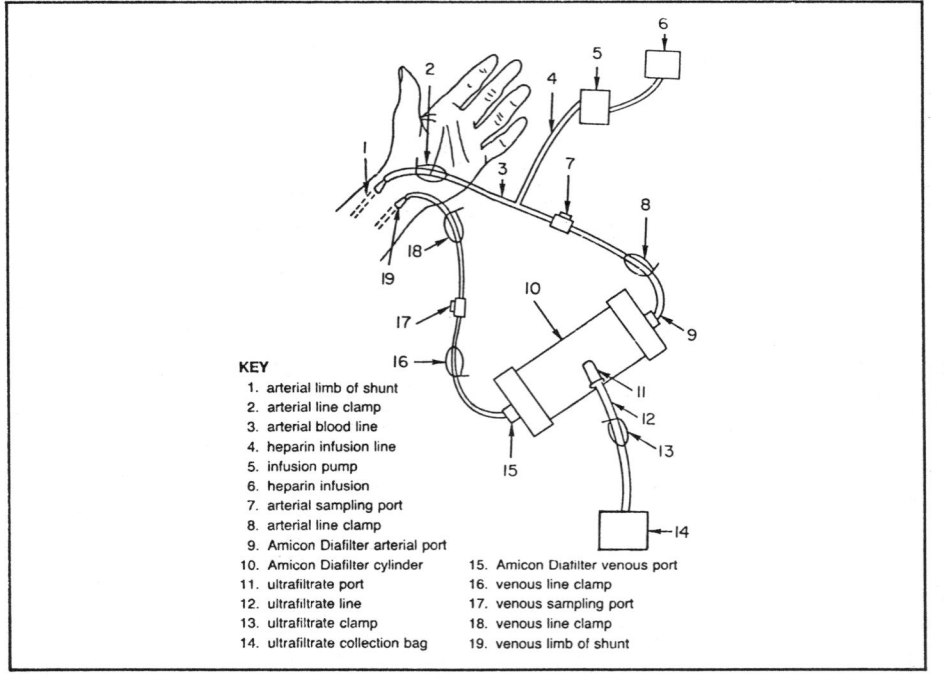

KEY
1. arterial limb of shunt
2. arterial line clamp
3. arterial blood line
4. heparin infusion line
5. infusion pump
6. heparin infusion
7. arterial sampling port
8. arterial line clamp
9. Amicon Diafilter arterial port
10. Amicon Diafilter cylinder
11. ultrafiltrate port
12. ultrafiltrate line
13. ultrafiltrate clamp
14. ultrafiltrate collection bag
15. Amicon Diafilter venous port
16. venous line clamp
17. venous sampling port
18. venous line clamp
19. venous limb of shunt

Figure 4–17. Basic hemofiltration schematic. *(From Williams, V., & Perkins, L. Continuous ultrafiltration: A new ICU procedure for the treatment of fluid overload. Critical Care Nurse, 1984, 4(4), 45, with permission.)*

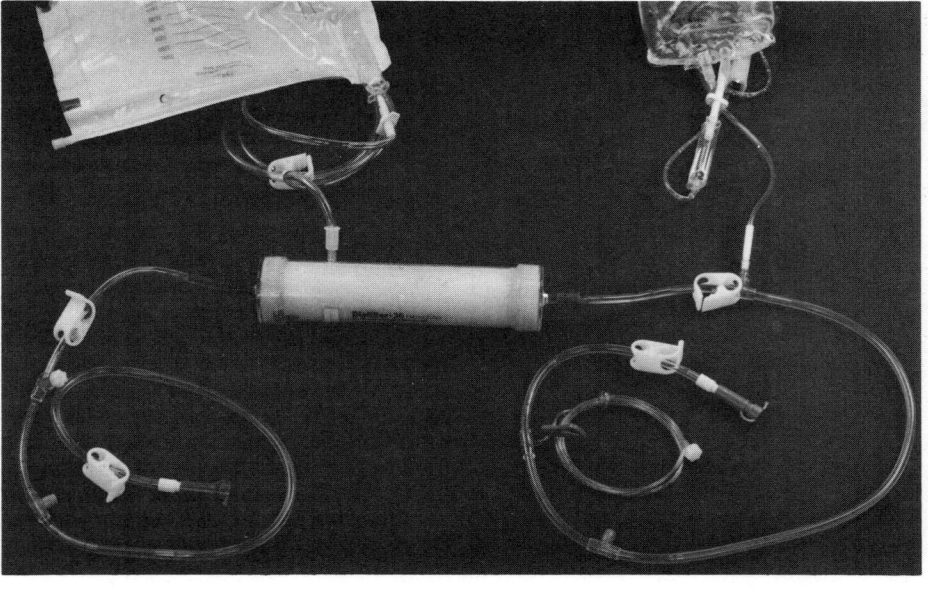

Figure 4–18. Hemofiltration equipment (filter and tubing).

Care of the Patient After Renal Transplant

NURSING DIAGNOSIS	RATIONALE	DEFINING CHARACTERISTICS	EXPECTED OUTCOME
Injury, potential for	Kidney transplantation has been employed as a treatment modality for end stage renal disease (ESRD) patients since the 1950s with variable success. With recent medical advances in immunology and immunosuppressive medication therapy, transplantation is becoming a more viable alternative in terms of longevity and offers the patient a less restrictive lifestyle in terms of therapeutic regimens and machine dependency. Although the critical care nurse will be concerned with the normal activities of postsurgical intervention, one of the primary areas of responsibility remains observation of patient status with reference to assessment of, and intervention for, rejection	The nurse must be aware that three types of rejection exist: (1) hyperacute rejection, in which antibodies immediately attack the kidney (intraoperatively or within a few hours), necessitating graft removal, (2) acute rejection, which may occur a few days after surgery and which may respond successfully to antirejection treatment, and (3) chronic rejection, which occurs months to years after the transplant and is probably indicative of eventual failure of the graft. The critical care nurse will most likely see acute rejection, as manifested by Edema, tenderness, or erythema over transplant site Elevated temperature WBC count elevation Decreased urine output Elevated BUN and creatinine levels Acute onset of hypertension Sudden weight gain Increased urine protein levels	No injury will occur to the transplanted kidney

NURSING INTERVENTIONS

1. Vital signs will be checked q15min for 4 hours, then q30min for 4 hours, then q1h immediately postoperatively, then q4h
2. CVP will be checked q30min for 4 hours, then q1h
3. Weight will be checked on arrival to the unit, then daily thereafter
4. Continuous ECG monitoring
5. Institute ventilatory assistance as ordered; institute pulmonary toilet as ordered
6. Urine will be checked q1h
7. Monitor electrolyte values as ordered, with particular reference to potassium
8. The abdominal girth will be measured q2h
9. The transplant site will be observed q2h
10. Administer immunosuppressant medications as ordered, such as azathioprine, corticosteroids, cyclophosphamide, antilymphocytic serum, cyclosporin
11. Assist in preparing the patient for specialized procedures to decrease host rejection (e.g., thoracic duct drainage, local irradiation to the transplant)
12. Promote the establishment of trust between the patient and nurse

1. Pulse will remain ± 20 measurements of baseline
   Temperature will remain below 100°F
   Respirations will remain between 5 and 10 measurements of baseline
   Blood pressure will remain between 40 systolic and 20 diastolic mm Hg of baseline
2. CVP will remain between 4 and 10 cm H_2O
3. Weight will remain at ± 1½ pounds of baseline
4. Cardiac dysrhythmias detected will be promptly identified and interventions initiated
5. Complications associated with impaired respiratory status will be minimized
6. Output will remain at least 30 cc/hr or more
7. Electrolyte imbalances, specifically hyperkalemia, will be promptly identified
8. Abdominal rigidity or increasing abdominal girth suggestive of mechanical loss of vascular or ureteral anastomosis will be promptly noted and interventions initiated
9. Erythema or localized tenderness at the transplant site will be noted
10. Immunosuppressive medication will be administered in an appropriate and timely fashion. Appropriate personnel will be notified of side effects and inability to administer medications
11. Patient will verbalize understanding and acceptance of the procedure
12. The patient will feel free to verbalize fears and anxieties to the nurse

The following will be noted, preferably on a specialized flowsheet (Fig. 4–19).

- Vital signs as ordered
- CVP readings as ordered
- Weight on arrival to unit, then daily
- Any ECG abnormalities (represented by rhythm strip), then q8h
- Ventilatory settings and time and patient response; pulmonary toilet initiated and patient tolerance
- Intake and output q1h
- Electrolyte determinations drawn, with results
- Assessment of abdominal status
- Observation of transplant site
- Any side effects or inability to administer medications
- Initiation of teaching, patient's verbalizations of understanding and knowledge deficits
- Patient's verbalization of fears and anxieties

Note: Any abnormality notation will include notification of physician, intervention taken, and patient response to therapy.

Protocol

Differing antirejection protocols will exist from institution to institution. The critical care nurse who is likely to care for renal transplant patients is strongly encouraged to become familiar with the protocols (medications and procedures) for her or his institution.

Occasional recurrence of the underlying renal disease will occur in the graft, and the nurse and the patient must be prepared for this possibility.

Transplant ATN

The nurse should be aware that a form of transplant acute tubular necrosis (ATN) exists, probably due to warm ischemia time in transferring the kidney to the recipient. This may resolve with treatment over a period of weeks.

PATIENT_____

TRANSPLANT DATE_____

RENAL TRANSPLANT FLOWSHEET

		OUTPUT		INTAKE		VITAL SIGNS			LABORATORY												
DATE	POST-OP DAY	URINE	OTHER	ORAL IV	WEIGHT	T P R	B/P	CVP	BUN	CR	Na	Ct	K	CO_2	Hgb	Hct	WBC	MEDICATIONS	OTHER	TX

Figure 4–19. An example of a renal transplant flowsheet.

Glossary

Anuria: Absence of urine formation (specifically, less than 50 cc/24 hr).

ARF (acute renal failure): A rapid decrease in renal function over a period of hours or days (frequently reversible).

Arginine: A basic amino acid, a by-product of protein hydrolysis.

Arginine hydrochloride: A form of arginine, administered intravenously in the treatment of hepatic encephalopathies and ammoniacal azotemia.

ATN (acute tubular necrosis): The most common cause of acute renal failure; a specific injury to the tubular section of the nephron.

Azotemia: An increased level of nitrogenous waste products in the blood.

CRF (chronic renal failure): A gradual decrease in renal function, usually over a period of months to years (usually irreversible).

Dysuria: Difficulty or pain on urination.

Ethylene glycol: Frequently used inhalant anesthetic.

Frequency: Urination at short intervals (usually smaller than normal volumes).

GFR (glomerular filtration rate): Rate of clearance of substances into the urine.

Hematuria: Condition in which the urine contains blood or red blood cells.

Hyperuricemia: Increased serum concentrations of uric acid.

Lysine: An alpha-amino acid common in many proteins.

Mesangial cells: Cells forming the mesangium, a part of the glomerulus between capillaries; cells in this area serve a phagocytic function.

Methanol: Methyl alcohol.

Nocturia: Urinating at night, often because of increased nocturnal secretion of urine (frequently seen in renal insufficiency because of decreased ability to concentrate urine at night).

Oliguria: Scanty urination (less than 400 cc/24 hr or less than 30 cc/hr).

Osteomalacia: Failure of osteroid tissue to calcify; may be mediated by renal tubular dysfunction; more common in females.

Polyuria: Excessive excretion of urine (true volume increase of more than 1500 cc/24 hr, as opposed to more frequent urination of small volumes).

Proteinuria: The presence of protein in urine in concentrations greater than 0.3 g in a 24-hour urine collection or greater than 1 g/L in a random urine collection.

Rhabdomyolysis: Destructive disease of skeletal muscle, acute and potentally fatal; manifestations include myoglobinuria and myoglobinemia.

Uremia: An excess of urea and other nitrogenous waste in the blood.

Urgency: A sudden sensation of needing to urinate.

Bibliography

Bononuni, V., Stefoni, S., & Vangelista, A. Long-term patient and renal prognosis in acute renal failure. *Nephron,* 1984, *36*(3), 169–172.

Earle, D. *Manual of clinical nephrology*. Philadelphia: Saunders, 1982.

Erlich, L., & Powell, S. Care of the patient with a Gore-Tex peritoneal dialysis catheter. *Dialysis and transplantation*, 1983, *12*(8), 572–574.

Fleming, L., & Kane, J. Step-by-step guide to safe peritoneal dialysis. *RN,* 1984, *47*(2), 44–47.

Gutch, C. F., & Stoner, M. *Review of hemodialysis for nurses and dialysis personnel.* St. Louis, Mo.: Mosby, 1983.

King, I. Effectiveness of nursing care: Use of a goal oriented nursing record in end stage renal disease. *Journal of the American Association of Nephrology Nurses and Technicians,* 1984, *11*,(2), 11–17.

Lancaster, L. Renal failure: Pathophysiology, assessment and intervention. *Nephrology Nurse,* 1983, *5*(2), 38–51. (vol. 5, 2)

Larson, E., Lindbloom, L., & Davis, K. *Development of the clinical nephrology practitioner*. St. Louis, Mo.: Mosby, 1982.

Levine, D. *Care of the renal patient*. Philadelphia: Saunders, 1983.

Luckenbaugh, P. An overview of nursing diagnosis and suggestions for use with chronic hemodialysis patients. *Nephrology Nurse,* 1983, *5*(6), 58–61.

Mars, D., & Treloar, D. Acute tubular necrosis—Pathophysiology and treatment. *Heart and Lung,* 1984, *13*(2), 194–201.

Norris, M. K. Management of acute conditions in chronic renal failure. *Dimensions in Critical Care Nursing,* 1983, *2*(6), 328–337.

Parisi, B., & Schrichs, M. Nursing diagnosis: Application for renal nurses. *Dialysis and transplantation,* 1983, *12*(5), 362–371.

Ramirez, G., Bruggemeyer, C., & Newton, J. Cardiac arrhythmias on hemodialysis in chronic renal failure patients. *Nephron,* 1984, *36*(4), 212–221.

Reed, S. Giving more than dialysis. *Nursing '82* 1982, *12*(4), 58–63.

Schrier, R. *Manual of nephrology: Diagnosis and therapy*. Boston: Little, Brown, 1981.

Sims, T. Successful utilization of subclavian catheters for hemodialysis and apheresis access. *Journal of the American Association of Nephrology Nurses and Technicians,* 1983, *10*(7), 41–44.

5

GASTROINTESTINAL SYSTEM

Imelda Clare Otte

Assessment of the Pertinent Gastrointestinal History

Assessment of the Gastrointestinal System by Inspection

Assessment of the Gastrointestinal System by Auscultation

Assessment of the Gastrointestinal System by Percussion

Assessment of the Gastrointestinal System by Palpation

Assessment of Pertinent Laboratory Data

Assessment of the Patient Receiving Total Parenteral Nutrition

Care of the Patient Receiving Total Enteral Nutrition

Care of the Patient Requiring Gastric Lavage

Care of the Patient Requiring a Sengstaken–Blakemore Tube

Assessment of the Pertinent Gastrointestinal History

RATIONALE

Often one can formulate a diagnosis from history alone. The history lends direction to the physical examination and may identify familial tendencies toward a disease process. A comprehensive patient profile will elicit information regarding any patterns in activities of daily living that may influence or may be influenced by an occult disease process.

PARAMETERS	FINDINGS	IMPLICATIONS FOR NURSING CARE
1. Family history	1. Esophageal disease Ulcer disease Liver disease Gallstones Inflammatory bowel disease Diabetes Bleeding dyscrasias	1. Strong familial history of gastrointestinal disease may identify the patient at risk for developing similar dysfunctions. The meaning and uses of food in the family should also be investigated. Ineffective methods of stress management may manifest as gastrointestinal disease. Teaching–learning needs may be identified

2. Past health history	2. A. Esophageal disease
	  a. Esophageal varices
	
	  b. Esophageal obstruction
	    Esophagitis with stricture
	    Tumor
	B. Ulcer
	
	C. Liver disease
	  a. Hepatitis
	  b. Cirrhosis
	
	D. Inflammatory bowel disease
	
	E. Abdominal surgeries or trauma
	
	F. Transfusions with blood or blood products
		2. A. a. Patients presenting with gastrointestinal bleeding may be experiencing a recurrence of previous variceal problems. Passage of a nasogastric tube should be performed only by experienced personnel
		  b. Esophageal obstruction may result from previous trama with scarring, from strictures following an inflammatory process, or from displacement related to a mass. Oral intake of both solids and liquids may be impaired
		B. Males are more likely to develop duodenal ulcers whereas females will develop gastric ulcers. This recurrent disease process may be exacerbated by the stress of the critical care environment. Dietary modifications may be required
		C. a. Abnormal liver function studies may reveal previously undiagnosed hepatitis. Reassessment may be required to determine the source of infection
		  b. A destructive process resulting in fibrotic and structural changes, cirrhosis is, in fact, a *group* of chronic liver diseases with multiple etiologies
		    Ingestion of alcohol results in indirect, dose-related hepatotoxicity
		    With any degree of liver impairment, hepatic clearance of medications should be carefully assessed
		D. Several conditions, such as ulcerative colitis, Crohn's disease, and diverticulitis are chronic, recurrent, and of uncertain etiology. Special attention should be paid to patients experiencing exacerbations
		E. Elective surgical procedures or trauma involving resection or reconstruction of the gastrointestinal system may result in alterations in oral ingestion, absorptive capabilities, or elimination patterns
		F. Transfusion with blood or blood products may result in transmission of hepatitis B as well as hepatitis non-A, non-B

3. Patient profile	3. A. Medications a. Salicylate-containing compounds	3. A. a. Although in certain individuals ingestion of aspirin may cause gastrointestinal hemorrhage, salicylate-induced gastric bleeding may be painless, with blood loss reflected only in the stool. Aspirin inhibits platelet aggregation and prolongs clotting

time. Patients may deny use of aspirin, unaware that such products as Anacin, Ascriptin, and Bufferin contain this compound

b. Nonsteroidal anti-inflammatory (NSAI) agents, such as sulindac (Clinoril), indomethacin (Indocin), naproxen (Naprosyn), and others

b. Nonsteroidal anti-inflammatory agents can interfere with diagnostic testing, such as clotting studies and liver function tests. Adverse gastrointestinal symptoms may be manifest

c. Substance abuse

c. A variety of illegal drugs may prove toxic to the liver, resulting in hepatocellular necrosis and even death. Infectious agents, such as hepatitis virus, may be introduced parenterally by patients who abuse drugs

Patient self-treatment with over-the-counter (OTC) medications, such as vitamins, acetaminophen, and laxatives, may result in significant gastrointestinal dysfunction. Manifestations include altered liver function and increased bowel motility

d. Antimetabolites and related compounds

d. Direct or indirect hepatotoxins, such as methotrexate or tetracycline, adversely affect metabolic and secretory liver cell functions

All medications identified should be promptly noted on the nursing care plan.

B. Toxins

B. Industrial chemicals, such as carbon tetrachloride, the arsenicals, and phosphorus-based compounds, not only may alter the gastric defense mechanisms but may also cause hepatocellular necrosis. Treatment is supportive after removal of the offending agent

C. Diet
   a. Malnutrition

C. a. Signs and symptoms of malnutrition, such as cachexia or severe dehydration, require further assessment. Occult eating disorders may be responsible. In addition, knowledge deficits and teaching–learning needs may be identified

   b. Protein intolerance

b. Chronic hepatic insufficiency may result in impaired protein clearance. Strict limitation of ingested protein load may be indicated

   c. Wheat intolerance

c. Sensitivity to gluten, a protein found in several grains and vegetables as well as in ice cream and instant coffee, is known as *celiac sprue disease*. Severe dietary restriction requires supplementation with folate, iron, calcium, and vitamins

   d. Lactose intolerance

d. Common in the black and Oriental population, ingestion of lactose-containing foods may result in increased osmolality of the intestinal contents. Manifestations include bloating, flatus, and osmotic diarrhea. Dietary modifications significantly decrease the symptoms

D. Stress factors

D. Work-related and family-related stress factors may precipitate gastrointestinal disease

E. Travel

E. With travel, there may be exposure to bacteria and parasites affecting the gastrointestinal system. Examples include amebiasis, giardiasis, and salmonellosis

4. Present problem

4. A. Abdominal pain

4. A. Abdominal pain in the critical care setting demands skilled nursing assessment. Evidence may be gathered regarding the five mechanisms of abdominal pain: (1) perforation, (2) obstruction, (3) ischemia, (4) inflammation, and (5) hemorrhage

B. Trauma

B. Any patient with abdominal trauma, blunt or penetrating, must be evaluated for presence of intra-abdominal bleeding as a result of organ laceration. Such bleeding may be massive but produce minimal findings. The potential for peritoneal infection is high after abdominal trauma, particularly if it is the result of a penetrating wound

C. Gastrointestinal bleeding

C. Significant gastrointestinal bleeding demands prompt recognition of the problem and stabilization of the patient. Maintenance of blood volume and immediate volume replacement are primary goals. A large bore IV route (14–18 gauge) should be inserted for rapid volume expansion

(continued)

PARAMETERS	FINDINGS	IMPLICATIONS FOR NURSING CARE
5. Review of systems	**5. A.** Gastrointestinal **B.** Central nervous system **C.** Cardiovascular	**5. A.** Nutrition, alteration in: less than body requirements Bowel elimination, alteration in Injury, potential for **B.** Comfort, alteration in: pain Self-care deficit: feeding **C.** Fluid volume, deficit, potential

Assessment of the Gastrointestinal System by Inspection

RATIONALE Usually, several clinical impressions are gained after taking a patient history. The technique of inspection is the first step in clarifying and refining those data. Vital clues to underlying dysfunction of the gastrointestinal system may be obtained by assimilating pertinent observations made during the course of routine patient care.

PARAMETERS	FINDINGS	POSSIBLE ETIOLOGIES	DOCUMENTATION
1. Skin	1. **A.** Pallor **B.** Ecchymosis **C.** Jaundice **D.** Spider nevi **E.** Dryness, rash **F.** Decreased turgor	1. **A.** Gastrointestinal bleeding with significant blood loss results in decreased levels of circulating hemoglobin **B.** Altered bleeding and clotting mechanisms **C.** Impaired bilirubin metabolism resulting in the deposition of the yellow bile pigment in the skin and mucous membranes **D.** May appear with liver disease **E.** Impaired nutritional status; multiple causes, such as prolonged illness, malabsorption syndromes, poor management **F.** Dehydration, may be related to decreased intake or excessive output as with severe vomiting or diarrhea	1. Pallor, bruises, spider nevi, dryness, rash, and turgor
2. Eyes	2. **A.** Conjunctival icterus (scleral icterus) **B.** Mucous membrane pallor	2. **A.** Impaired bilirubin metabolism resulting in deposition of the yellow bile pigment in the skin and mucous membranes **B.** Anemia related to decreased levels of circulating hemoglobin; may be from actual loss or absorptive defects	2. Icterus and pallor
3. Oropharynx	3. **A.** Pallor **B.** Jaundice **C.** Beefy, red tongue	3. **A.** Anemia related to decreased levels of circulating hemoglobin; can be a result of actual loss or from absorptive defects **B.** Impaired bilirubin metabolism resulting in deposition of yellow bile pigment in the skin and mucous membranes **C.** Malnutrition	3. Color

4. Abdomen	4. **A.** Contour
	  a. Scaphoid
	  b. Distention
	  c. Asymmetry
	
	B. Movement
	  a. Peristalsis
		4. **A.** **a.** Malnutrition
		  b. Ascites, hemoperitoneum, obstruction, tumor, pregnancy, obesity, starvation
		  c. Mass or tumor may distort asymmetrically; wall defects such as inguinal hernias (more common in males) or femoral hernias (more common in females)
		B. **a.** Normally not observable but does occur from right to left
		    Reverse peristalsis (left to right) is a
			4. **A.** **a.** Concavity
			  b. Convexity
			
			  c. Masses including shape, size, location
			
			B. Presence, absence, location observed

	classic manifestation of pyloric stenosis Absent peristalsis may indicate intestinal obstruction	
b. Pulsation	**b.** Abdominal aneurysm, tumor; may also indicate obstruction of the vena cava	
C. Skin **a.** Scars	**C. a.** Previous surgeries or trauma (more recent scars are pink or bluish, those of older origin are silvery in color)	**C. a,b.** Presence, absence, size, location, color, healing status
b. Striae	**b.** Weight loss, Cushing's disease, previous pregnancies	
c. Grey Turner's sign	**c.** Extravasation of blood within the abdominal cavity	**c,d.** Presence or absence
d. Superficial vessels	**d.** Normal until puberty. Persistence after this time, accompanied by distention may indicate a partial obstruction. Caput Medusa may indicate portal hypertension (Fig. 5–1)	
D. Umbilicus **a.** Inverted	**D. a.** Obesity	**D.** Color, condition, presence or absence of nodules
b. Everted	**b.** Ascites	
c. Cullen's sign	**c.** A bluish umbilicus, indicating possible intra-abdominal hemorrhage	
d. Sister Mary Joseph's Nodule: A nodular area surrounding the umbilicus	**d.** May be indicative of an abdominal malignancy	
E. Fistula	**E.** Infection, inflammatory bowel disease, recent surgery or trauma	**E.** Location Quantity and characteristics of drainage
F. Tubes or drains	**F.** T-tube, gastrostomy, and so on. Size, type, and wound location may influence the choice of drain system. Expected quantity of drainage is also to be considered	**F.** Location and type Connection to suction or drainage device Quantity and characteristics of drainage
5. Extremities		
5. A. Palmar erythema	**5. A.** Abnormal metabolism of hormones in liver disease	**5. A.** Pronounced redness of thenar or hypothenar eminence
B. Asterixis	**B.** Abnormal protein metabolism in liver disease may result in peripheral neuromuscular weakness	**B.** Presence or absence of finding
C. Edema	**C.** Venous obstruction or decreased serum albumin, as in tumor, cirrhosis, or malabsorption syndromes	**C.** Degree of edema, location, pitting or nonpitting

POSSIBLE NURSING DIAGNOSES

- Bowel elimination, alteration in
- Fluid volume, deficit, potential
- Skin integrity, impairment of actual and potential
- Nutrition, alteration in: less than body requirements
- Nutrition, alteration in: more than body requirements
- Tissue perfusion, alteration in: gastrointestinal
- Tissue perfusion, alteration in: peripheral
- Comfort, alteration in: pain

SPECIAL NOTE

Abdominal Drains

Some drains are used interchangeably dependent upon the preference of the surgeon. There are, however, several important nursing responsibilities to be addressed.

- During the recovery and immediate postoperative period, verify the results of assessment by inspection with operative records. Number of drains found should equal number of drains recorded as inserted
- Some drainage may be expected to appear on fresh surgical dressings. Unexpected drainage or saturation should be promptly investigated. It may indicate dislodgment of the drain
- Unusually large amounts of drainage, greater than expected in a particular situation, should be investigated promptly
- Complications associated with the use of abdominal drains may occur and may become the basis for litigation. Accurate documentation regarding type, size, numbers, and location of drains, the quantity and characteristics of drainage, and all related nursing interventions is essential

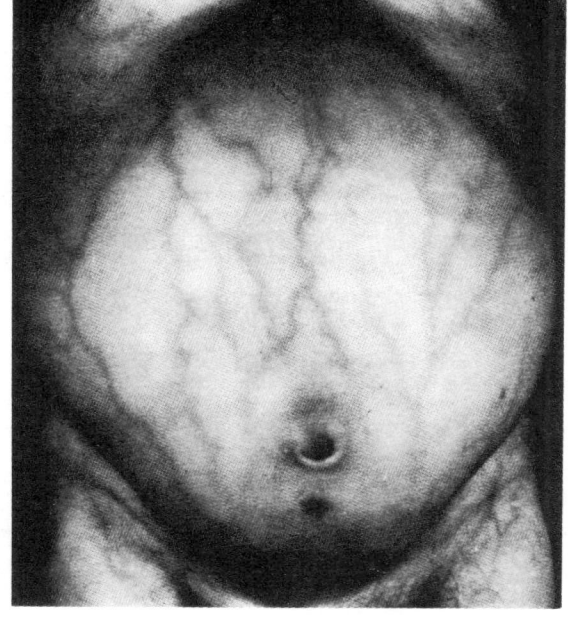

Figure 5–1. Caput Medusa. *(From Sherman, J. L., & Fields, S. K. Guide to patient evaluation (3rd ed.). Garden City, N. Y.: Medical Examination Publishing, 1978, p. 203, with permission.)*

Assessment of the Gastrointestinal System by Auscultation

RATIONALE

Those organs of the gastrointestinal system contained within the abdominal cavity may produce distinctive sounds (Fig. 5–2). Auscultation with the stethoscope is the technique by which certain sounds are assessed. Auscultation in all four quadrants should precede percussion and palpation, since bowel sounds may be altered by percussion and palpation.

PARAMETERS	FINDINGS	POSSIBLE ETIOLOGIES	DOCUMENTATION
1. Peristaltic sounds. Peristaltic sounds are assessed using the diaphragm on the abdomen with only light pressure (Figs. 5–3 to 5–6)	1. A. Normal B. Hypoactive C. Absent D. High pitched	1. A. Normal movement of fluid and air in the bowel produces soft gurgling sounds occurring in an irregular pattern q5–15sec. Borborygmi is the term describing hyperperistaltic stomach growling B. Associated with the slow phase of digestion. Electrolyte disturbance and certain medications, particularly analgesics, may produce this finding C. Paralytic ileus, which may occur in the postoperative period, results in loss of motility but lumen patency D. Obstruction of bowel alters the lumen diameter, with resultant increase in pitch. May be correlated with other findings, such as diarrhea or abdominal pain or cramping	• Quandrant auscultated • Sound quality
2. Vascular sounds. Vascular sounds are heard best by using the bell. A slightly firmer pressure may be applied	2. A. Bruit and murmurs: A bruit is a low-pitched, soft blowing sound. Normal pulsation is extended and may have a swishing quality. Best heard over the epigastrium or major arteries B. Venous hum: A venous hum is of medium tone, continuous through systole–diastole, and slightly higher pitched than a bruit. Most likely heard over the umbilicus and liver C. Friction rub: Friction rubs, because of the softness and subtlety of tone, may be mistaken for breath sounds. Usually heard over the liver or spleen	2. A. Sounds produced by turbulent blood flow; may be heard normally in a very thin person. Abdominal aortic aneurysms, renal artery stenosis, or increased blood flow to a vascular tumor may also produce this finding B. May be present in liver tumor, in veno-obstructive processes, or in cirrhosis. Umbilical vein abnormalities may also produce this sound C. May accompany peritoneal inflammation, as in cholecystitis, splenic inflammation, or infarct. Also heard with hepatic tumors	

- Bowel elimination, alteration in
- Tissue perfusion, alteration in: gastrointestinal
- Tissue perfusion, alteration in: renal

SPECIAL NOTE

Secussion Splash

Secussion splash is a sound produced during performance of a specific maneuver. It may be elicited by gently grasping the hips of the supine patient and rocking him back and forth. The sound of fluid splashing, as in a closed container, may be heard if the patient has a large collection of fluid and air in a hollow organ, such as in gastric outlet obstruction.

Gastric Outlet Obstruction

Gastric outlet obstruction is a complication associated with peptic ulcer disease or tumor. Obstruction of the outlet may be manifested by severe nausea and vomiting of partially digested food. Aspiration of 400 cc or more in 30 minutes and a secussion splash may indicate pyloric obstruction.

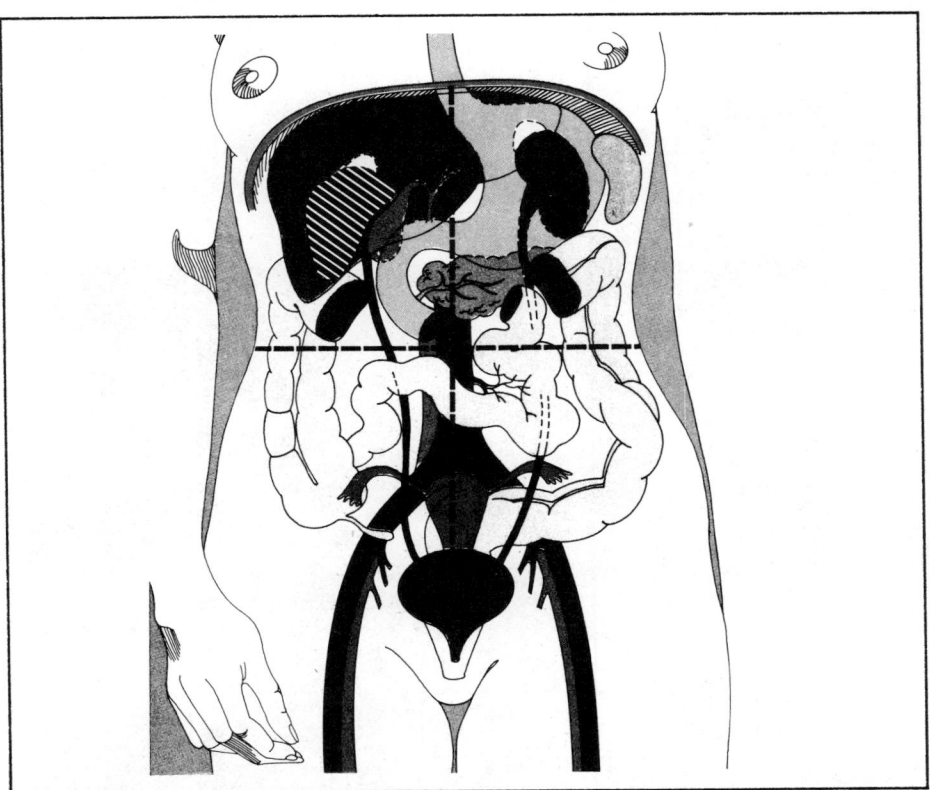

Figure 5–2. The abdomen divided into quadrants, showing placement of the organs in each quadrant. *(From Barisonek, K., Newman, E., & Logio, T. "My stomach hurts." Nursing 84, 1984, 14(11), 38, with permission.)*

(continued)

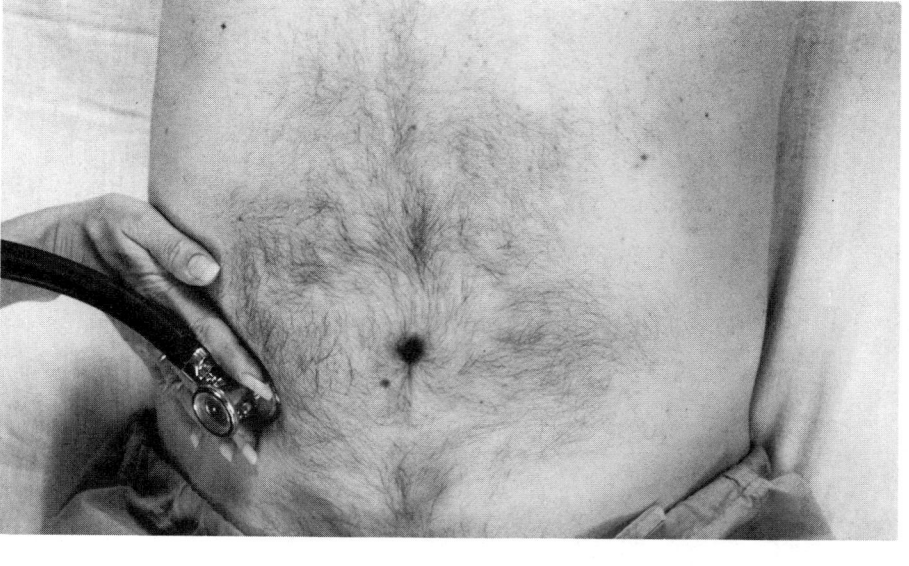

Figure 5–3. Auscultation of the right lower quadrant.

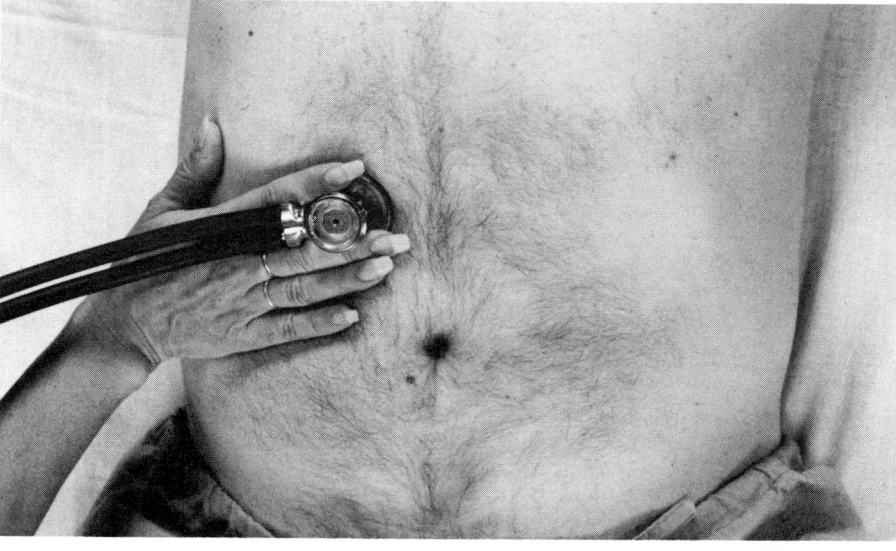

Figure 5–4. Auscultation of the right upper quadrant.

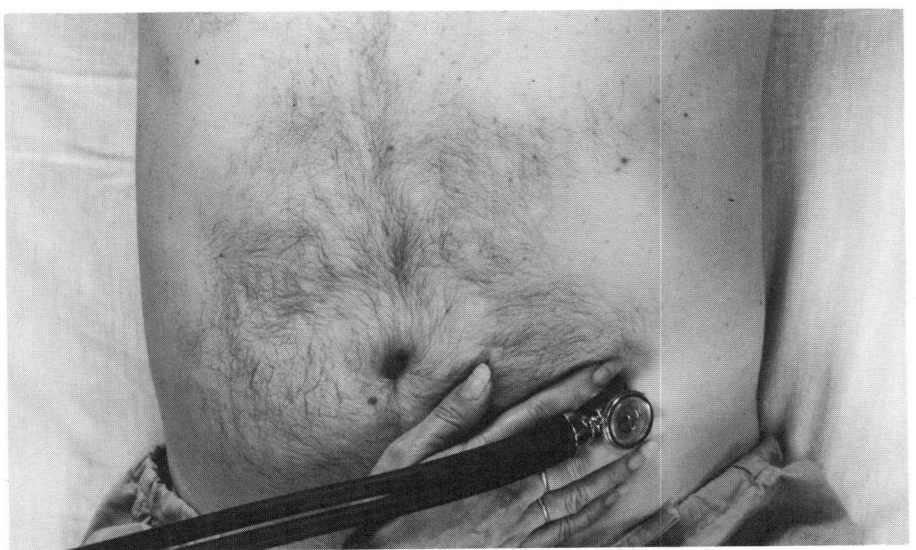

Figure 5–5. Auscultation of the left lower quadrant.

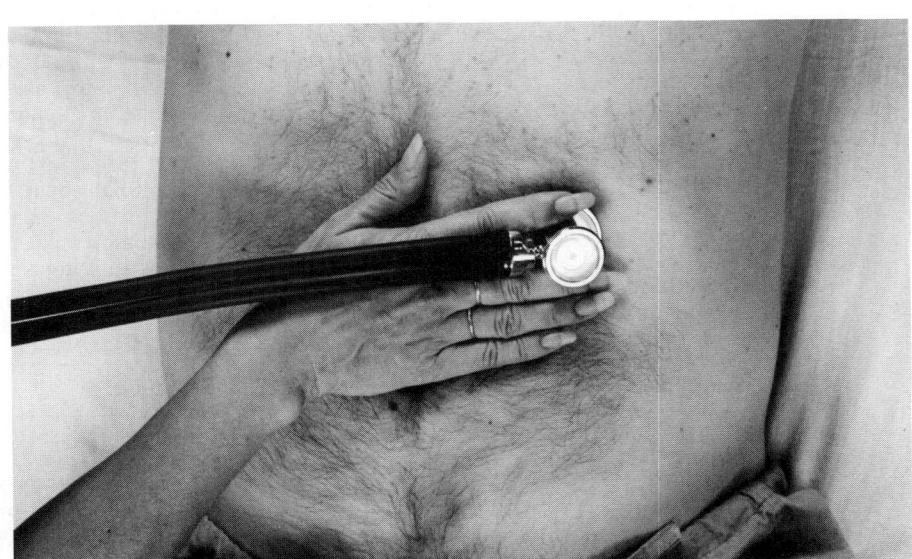

Figure 5–6. Auscultation of the left upper quadrant.

Assessment of the Gastrointestinal System by Percussion

RATIONALE

Percussion enhances auscultation and precedes palpation. Percussion is a technique by which sounds are produced as the examiner manually outlines organs or masses of differing densities. Recognition of alterations in the percussed notes is of the utmost importance. Percussion should be performed over all four quadrants using anatomical landmarks as guides (Fig. 5–7).

PARAMETERS	FINDINGS	POSSIBLE ETIOLOGIES	DOCUMENTATION
1. Dullness	1. Outlines a solid organ, such as liver or spleen. Normally, the liver is percussed in the right upper quadrant in the midclavicular line. Upper border found at the fifth to seventh intercostal space; lower border at the right costal margin. On held inspiration or expiration, border identification may vary by two finger-widths (Fig. 5–9)	1. Extended borders may indicate hepatomegaly The spleen is not normally identifiable by percussion, but with moderate splenomegaly, it may be detected below the left costal margin on deep inspiration (Fig. 5–8) Left lower quadrant dullness may indicate stool in the bowel Dullness above the symphysis pubis indicates bladder distention Free fluid in the abdomen, usually associated with ascites, is indicated by shifting dullness. It may be detected as flank dullness as the patient is repositioned. A fluid wave may also be present in ascites	• Organ percussed • Anatomical location of borders • Sound elicited, e.g., Liver dullness at right sixth intercostal space Splenic dullness over left costal margin • Performance of shifting dullness maneuver • Anatomical landmarks identified, e.g., No flank dullness identified No fluid wave present • Location of tympany, e.g., Mild upper abdominal distention, gastric bubble tympanic
2. Tympany To perform the technique of percussion, stand on the patient's right side. Place your left middle finger flat on the patient's abdomen and apply only slight pressure. Tap the distal joint of the finger of your left hand with the flexed middle finger of your right hand. Lightly percuss all four quadrants to assess any disproportionate dullness or tympany. Proceed then to assess each parameter (Figs. 5–11, 5–12, and 5–13).	2. Outlines air-containing organs, such as stomach or intestines. Tympany may be heard most commonly over air-containing organs, such as the stomach or intestines	2. Increase in the size of the gastric bubble associated with gastric distention (Fig. 5–10)	

- Fluid volume, alteration in: excess
- Bowel elimination, alteration in

SPECIAL NOTE

Shifting Dullness

Movement of free abdominal fluid as the patient is repositioned produces the finding of shifting dullness. To percuss for the presence of free fluid in the abdominal cavity (ascites), perform the test for shifting dullness as follows:

1. Place the patient in a supine position. Free fluid will migrate to the flanks and produce dullness laterally
2. Percuss the abdomen
3. Draw a line to mark the level of dullness
4. Reposition the patient on one side
5. Again percuss the abdomen
6. Mark the level of dullness

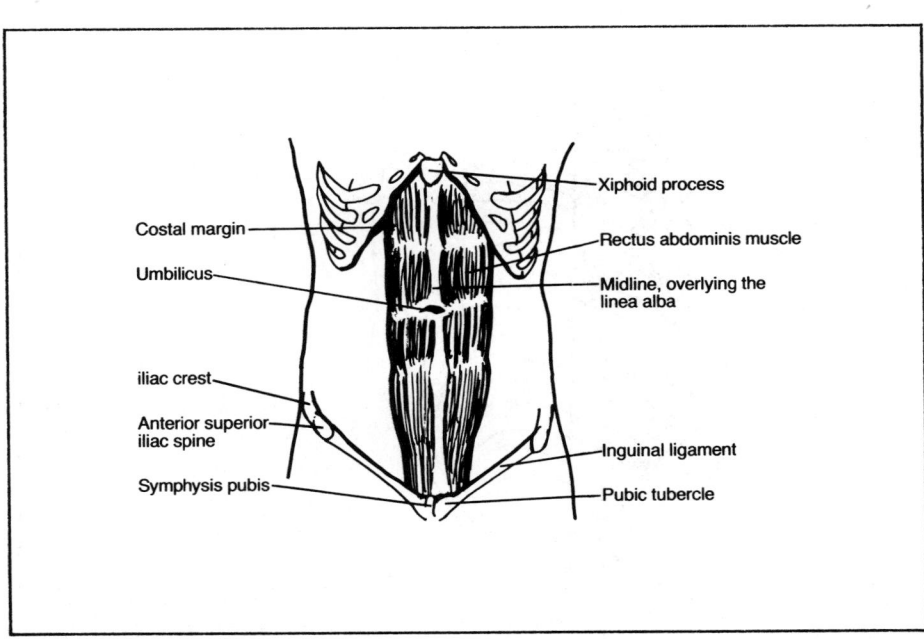

Figure 5–7. The abdomen with anatomical landmarks highlighted.

(continued)

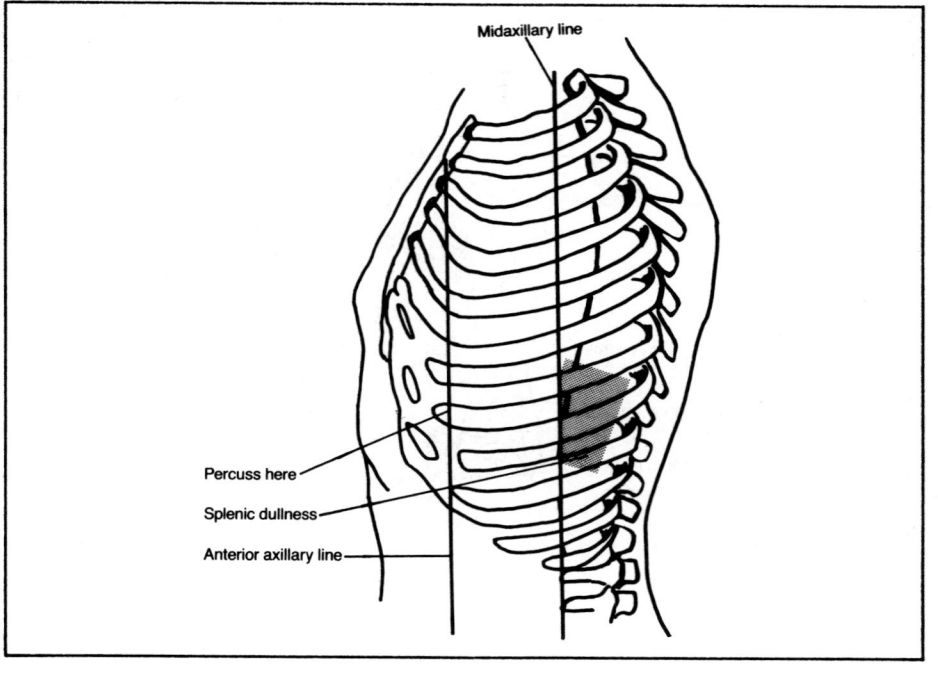

Figure 5–8. Percussion of the spleen tip.

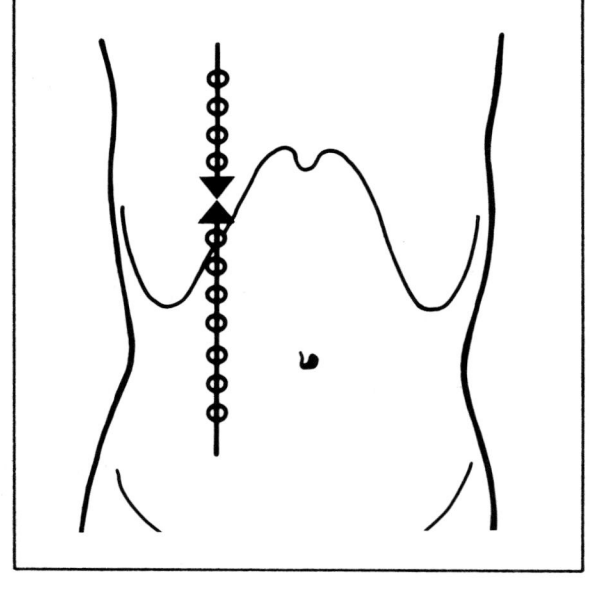

Figure 5–9. The upper border of the liver is located at the 5th to 7th intercostal space. The lower border is located at the right costal margin.

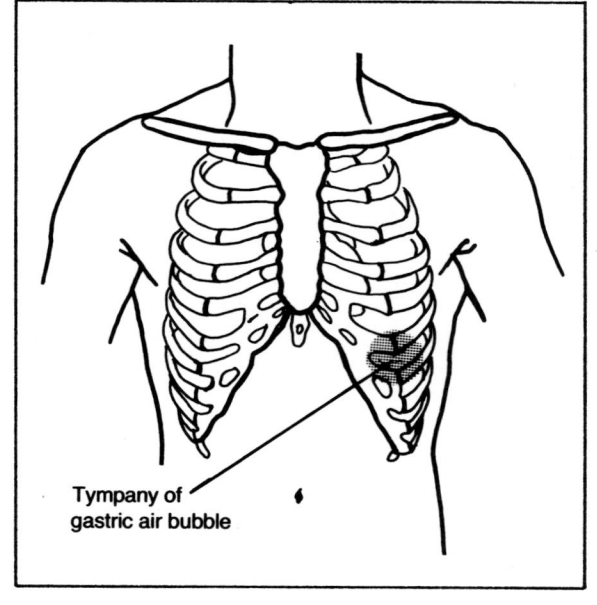

Figure 5–10. Percussion of the gastric bubble.

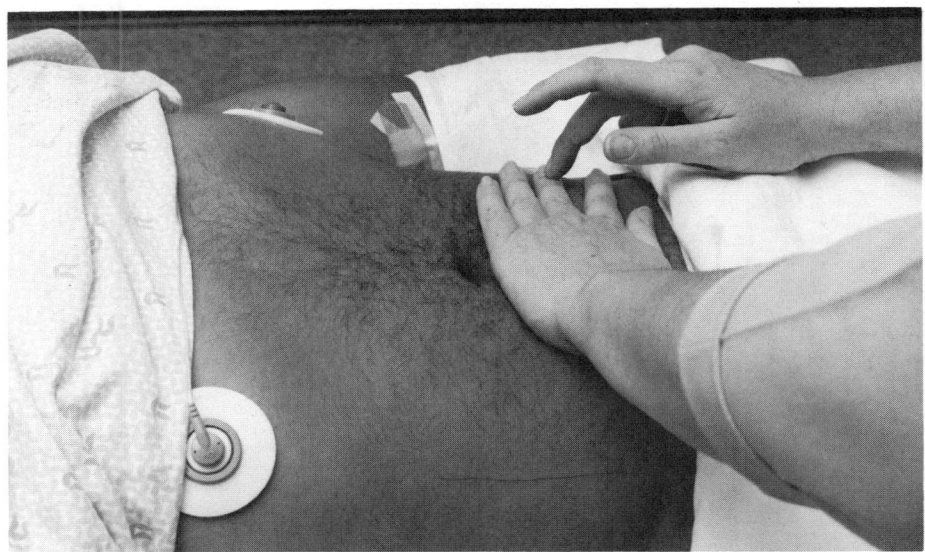

Figure 5–11. Percussion of the spleen tip.

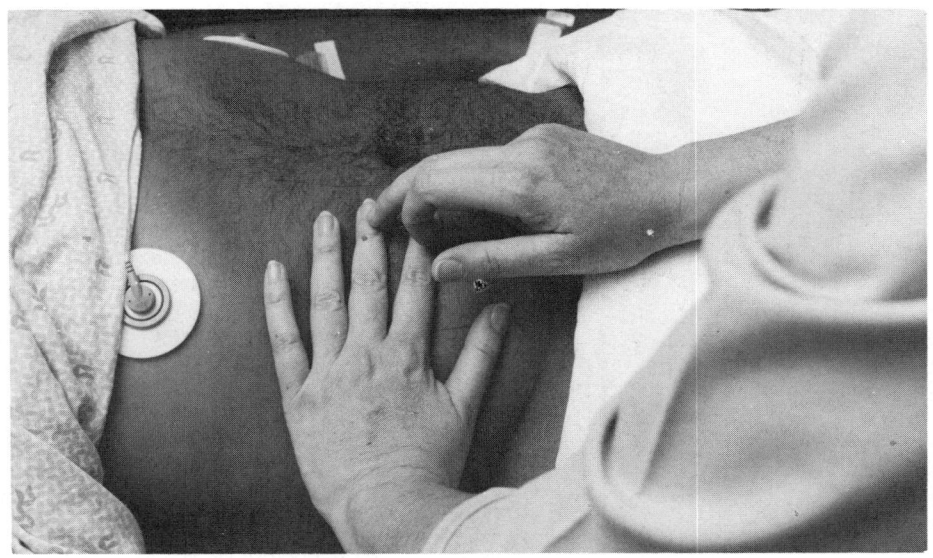

Figure 5–12. Percussion of the liver.

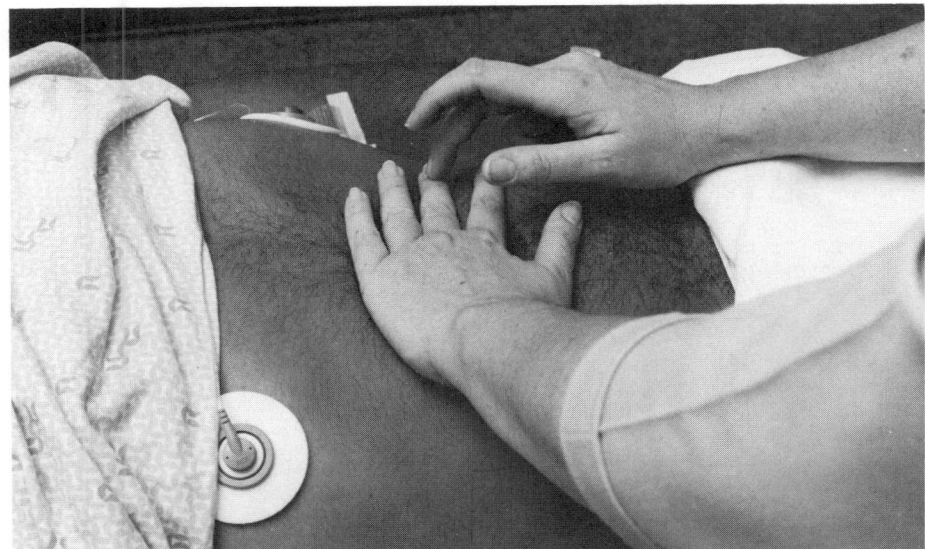

Figure 5–13. Percussion of the gastric bubble.

Assessment of the Gastrointestinal System by Palpation

RATIONALE

Palpation of the abdomen may reveal information not gained by inspection, auscultation, or percussion. Palpation shall be performed after the other techniques and with the patient in the supine position with the knees slightly flexed. Information may be obtained regarding the size and characteristics of an organ as well as associated tenderness.

PARAMETERS	FINDINGS	POSSIBLE ETIOLOGIES	DOCUMENTATION
	Superficial palpation is performed lightly by gently pressing with the fingertips on the abdomen. Deep palpation is performed by placing one hand atop the other and firmly pressing with the fingertips. Rebound tenderness is elicited by abrupt withdrawal of pressure from deep palpation. Painful areas should be examined last (Figs. 5–14 to 5–17).		• Presence or absence and characteristics of associated tenderness • Location of an organ or mass using anatomical landmarks • Presence or absence of any abdominal tenderness • Presence or absence of rebound tenderness • Unusual placement of umbilicus • Umbilical nodularity
1. Right upper quadrant (RUQ)	1. Liver A. Location	1. A. Normally located in the RUQ, 4–8 cm in the midsternal line and 6–12 cm in the midclavicular line. May be palpated at the right costal margin. Enlargement should be carefully documented by both palpation and percussion	
	B. Edge	B. Normally smooth. Nodules or an irregular border may indicate cirrhosis or malignancy	
	C. Elongated right lobe	C. A normal anatomical variation in tall, thin patients, this may be a shape change rather than a size change	
	D. Consistency	D. Suspected enlargement may be, in fact, due to a downward displacement of the diaphragm, common in patients with emphysema; not only hepatomegaly	
2. Left upper quadrant (LUQ)	2. Spleen A. Location	2. A. Normally may be palpated under the left costal margin during deep inspiration with the patient in the lateral decubitus position	
	B. Tip	B. With moderate enlargement, may be palpated below the left costal margin Marked enlargement, may be palpated in the lower left quadrant Massively enlarged, the spleen may cross the midline	
	C. Shape	C. Will distinguish enlarged spleen from an enlarged kidney	

3. Right lower quadrant (RLQ)	**3.** Kidneys
	  A. Location
	  B. Edge
		3. A. Normally located bilaterally below the costal margins but above the iliac crests
		  B. May be indicative of polycystic kidney disease, neoplasm, or hydronephrosis

4. Left lower quadrant (LLQ)	**4.** Tenderness
	  A. Murphy's sign
	  B. McBurney's point
	
	  C. Midline
	
	  D. Visceral
	  E. Inflammatory
		4. A. RUQ tenderness associated with acute cholecystitis
		  B. RLQ tenderness associated with acute appendicitis
		  C. Epigastric tenderness associated with acute pancreatitis
		  D. May be associated with hepatomegaly
		  E. May be related to bladder distention or may be related to pleuritic inflammation

5. Midline	**5.** Umbilicus
	  A. Placement
	
	  B. Texture
		5. A. May be displaced upward by pregnancy, off midline by trauma or surgical scars, everted with ascites
		  B. Pouching may indicate an umbilical hernia Nodularity (Sister Mary Joseph's nodule) may indicate metastasis from an intra-abdominal neoplasm

POSSIBLE NURSING DIAGNOSES

- Comfort, alteration in
- Nutrition, alteration in: less than body requirements
- Tissue perfusion, alteration in: gastrointestinal

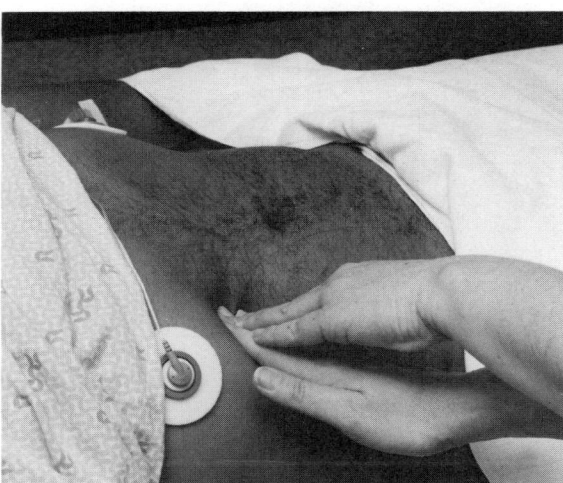

Figure 5–14. Hand position; right upper quadrant for organ palpation.

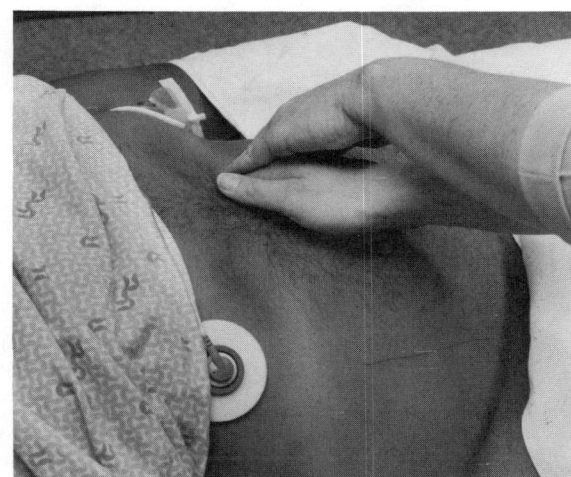

Figure 5–15. Hand position; left upper quadrant for organ palpation.

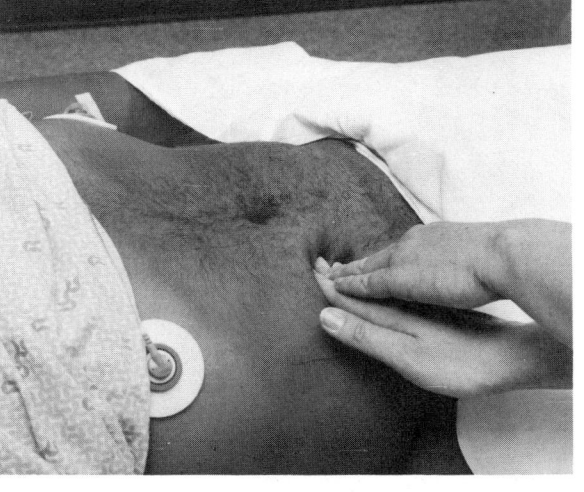

Figure 5–16. Hand position; right lower quadrant for organ palpation.

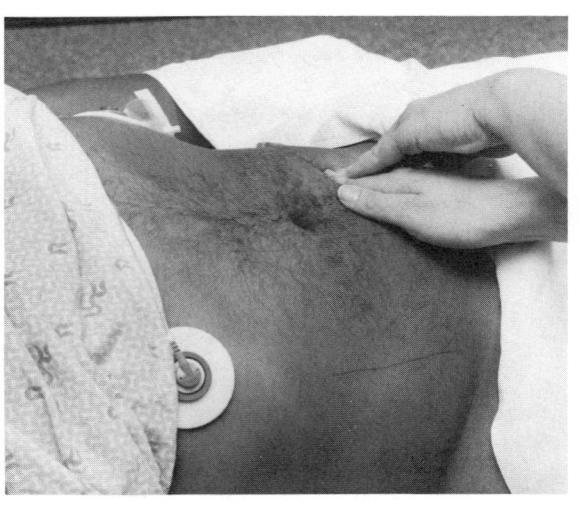

Figure 5–17. Hand position; left lower quadrant for organ palpation.

Assessment of Pertinent Laboratory Data

RATIONALE   Laboratory data are meant not to replace but to complement history and physical examination for diagnosis and follow-up. Changing laboratory data may occasionally be the first indication of gastrointestinal bleeding, hepatic dysfunction, or pancreatitis. Such laboratory indicators are of particular importance in patients in ICU, who often cannot communicate their problems. Early recognition, correlation, and intervention may avert life-threatening situations, such as gastrointestinal hemorrhage.

PARAMETERS	FINDINGS	POSSIBLE ETIOLOGIES	DOCUMENTATION
	The values listed are normal ranges.		• Manner in which the specimen was obtained
1. Hemoglobin (Hgb)	1. Male, 14–18 g/dl; female, 12–16 g/dl	1. Decrease may be a reflection of blood loss from occult or acute gastrointestinal bleeding	• Delivery to the laboratory • Results recorded accurately and sequentially
2. Hematocrit (HCT)	2. Male, 41–51%; female, 37–47%	2. Unchanged or elevated or decreased; may be a reflection of hemoconcentration or blood loss	• Communication of results to the appropriate personnel
3. White blood cell (WBC) count	3. 6000–10,000/μl	3. Elevation may be indicative of inflammation, such as appendicitis	
4. Prothrombin time (PT)	4. 9.6–12.1 second	4. If prolonged, may be indicative of liver disease, reflecting inability of the liver to synthesize clotting factors	
5. Platelet count	5. 150,000–400,000/μl	5. If decreased, may be indicative of liver disease, reflecting inability of the liver to synthesize clotting factors	
6. Blood urea nitrogen (BUN)	6. 8–24 mg/dl	6. Elevation may be indicative of bleeding into the gastrointestinal tract as the by-products of protein (blood) breakdown are absorbed	
7. Creatinine	7. 0.5–1.5 mg/dl	7. If unchanged or elevated, may be indicative of decreased renal perfusion that may occur with massive gastrointestinal bleeding	
8. Potassium (K$^+$)	8. 3.5–5.0 mEq	8. Decrease may be indicative of volume depletion related to watery diarrhea, excessive vomiting, or nasogastric suction	
9. Calcium (Ca^{2+})	9. 8.7–10.7 mg/dl	9. Decrease may be indicative of saponification, as in pancreatitis	

10. Bilirubin
   A. Total
   B. Direct
	10. 0.2–1.2 mg/dl	10. Elevation is indicative of altered bilirubin metabolism	

11. Alkaline phosphatase	11. 25–100 mg/dl	11. Abnormalities, typically elevations, may be seen during spurts of bone growth, as in adolescents, or in the presence of biliary tract disease	
12. Serum glutamic-pyruvic transaminase (SGPT)	12. 5–35 mIU/ml	12. Elevation may be indicative of cellular destruction in liver disease	
13. Serum glutamic-oxalo-acetic transaminase (SGOT)	13. 5–30 mIU/ml	13. Elevated, often higher than the SGPT, in alcoholic liver disease	
14. Albumin	14. 3.5–5.1 g/dl	14. Abnormalities, usually decreased, reflect the inability of the liver to synthesize proteins	
15. Serum protein	15. 6.8–8.4 g/dl	15. Abnormalities, usually decreased, reflect the inability of the liver to synthesize proteins	

POSSIBLE NURSING DIAGNOSES

- Fluid volume, deficit, potential
- Gas exchange, impaired
- Nutrition, alteration in: less than body requirements
- Tissue perfusion, alteration in: gastrointestinal

Assessment of the Patient Receiving Total Parenteral Nutrition

RATIONALE

Total parenteral nutrition (TPN) is also known as *hyperalimentation*. It is the administration of a solution containing protein hydrolysates, electrolytes, and dextrose supplemented with a fat emulsion to provide adequate caloric intake. Trace elements and multivitamins may be included. Hyperalimentation is advantageous when increased metabolic requirements exceed the oral intake and the gastrointestinal tract is nonfunctional, as in malabsorption or intestinal obstruction. Traditionally TPN is administered through a central venous access site, but recent pharmacological advances have provided the option of using a peripheral vein, thus minimizing risks and allowing oral nutritional intake to begin. Each of the major components of the solution performs a vital function. Complication-free administration rests heavily on the nurse's ability to adequately assess the actions of each component and its effect on the client.

PARAMETERS	FINDINGS	POSSIBLE ETIOLOGIES	DOCUMENTATION
1. Carbohydrates	1. **A.** Hyperglycemia 　　Alteration or decrease in the level of consciousness 　　Blood glucose of 200 mg/dl or greater 　　Glycosuria of 2+ or greater **B.** Hypoglycemia 　　Restlessness 　　Confusion, disorientation 　　Diaphoresis 　　Blood glucose below 60 mg/dl	1. **A.** May be related to change in rate of administration, sepsis, dehydration, or HHNK **B.** May be related to abrupt cessation of administration without adequate replacement therapy	1. Neurovital signs and Glasgow coma scale scores q4h Restlessness, confusion, and disorientation
2. Amino acids	2. **A.** Positive nitrogen balance (desired state) 　　Absence of urine ketones **B.** Negative nitrogen balance 　　Weight loss 　　Proteinuria 　　Ketonuria	2. **A.** Protein synthesis occurring at a rate equal to or greater than protein use **B.** Rate of use exceeds rate of protein synthesis	2. Weight preadministration and daily thereafter
3. Electrolytes 　A. Sodium	3. **A. a.** Hypernatremia 　　Serum sodium above 145 mEq/L 　　Thirst 　　Decreased urine output 　　Increased specific gravity 　　**b.** Hyponatremia 　　Serum sodium below 135 mEq/L 　　Mild weakness 　　Confusion 　　Muscle twitching	3. **A. a.** Occurs when water is lost in excess of salt. Hypernatremia due to salt gain is rare. Loss of intracellular water in excess of loss of third space water may occur with administration of high-protein feedings 　　**b.** May be dilutional from inadequate loss replacement. May be defective urine dilution, as in cirrhosis	3. Muscle testing describing the quality of weakness and the groups tested Cardiac dysrhythmias with a rhythm strip present when indicated Abdominal assessment, including measurement of abdominal girth, describing the anatomical landmarks for placement of the measuring tape

B. Potassium	**B.** **a.** Hyperkalemia Potassium above 4.5 mEq/L Impaired neuromuscular function Widening QRS complex Ventricular irritability Abdominal distention **b.** Hypokalemia Potassium below 3.5 mEq/L Impaired skeletal muscle function ST segmental depression Flattened T-waves Increased sensitivity to digitalis preparations Polyuria Impaired smooth muscle function	**B.** **a.** Decreased excretion may indicate impaired renal function, as in acute renal failure or renal insufficiency. Severe acidosis or increased tissue breakdown results in increased release of intracellular potassium **b.** Most common with severe nausea, vomiting, nasogastric suction, diarrhea	
C. Calcium	**C.** **a.** Hypercalcemia Calcium above 10.7 mg/dl Neuromuscular weakness Muscle flaccidity Increased cardiac contractility Shortened QT interval Heart block Nausea, vomiting Constipation **b.** Hypocalcemia Calcium below 8.7 mg/dl Neuromuscular irritability Carpopedal spasm, muscle twitching Prolonged QT intervals Inverted T-waves Dyspnea Abdominal cramping Numbness, tingling in the extremities	**C.** **a.** May occur in presence of excess vitamin D or with calcium sensitivity and malignancies **b.** Administration of phosphates to correct hypophosphatemia without supplemental administration of calcium	
4. Hydration	**4.** **A.** Overhydration Elevated diastolic pressure Tachycardia Tachypnea Elevated CVP readings Increased urine output Edema Weight gain (excessive) **B.** Dehydration Decrease in cardiac output Decreased CVP readings Thickening of secretions Thirst	**4.** **A.** Fluid retention, too rapid administration, impaired renal function **B.** Inadequate volume administration, excessive fluid loss, electrolyte imbalances	**4.** Vital signs CVP reading Intake and output Weight daily Cardiac assessment Pulmonary assessment Skin integrity Edema: Presence, degree, location Secretions, noting tenacity Thirst

PARAMETERS	FINDINGS	POSSIBLE ETIOLOGIES	DOCUMENTATION

5. Fatty acids	Poor skin turgor
	Dry skin
	Elevated BUN and creatinine
	5. A. Fatty acids, balanced
	  Absence of hyperglycemia
	  Absence of hyperosmolar hyperglycemic nonketotic coma (HHNK)
	  Absence of hyperinsulinemia
	B. Fatty acids, excessive
	  Exacerbation of preexisting conditions, such as
	    Pulmonary dysfunctions
	    Liver disease
	    Anemia
	  Fat emboli
	C. Fatty acids, inadequate
	  Weight loss
	  Hair loss
	  Skin dryness
		5. A. Balanced administration of fatty acids
		
		B. Excessive administration of fatty acids
		
		C. Absent or inadequate administration of fatty acids for an extended period
			5. Neurovital signs and Glasgow coma scale scores
			Indications of vascular occlusion (emboli)
			Skin integrity
			
			Documentation shall reflect timely, accurate, and sequential recording of all laboratory data. Other laboratory data periodically recorded should include Hgb, Hct, magnesium, phosphorus, SGOT, SGPT, and alkaline phosphatase. Recognition of changes, trends, and interventions shall also be recorded.

POSSIBLE NURSING DIAGNOSES

- Nutrition, alteration in: less than body requirements
- Nutrition, alteration in, potential for: more than body requirements
- Fluid volume, alteration in: excess
- Fluid volume, deficit, actual
- Fluid volume, deficit, potential

SPECIAL NOTE

Nitrogen Balance

Nitrogen balance is a measure of net changes in total body protein mass. Increased protein metabolism occurs in disease states: fever, trauma, burns, and many other conditions. If breakdown occurs more rapidly than synthesis, a negative nitrogen balance exists. If synthesis occurs at a rate equal to or greater than breakdown, a positive nitrogen balance exists. Hyperalimentation or parenteral alimentation has offered an alternative means to achieve a positive nitrogen balance when there is impairment of the integrity of the gastrointestinal tract.

Administration

The hypertonic solutions of hyperalimentation must be administered through a subclavian catheter. These concentrated solutions are not tolerated by peripheral veins. Maintenance of aseptic technique is of prime importance. Addition of any mixtures to the prepared solution is prohibited. Coadministration of fat emulsions or medications is accomplished by administration below the final filter (Fig. 5–18) or by using a multilumen catheter.

Peripheral Alimentation

The solutions used in peripheral alimentation are more nearly isotonic than those administered centrally, and they may be used for a shorter time span when oral nutrition is not tolerated or is undesirable.

Intralipids

Fat emulsions provide essential fatty acids and high caloric density, thus providing the option to supply total caloric intake with lessened dependence on the carbohydrate concentrations in 50% dextrose solutions.

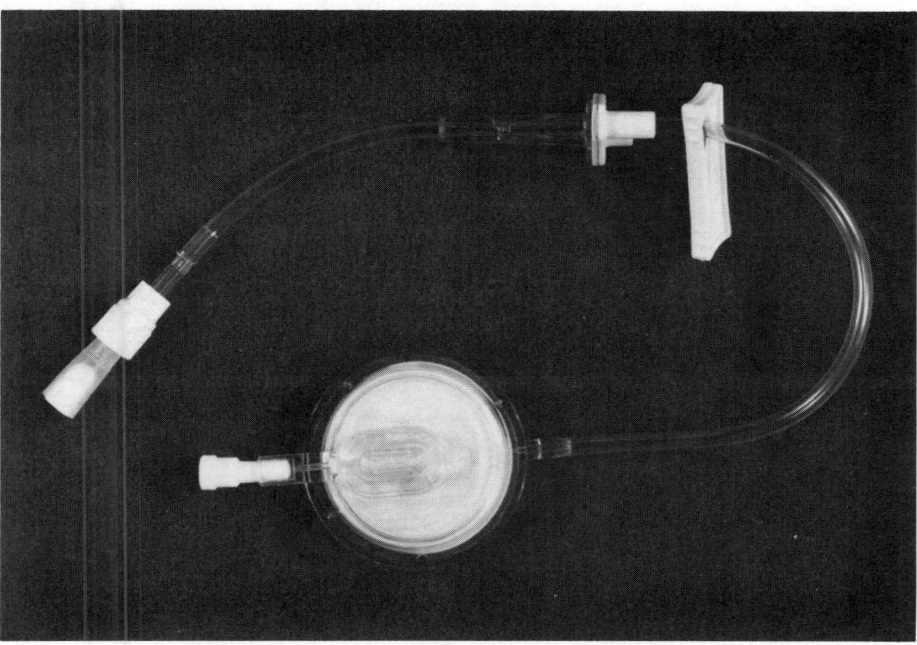

Figure 5–18. Final filter.

Care of the Patient Receiving Total Enteral Nutrition

NURSING DIAGNOSES	RATIONALE	DEFINING CHARACTERISTICS	EXPECTED OUTCOME

1. Nutrition, alteration in: less than body requirements	Nutritional support is often overlooked in deference to other life-threatening situations. Once the patient is stabilized, however, it is important to implement nutritional support. The patient in a critical care environment has increased metabolic needs and may require nutritional supplement. If the intestinal mucosa is intact and there is no evidence of obstruction, oral or enteral nutritional supplements should be instituted. Such nutritional supplements may be given orally or through a nasogastric, gastrostomy, or jejunostomy tube	1. **A.** Physical
		    a. General
		        Muscle wasting
		        Peripheral or sacral edema
		        Poor wound healing
		        Fistula present
		    b. Integument
		        Poor skin turgor
		        Dry, scaling skin
		        Rash
		    c. Cardiovascular
		        Tachycardia
		        Dysrhythmias
		    d. Pulmonary
		        Tachypnea
		    e. Oral cavity
		        Cheilosis
		        Magenta tongue
		    f. Abdomen
		        Scaphoid
		        Striae
		        Hepatomegaly
		    g. Central nervous system
		        Altered mental status
		        Depressed level of consciousness
		B. Metabolic
		    a. Laboratory data
		        Decreased serum albumin
		        Decreased total protein
		        Ketonuria
		        Proteinuria
			1. Patient's metabolic (caloric) requirements will be met

2. Injury, potential for:
A. Aspiration
 	
B. Pressure necrosis
		2. **A.** Emesis
		    Pulmonary secretions, congestion
		    Infiltrates or consolidation on chest x-ray
		    Fever
		B. Redness
		    Skin irritation
		    Skin breakdown
			2. No complications associated with enteral nutritional support will occur

C. Tube displacement		C. Coughing Choking Gagging Feeding does not flow	

Nutrition, alteration in: less than body requirements:

1. Physical
   A. Assess muscle strength and reflexes q8h
      Perform passive–active exercises q4h
      Evaluate lower extremities for the presence of edema q8h
      Evaluate for presence of sacral edema q8h
      Elevate extremities and apply support hose as necessary
      Perform skin and wound care as necessary
      Monitor quality and quantity of fistula drainage q4h
      Assess integrity of skin and tissue surrounding fistulas q4h
   B. Assess skin turgor q8h
      Monitor intake and output, including insensible loss, q8h
      Assess the skin for dryness and scaling q8h
      Perform skin care as necessary
      Inspect the skin, particularly the buttocks and groin, for the presence of a rash q8h
      Keep areas clean and dry at all times
   C. Assess cardiac rate and rhythm q4h
      Note the presence of jugular venous distention (JVD) q4h
   D. Assess the respiratory rate, rhythm, and breath sounds q4h
   E. Inspect oral cavity, noting color and integrity of mucous membranes and tongue and the presence of cheilosis
      Mouth care as needed
   F. Perform inspection, auscultation, percussion, and palpation of the abdomen q8h or more often as necessary
   G. Perform neurological evaluation by employing the Glasgow coma scale q4h
      Assess appropriateness of verbal and behavioral responses q4h
2. Metabolic
   A. The critical care nurse will be aware of laboratory data, will recognize changes and trends, and will report same to appropriate personnel

Injury, potential for:

1. Aspiration
   A. For continuous tube feeding, the patient will be maintained in reverse Trendelenburg's position. For intermittent or bolus feeding, the patient will be maintained in a semi-Fowler's position 30 minutes before and at least 2 hours after each feeding
   B. During continuous tube feeding, inflation of the endotracheal cuff will be maintained. Deflate only as necessary to prevent tracheal injury. During intermittent tube feeding, the endotracheal cuff will be inflated before and maintained for at least 2 hours after each feeding (Fig. 5–19)

(continued)

C. Verification of tube placement prior to the initiation of feeding will be accomplished by
    X-ray
    Instillation of a bolus of air through the feeding tube while listening with a stethoscope over the epigastrium (Figs. 5–20 and 5–21)
D. Aspiration for residual gastric contents every shift or prior to each feeding
2. Pressure necrosis
    A. Inspect face and nares for signs of irritation q4h
    B. Reposition feeding tube as necessary
    C. Replace with a smaller bore tube as necessary
    D. Mouth care at least q4h
    E. Nares and facial skin care at least q4h
3. Tube displacement
    A. Inspect oral cavity to detect tube coiled or dislodged during insertion
    B. Inspect oral cavity q4h, since tube may become displaced following prolonged coughing or emesis
    C. Secure tube with tape (Figs. 5–22 and 5–23)

OUTCOME CRITERIA

Nutrition, alteration in: less than body requirements:

1. Physical
    Muscle strength and reflexes will be maintained or improved
    Muscle contractures will be absent or minimized
    Peripheral edema will be minimized
    Wounds will heal in a timely fashion
    Undue skin excoriation will be prevented
    Skin integrity will be maintained
    Complications associated with fluid overload will be minimized or avoided
    Pulmonary aspiration or infection will be minimized or avoided
    Integrity of the oral cavity will be maintained
    Complications will be promptly recognized and treated
    Changes in level of responsiveness will be recognized and appropriate interventions initiated
2. Laboratory data: Changes and trends will be identified and appropriate interventions initiated

Injury, potential for:

1. No aspiration will occur
2. No pressure necrosis or dental caries will occur
3. Tube displacement will be recognized and corrected

DOCUMENTATION

Nutrition, alteration in: less than body requirements:

1. Physical
    Activity, muscle strength, and reflexes
    Presence or absence of peripheral or sacral edema
    Location and condition of wounds or fistula. Type and amount of drainage; frequency of wounds or fistula care. Add the amount of wound or fistula drainage into the total output
    Skin integrity
    Cardiac rate and rhythm; a rhythm strip will be placed on the chart when indicated and at least each shift. Presence or absence of JVD
    Findings of pulmonary assessment
    Integrity of the oral mucosa, tongue, nares, and facial skin

Findings of abdominal assessment
Alterations in mental status, interventions initiated, and responses to same
Glasgow coma scale and neurological vital signs q4h
2. Laboratory data
Type and time the specimen was obtained
Disposition of the specimen
Results
Data must be accurate and sequential
Changes and trends identified and reported to the appropriate personnel

Injury, potential for:

1. Aspiration
Position of patient and bed before and after feedings
Inflation and deflation of endotracheal cuff, including amount of air (in cc) and the time in relation to feedings
Time and method for tube placement verification
Quantity and quality of gastric residual aspirated
2. Pressure necrosis
Tube placement, position, and size
Frequency of oral hygiene
Condition of the oral mucosa
Integrity of facial skin and nares
Frequency of skin care
3. Tube displacement
Inspection of the oral cavity
Assessment of the abdomen
How and where the feeding tube is anchored, noting any marks or length indicators

SPECIAL NOTE

Feeding Interruptions

If the tube feeding is interrupted in preparation for testing, such as an upper gastrointestinal endoscopy or an arteriogram, the feeding tube should be flushed with at least 60 ml of water prior to being clamped. If the patient is receiving medication dependent upon intake, e.g., insulin, notify appropriate personnel that the feeding is being held and request recommendations regarding therapy.

Guidewire

Many of the newer, small-bore diameter, nasogastric tubes have a guidewire to facilitate insertion. It is not recommended that the guidewire be reinserted when the tube is in the patient even if the tube is displaced. The tube should be removed, the guidewire reinserted, and the tube then reinserted.

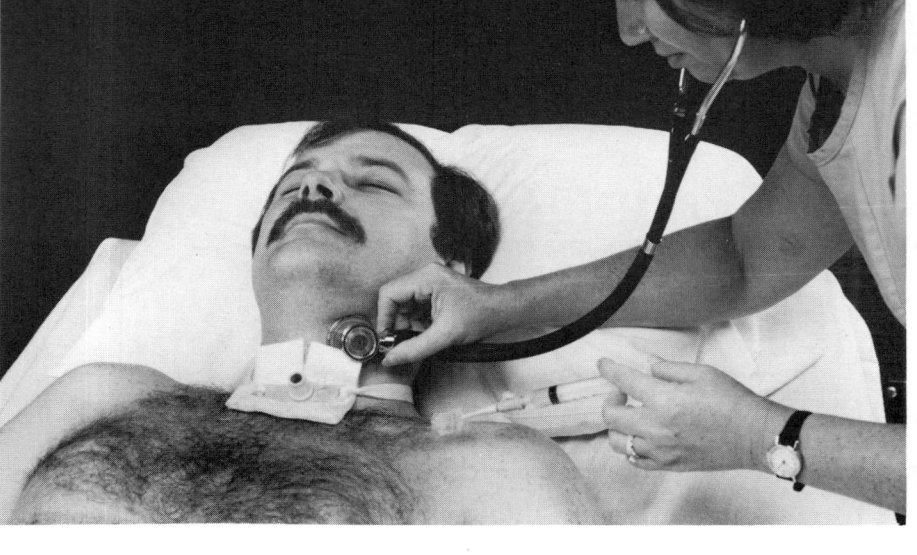

Figure 5-19. Nurse inflating cuff of tracheostomy tube.

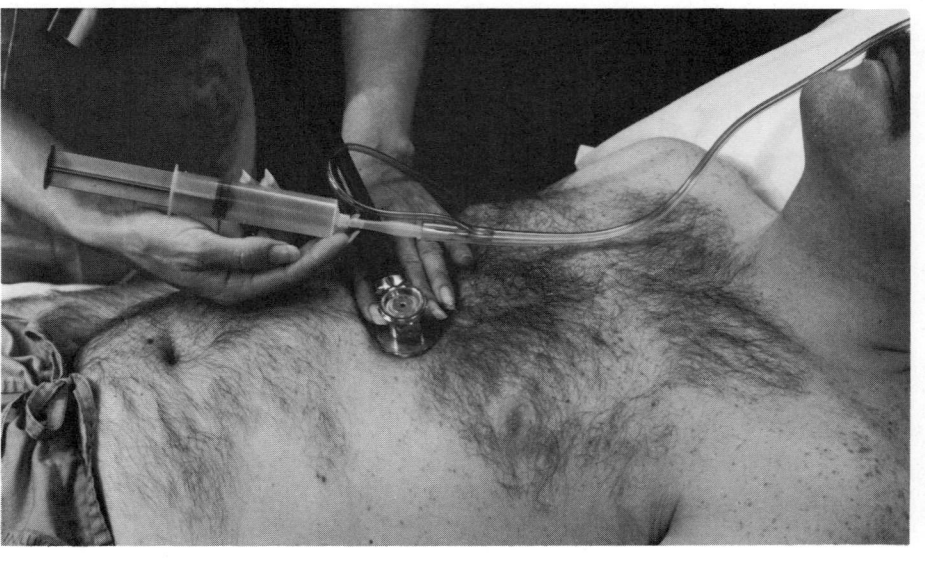

Figure 5-20. Instillation of air for verification of tube placement.

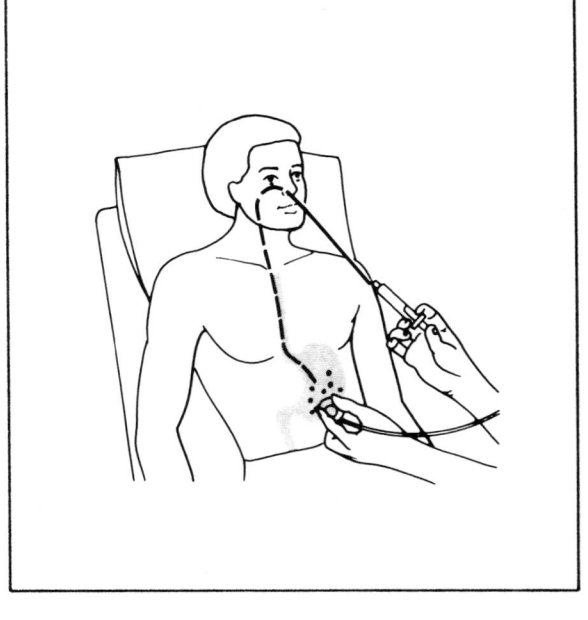

Figure 5-21. Placement of nasogastric tube. *(From Brill, E. L., & Kilts, D. F.* Foundations for nursing. *Norwalk, Conn.: Appleton-Century-Crofts, 1980, p. 528, with permission.)*

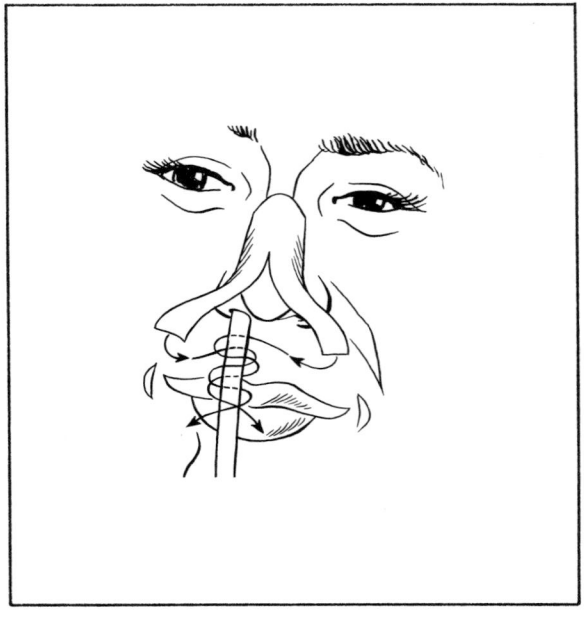

Figure 5-22. Taping of nasogastric tube (one method). *(From Norton, B. A., & Miller, A. M.* Skills for professional nursing practice. *Norwalk, Conn.: Appleton-Century-Crofts, 1986, p. 577, with permission.)*

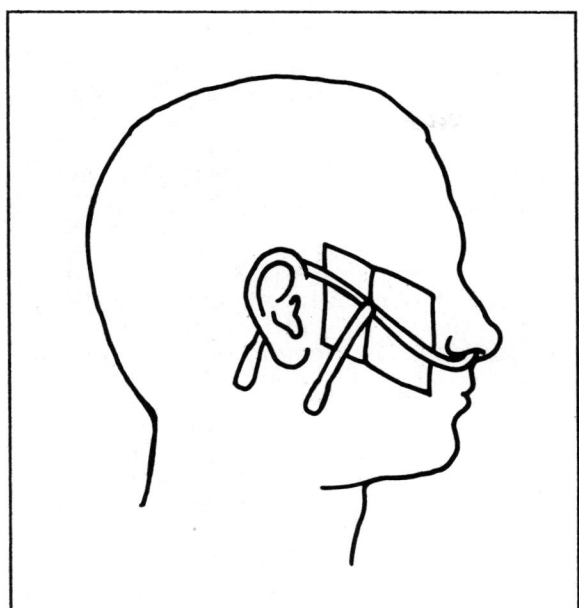

Figure 5–23. Taping of nasogastric tube (second method).

Care of the Patient Requiring Gastric Lavage

NURSING DIAGNOSES	RATIONALE	DEFINING CHARACTERISTICS	EXPECTED OUTCOME
1. Fluid volume deficit, potential for	1. Gastric lavage is a very effective way to decrease or stop upper gastrointestinal bleeding. Since the source of most gastrointestinal bleeding is above the ligament of Treitz, such intervention will be of benefit in most cases. Use of a large-bore tube for gastric lavage not only may stop bleeding but also may clean the stomach of clots, thus enabling further diagnostic and therapeutic measures to be instituted.	1. Hematemesis	1. Upper gastrointestinal bleeding will be effectively controlled
2. Injury, potential for: poisoning	2. Gastric lavage soon after the ingestion of a toxic substance decreases the amount of such substance to be absorbed, thereby minimizing the drug toxicity to the patient. With the tube in place, administration of chelating agents or cathartics is facilitated.	2. Known or suspected ingestion of a toxic substance	2. Absorption of an ingested toxin will be decreased

NURSING INTERVENTIONS

For all patients requiring gastric lavage:

1. Maintain patent airway at all times
2. Vital signs q1h
3. Neurovital signs and Glasgow coma scale q1h
4. Fluids administered as ordered
5. CVP monitoring q1h
6. Intake and output q1h
7. Gastric lavage
   A. Oropharyngeal insertion of 36 Fr tube (Figs. 5–24 and 5–25)
   B. Verification of tube placement by auscultation over the epigastric area during the instillation of a bolus of air through the lavage tube or by aspiration of gastric contents
   C. Continuous or intermittent lavage with an iced saline solution
8. Oral hygiene performed as needed
9. Prepare the patient for further diagnostic or therapeutic modalities

When known or suspected toxic ingestion has occurred, addiitonal interventions are indicated:

1. Procurement of specimens for toxicology studies, insuring proper technique, proper labeling, and protection of patient's right to privacy
2. Seizure precautions at all times
   Assess level of consciousness and mental status q1h
3. Administration of binding substances, cathartics, or antidotes

OUTCOME CRITERIA

For all patients requiring gastric lavage:

1. No compromise of the airway will occur
2. Bleeding will be controlled

When known or suspected toxic ingestion has occurred:

1. No compromise of the airway will occur
2. Minimal absorption of toxic substance will occur

DOCUMENTATION

For all patients requiring gastric lavage:

- Mechanism by which airway is maintained
- If an endotracheal tube is required, the size and amount of air instilled into the cuff, as well as verification of tube placement
- Tube care
- The quality and quantity of endotracheal aspirate
- Vital signs
- Neuro/vital signs and Glasgow coma scale scores
- Fluids and blood or blood products administered
- CVP measurements
- Intake and output
- Type and size of tube inserted
- Method of verification of tube placement
- Quantity and characteristics of aspirate
- Mechanism of lavage: Continuous or intermittent and the type and amount of fluid used
- Inspection of the oral cavity and frequency and type of mouth care
- Preparation and instructions regarding further treatment

When known or suspected toxic ingestion has occurred, additional documentation is indicated:

- Specimens obtained: Type, amount, time, and disposition
- When available, results should reflect accuracy and to whom communicated
- Measures instituted to prevent injury
- Substances administered as antidotes, chelating agents, or cathartics
- Patient's response to therapy

SPECIAL NOTE

Lavage Techniques

Gastric lavage may be performed by either of the following methods:

Continuous lavage. After insertion of the Ewald tube through the oropharynx into the stomach, the stem of a Y-connector is attached to the Ewald tube. One branch of the Y-connector is attached to a continuous drip apparatus and the other branch to a suction apparatus. Then, 200–300 cc of lavage solution is infused after clamping the suction tubing. The clamp is released from the suction tubing and applied to the lavage line. The stomach is then emptied. To ensure adequate lavage, it is best to reposition the patient from side to side q1h. The advantage of continuous lavage over intermittent lavage is that greater amounts of solution can be lavaged in a shorter period of time as compared to hand irrigation. This more efficiently controls bleeding and removes from the stomach both fresh and old blood.

Intermittent lavage. After insertion of the Ewald tube through the oropharynx and into the stomach, an irrigation syringe is used to instill irrigating solution and aspirate the gastric contents. The advantage of intermittent lavage over continuous lavage is that less equipment is required

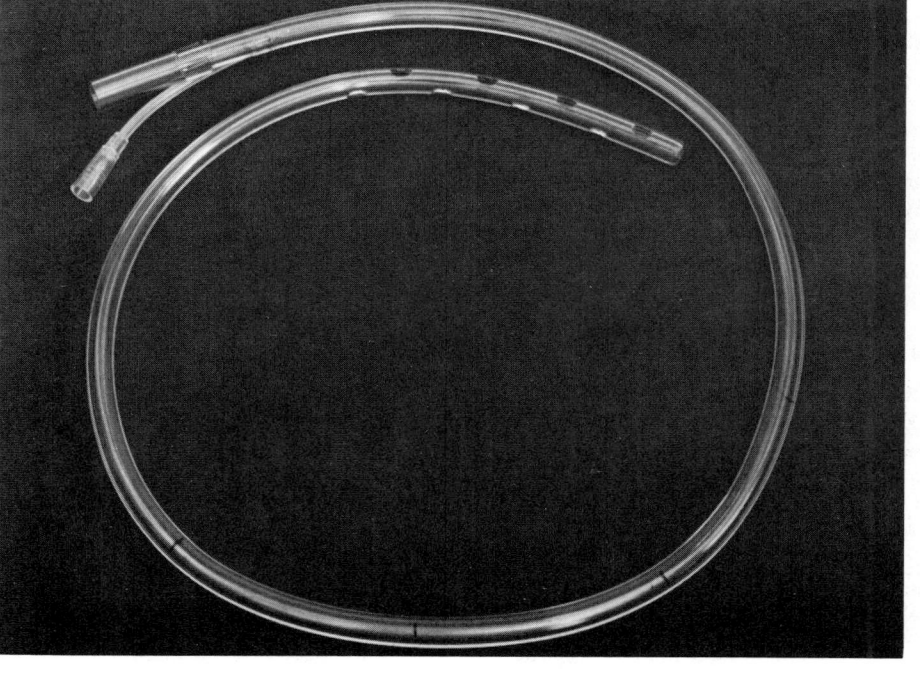

Figure 5–24. Ewald tube.

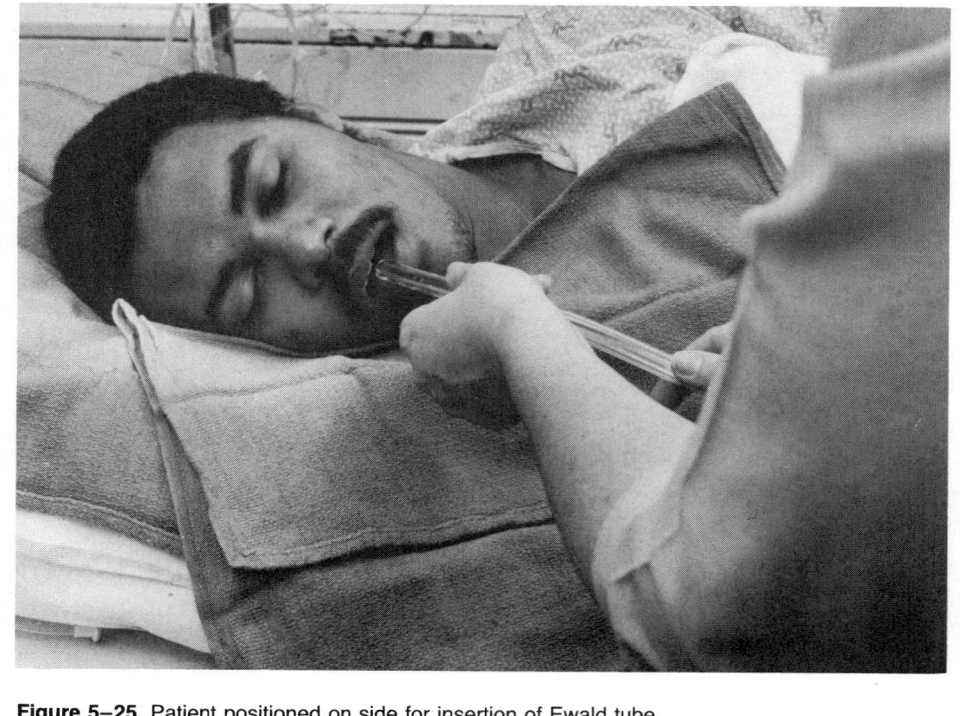

Figure 5–25. Patient positioned on side for insertion of Ewald tube.

Care of the Patient Requiring a Sengstaken–Blakemore Tube

NURSING DIAGNOSES	RATIONALE	DEFINING CHARACTERISTICS	EXPECTED OUTCOME
1. Fluid volume, deficit, actual	1–3. Massive upper gastrointestinal bleeding manifested by hematemesis may be related to bleeding esophageal varices. The Sengstaken–Blakemore tube (Fig. 5–26), which provides esophageal and gastric tamponade (Fig. 5–27), may control or stop the bleeding, thus avoiding more invasive techniques, such as surgery. However, there are risks associated with the use of this tube. Sudden airway occlusion may occur if there is migration of the tube. Esophageal necrosis or perforation may occur related to prolonged or excessive inflation of the balloon. Aspiration may occur if the esophagus is obstructed by the inflated balloon	1. Hypotension Tachycardia Tachypnea Pallor Cyanosis Altered mental status Confusion Disorientation Restlessness	1. Fluid volume will be restored
2. Airway clearance, ineffective		2. Coughing Choking Gagging Cyanosis Respiratory stridor	2. Airway will remain patent
3. Injury, potential for: A. Aspiration B. Airway obstruction C. Pressure necrosis		3. A. Emesis Decreased breath sounds Increased pulmonary secretions Consolidation or infiltrates on chest x-ray Fever B. Sudden, severe respiratory distress Acute cyanosis C. Nares reddened, irritated Skin breakdown Erosion or perforation of esophagus	3. Complications associated with the use of the Sengstaken–Blakemore tube will be absent or minimized

NURSING INTERVENTIONS

1. Fluid volume maintenance
   A. Continuous cardiac monitoring
   B. Vital signs q1h
      CVP readings
      Intake and output
   C. Assess tissue perfusion
      Check color and temperature of extremities
      Perform the capillary blanch test q2h
   D. Neurological assessment q2h

2. Airway patency
   A. Assess respiratory pattern q1h
   B. Check the security of the tape, connections, and weights during the initial assessment, then q1h (Fig. 5–28)
   C. Check the mercury pressure in the esophageal balloon q30min
   D. Scissors taped to head of the bed continuously (Fig. 5–29)
   E. Observe nailbeds and perioral area for evidence of cyanosis
3. Injury, potential for
   A. Aspiration
      a. Suction nasopharyngeal cavity q1h and as necessary
      b. Irrigate nasogastric tube q1h and as necessary
      c. Record quantity, characteristics of nasogastric drainage q4h
      d. Notify physician of changes in character of drainage
   B. Pressure necrosis
      a. Provide protective padding between skin and tube at all times (Fig. 5–30)
      b. Mouth care q1h and as necessary
      c. Nares and facial skin care q4h and as necessary
      d. Monitor balloon pressures q1h

OUTCOME CRITERIA

1. Fluid volume restoration
   A. Cardiac dysrhythmias will be recognized promptly and interventions initiated
   B. Patient will be maintained in a normotensive state
      CVP will be maintained between 4 and 10 mm of water pressure
      Urine output will be greater than 30 cc/h
   C. Adequate tissue perfusion will be maintained
   D. Changes in mental status will be recognized promptly and interventions initiated
2. Airway patency
   A. Evidence of tube migration will be recognized promptly and appropriate interventions initiated
   B. Connections will remain secure and without leaks
   C. Esophageal balloon pressure will be maintained between 35 and 40 mm Hg
   D. Emergency deflation of the tube will be accomplished when indicated
   E. Evidence of cyanosis will be recognized and interventions initiated
3. Injury, potential for
   A. Aspiration
      a. The nasopharyngeal cavity will remain free of secretions
      b. The nasogastric tube will remain patent
   B. Pressure necrosis
      a. Signs and symptoms of pressure necrosis will be absent or minimized
      b. Oral mucosa will remain free of irritation
      c. Nares and facial skin will remain free of irritation
      d. Changes in balloon pressures will remain within strict limits

DOCUMENTATION

- ECG pattern is described and tracings present when appropriate
- Vital signs, CVP, and urine output will be charted numerically
- Pulmonary assessment: Respiratory rate and rhythm, characterisitics of breath sounds, quantity and characteristics of aspirate
- Neurological assessment: Mental status, level of consciousness, Glasgow coma scale scores
- Security of tape, connections, and weights

(continued)

- Balloon pressures
- Availability and location of scissors
- Respiratory rate and rhythm
- Suctioning frequency, characteristics of aspirate obtained
- Irrigation frequency, quantity and characteristics of aspirate obtained
- Presence of protective padding
- Integrity of nares and facial skin and the frequency of skin care
- Integrity of oral mucosa and the frequency of mouth care

SPECIAL NOTE

Equipment

Tubes available for esophageal or gastric tamponade other than the Sengstaken–Blakemore are the Linton and the Davol Minnesota.

- Linton tube
  Three-lumen tube: two patent lumens, one balloon lumen
  The Linton tube provides only gastric tamponade but is thought by some experts to provide sufficient pressure to stop bleeding from esophageal varices and to carry a decreased incidence of complications associated with concomittant esophageal tamponade
- Davol Minnesota
  Four-lumen tube: two patent lumens, two balloon lumens
  The Davol Minnesota tube provides esophageal and gastric tamponade as well as esophageal and gastric suction, thus eliminating the need for a nasogastric tube

Vasopressin

In addition to the treatment modality of tamponade, bleeding esophageal varices may be treated by infusion of intravenous vasopressin. Remember that esophageal bleeding is venous not arterial! Vasopressin therapy may be used alone or in conjunction with tamponade

- Dosage: Vasopressin 100 units diluted in 500 cc 0.9% normal saline
- Rate: Approximately 0.2 U/min but must be titrated and should be decreased over 48–72 hours
- Special considerations
  Use of a volume control infusion pump is essential
  Vasopressin must be used cautiously in patients with vascular disease
  As the rate is decreased rebleeding may occur
  If there is infiltration of the IV containing vasopressin, tissue necrosis may occur

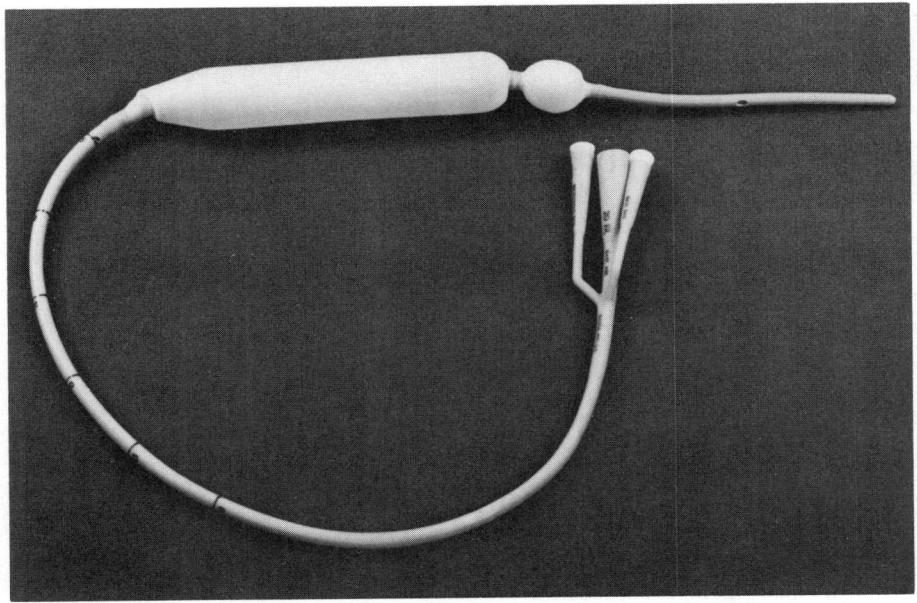

Figure 5-26. Sengstaken–Blakemore tube with balloon deflated.

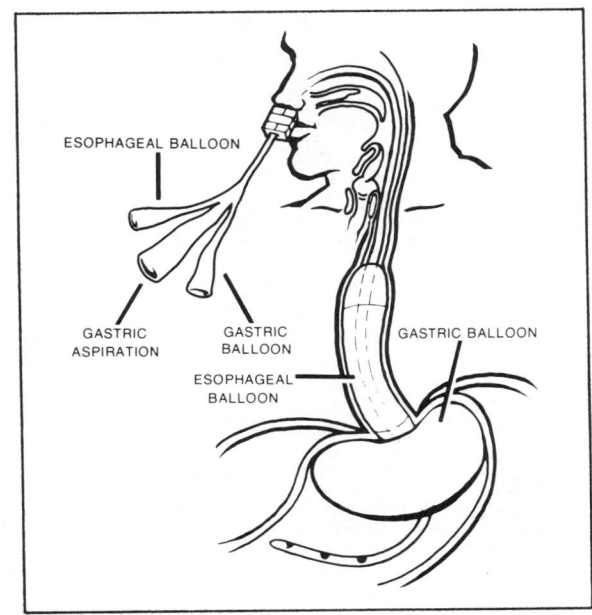

Figure 5-27. Anatomical cutaway showing Sengstaken–Blakemore tube in place. *(From Millar, S., Sampson, L. K., & Soukup, Sr., M. (Eds.). AACN procedure manual for critical care (2nd ed.). Philadelphia: Saunders, 1985, p. 370, with permission.)*

ESOPHAGEAL BALLOON

GASTRIC ASPIRATION

GASTRIC BALLOON

GASTRIC BALLOON

ESOPHAGEAL BALLOON

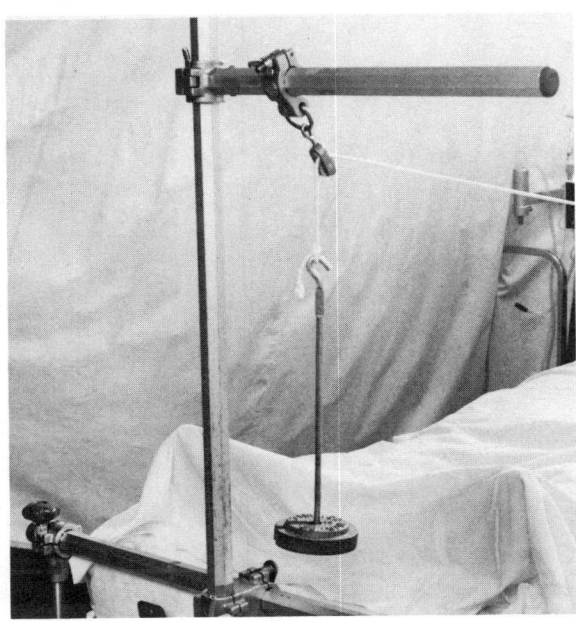

Figure 5-28. Weights and traction to maintain position of the Sengstaken–Blackmore tube.

(continued)

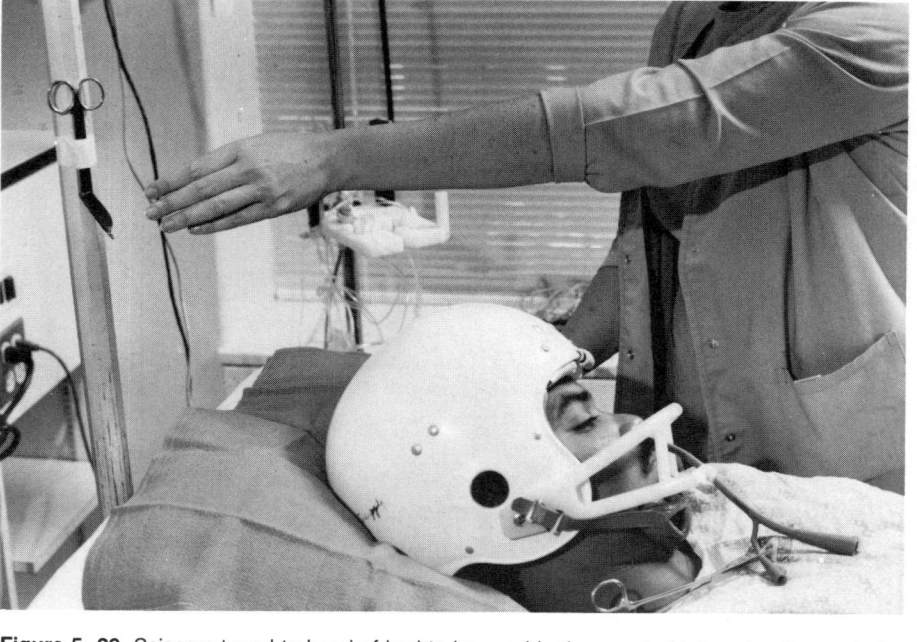

Figure 5–29. Scissors taped to head of bed to be used in the event of tube migration and signs and symptoms of airway obstructions.

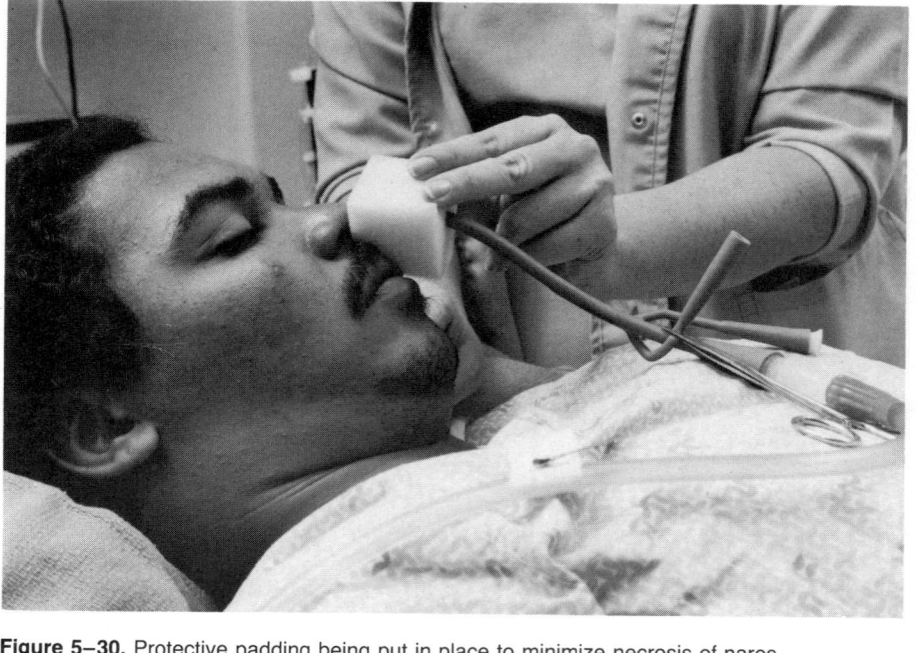

Figure 5–30. Protective padding being put in place to minimize necrosis of nares.

Amebiasis: An infectious disease acquired following the ingestion of food or fluid infested with amebic encysted forms. May be asymptomatic or manifest as mucosal colonic ulcers, hepatic abscesses, or dysentery.

Asterixis: Involuntary, flapping tremor, particularly of the hands. Elicited by having patient extend arms, dorsiflex wrists, and spread fingers. Seen in impending hepatic coma but also with other metabolic encephalopathies.

Borborygmi: Distant, rumbling, gurgling sounds produced as air passes through the intestines.

Caput Medusa: Distended veins radiating from the umbilicus, most likely related to portal hypertension.

Cheilosis: Redness and then fissures radiating outward from the corners of the mouth, a result of dietary deficiencies of riboflavin and the vitamin B complexes.

Chelation (agents): Substances of particular value for their chemical ability to bind molecularly with certain compounds and thus allow them to be excreted from the body.

Cirrhosis: A chronic liver disease resulting from any one of a number of etiologies. Architectural lobar changes including vascular derangement and fiberosis ultimately end in death. Specific types include alcoholic, biliary, cardiac, cryptogenic, and postnecrotic.

Concave: Depressed, hollow surface.

Conjunctiva: Mucous membrane lining the eyelid and anterior surface of the eyeball.

Convex: Evenly curved or bulging outward.

Cullen's sign: Periumbilical darkening of the skin from blood, associated with intraperitoneal hemorrhage and ruptured ectopic pregnancy.

Cushing's syndrome: Constellation of symptoms resulting from hypersecretion of glucocorticoids from the adrenal cortex. Manifestations include osteoporosis, capillary fragility, hirsutism, edema, and purplish striae.

Encephalopathy: Any disease of the brain.

Bilirubin encephalopathy: Kernicterus; severe form of icterus neonatorum; yellow pigment and degenerative lesions are found in multiple intracranial structures.

Hepatic encephalopathy (portal–systemic encephalopathy): Toxic nitrogenous substances pass from the hepatic to the systemic circulation, producing global disruption in CNS function from dementia to coma.

Korsakoff's encephalopathy: An amnesic psychosis characterized by severe memory impairment and confusion. Patients compensate by use of confabulation. Most likely due to the severe nutritional deficiencies accompanying chronic alcoholism. May coexist with Wernicke's syndrome.

Pancreatic encephalopathy: Intracranial lesions consisting of focal gliosis, perivascular bleeding, and capillary necrosis, seen with extensive pancreatic necrosis.

Wernicke's encephalopathy: Frequently found in chronic alcoholism; a result of thiamine deficiency. Manifestations include gaze palsies, nystagmus, ataxia, and tremors. Some symptoms are irreversible. May coexist with Korsakoff's syndrome.

Gastric outlet obstruction: A complication of peptic ulcer disease, occurs most often in those patients with duodenal ulcers in proximity to the pyloric channel. As the stomach is prevented from emptying, distention, severe nausea, and vomiting occur.

Gastrostomy: An artificially created opening into the stomach, most commonly for introduction of a feeding tube.

Giardiasis: Intestinal infestation by the protozoan parasite *Giardia lamblia*.

Gluten enteropathy (celiac sprue disease): Intolerance for gluten, an insoluble protein present in multiple grains. Small bowel biopsy will demonstrate absence of villi.

Grey Turner's sign: Large area of periumbilical ecchymosis, flanks and loins; a sign of extravasation of blood from the abdominal cavity; may be seen with acute hemorrhagic pancreatitis; not associated with trauma.

Hematemesis: Vomiting blood.

Hematochezia: Passing blood per rectum.

Hemoconcentration: Decreased plasma volume in relation to red blood cells; may be seen in dehydration.

Hydrolysate: A solution containing the products of hydrolytic cleavage; enzymes, acids and alkalies which act on complex compounds to reduce them to two or more simple compounds.

Icterus: Jaundice.

Jaundice: Yellow staining of the skin and mucous membranes resulting from increased serum concentrations of bile.

Jejunostomy: Creation of an artificial opening from the abdominal wall into the jejunum, most likely for insertion of a feeding tube.

Melena: Passage of dark or black stool of tarry consistency. Related to the presence of blood altered by the action of intestinal secretions.

Nevi (spider): Also called *arterial spider* or *vascular spider* or *spider angioma*. A superficial arteriole with spiderlike extending rays seen often in parenchymatous liver disease.

Petechiae: Minute, hemorrhagic, pin-sized spots on the skin.

Pseudocyst: A false or adventitious cyst.

Salmonellosis: Three forms occur in man during infestation with the bacterial genus *Salmonella*: (1) enteric fever (typhoid fever), (2) septicemia (*Salmonella choleraesuis*), and (3) acute gastroenteritis (*Salmonella enteritidis*).

Scaphoid: Hollow, boatlike shape, as the abdomen appears in cachexia.

Sclera: White fibrous tissue covering the white of the eye from the cornea to the optic nerve.

Telangiectasia: Dilation of the small, terminal vascular structures.

Thenar (eminence): Fleshy area on the palmar surface at the base of the thumb.

Trace elements: Essential for metabolism or compound formation; present in minute amounts. Examples include copper, zinc, cobalt, iodine, manganese.

Transferrin: AB, plasma globulin which acts as an iron-transporting protein.

Treitz (ligament of): Also known as *musculus suspensorius duodeni,* a tough band of smooth muscle and fibrous tissue connecting the duodenum at the jejunal junction to the right crus of the diaphragm.

Turgor: Fullness; related to hydration status, as in "skin turgor."

Varix: A dilated, tortuous artery or vein. (Singular of varices.)

Esophageal varices: Venous varices longitudinal in direction located at the lower end of the esophagus. Result from portal hypertension.

Bibliography

Barisonek, K., Newman, E., & Logio, T. Assessment under pressure: When your patient says "My stomach hurts." *Nursing 84, 14*(11), 34–41.

Bates, B. *A guide to physical examination* (3rd ed.). Philadelphia: Lippincott, 1983, 228–250.

DeGowan, E., & DeGowan, R. *Bedside diagnostic examination*. New York: Macmillan, 1976.

Hamilton, A. J. Critical care nursing skills. In *Total parenteral nutrition*. New York: Appleton-Century-Crofts, 1981, 243–256.

Hawker, K. J. (Ed.). *Clinical consultations in nutritional support. Les Nigro,* 1984, *4*(1), 1–15.

Kinney, M. R., Dear, C. B., Packa, D. R., & Voorman, D. M. N. (Eds.). *AACN's clinical reference for critical care nursing*. New York: McGraw-Hill, 1981.

Konstantinides, N. N., & Shronts, E. Tube feeding: Managing the basics. *American Journal of Nursing,* 1983, *3*(9), 1312–1326.

Morgan, J. Nutritional assessment of critically ill patients. *Focus on Critical Care,* 1984, *11*(3), 28–34.

Sherman, J. L., Jr., & Fields, S. K. *Guide to patient evaluation* (3rd Ed.). New York: Medical Examination Publishing Co., 1978.

Siskind, J. Handling hemorrhage wisely. *Nursing 84,* 1984, *14*(1), 34–41.

6

HEMATOLOGICAL SYSTEM

Marilyn B. Damato

Assessment of the Pertinent Hematological History

RATIONALE

Functions of blood components include transportation of oxygen and carbon dioxide for cellular consumption, mediation of the immunological defense mechanisms for response to infection, and regulation of the processes of coagulation and fibrinolysis for control of bleeding and clotting. The hematological history will identify the patient with actual alteration in various cellular components and may be of additional value in focusing attention on the patient at high risk for potential system dysfunction.

PARAMETERS	FINDINGS	IMPLICATIONS FOR NURSING CARE

1. Family history	1. Hereditary factor deficiencies
	  A. Factor VIII: Classical hemophilia A
	  B. Factor IX: Christmas disease (hemophilia B)
	
	  C. Factor VIII deficiency and platelet adhesion: von Willebrand's disease
	  Hereditary platelet disorders
	  D. Essential thrombocytopenia
	
	  E. Hereditary thrombocytopenia
	  Congenital hemolytic anemia
	  F. Sickle cell disease
		1. **A.** The most commonly occurring coagulation factor defect, classic hemophilia (Factor VIII deficiency) results in a circulating Factor VIII less than 2%
		
		  B. Sex-linked (female carriers and male bleeders) as with Factor VIII. Bleeding into the central nervous system (CNS) may occur. Treatment is similar to that for deficient Factor VIII
		  C. Equally manifest by male and female. Cryoprecipitate administration is recommended rather than platelet transfusion
		
		  D. Platelet count elevated to over 1 million. May be associated in patients over age 30 with splenomegaly. Acetylsalicylic acid (ASA) may reduce aggregation. Anticoagulant therapy may control formulation of thrombin
		  E. Five types have been identified, but all are considered rare
		
		  F. A hereditary, chronic, hemolytic anemia. RBC survival time is decreased, and mechanical fragility is increased. Occurs as trait in about 10% of American blacks; occurs as sickle cell anemia in 1:625 American blacks. Care should be taken to prevent hypoxia, which precipitates a crisis with severe pain from clumping. Crises can be fatal

2. Past health history	2. **A.** Any previously diagnosed blood dyscrasia
	
	  B. Neoplastic disease (specific)
	    Leukemias
	    Lymphomas
	    Multiple myeloma
	
	  C. Neoplastic disease (general)
	
	  D. Hepatic disease
		2. **A.** Any treatment will depend upon the individual dysfunction identified. Etiology and reversibility vary with the severity of the defect. Any previously well-controlled condition may become unstable with the stress of critical illness or injury
		  B. Malignant disease of the bone marrow, lymphatic system, and spleen; about 6% of all neoplasms. Results in abnormal then decreased production of RBCs, WBCs, and platelets
		  Malignant tumors of the reticuloendothelial system. Hodgkin's and non-Hodgkin's varieties
		  Infiltrative neoplastic disease resulting in destruction of bone and bone marrow
		  C. Use of chemotherapeutic agents and radiation therapy for the control of neoplastic disease predisposes the patient to bone marrow suppression and alteration in production of various blood components. Normal immune response mechanism may be impaired or absent
		  D. Eleven of the twelve clotting factors (exception, Factor VIII) are synthesized in the liver. Impairment of hepatic function affects the coagulation system. Bleeding may be disproportionate to the injury, e.g., venipuncture or IV insertion, or may occur spontaneously

	E. Major trauma involving the chest or abdomen	**E.** Crushing, lacerating, shearing, or stellate injuries to thoracic or abdominal structures may result in massive blood loss requiring replacement or surgically irreparable injury requiring organ removal. Dilutional or acquired coagulopathies may result
	F. Major cardiothoracic or abdominal surgery	**F.** Implantation of synthetic cardiac valvular prosthesis may require long-term anticoagulant management. Less problematic with bioprostheses. Intracerebral hemorrhage may be a complication. Duodenal excision may severely impair absorption of iron, resulting in iron deficiency anemia. Dietary modifications may be necessary
	G. Gastrointestinal disease	**G.** Malabsorptive disorders and achlorhydria may predispose to hematological dysfunction due to deficient supply of vitamin B_{12} and vitamin K
	H. Transfusion history	**H.** Any incident requiring multiple transfusions may result in hematological impairment from dilution of available clotting factors, predisposing the patient to excessive bleeding. Previous transfusion reactions may result in antibody formation and increased patient sensitivity, complicating any future crossmatching. Investigate the transfusion history carefully
3. Patient profile	**3. A.** Gender	**3. A.** Two of the most common congenital blood dyscrasias are sex-linked, with a specific carrier–manifester presentation. Of note are Factor VIII and Factor IX deficiencies. Other dyscrasias are autosomal dominant or autosomal recessive and statistically may affect one sex more frequently than the other
	B. Dietary habits	**B.** Dietary habits, preferences, or abstentions may result in intake inadequate in vitamin B_{12}, vitamin K, or folic acid. As these substances are vital to RBC production, covert anemic states may result in their absence
	C. Occupations involving exposure to toxins	**C.** Exposure to heavy metals and some toxic radioactive substances as well as to petrochemicals may result in a toxic insult sufficient to produce hematological dysfunction not readily apparent on admission
	D. Alcohol intake: Quantity and frequency	**D.** Production and synthesis of multiple coagulation factors by the liver can be seriously impaired if hepatic function is compromised from methanol abuse
	E. Medications	**E.** Multiple classifications of pharmacological agents can result in impairment of hematological function. Not all drugs in all classes produce these side effects. Among the more common drugs that may produce these effects are antibiotics, anticonvulsants, antihypertensives, anti-inflammatory agents, antibacterial drugs, antifungal agents, immunosuppressants, diuretics, antipyretics, and oral contraceptives, as well as specific anticoagulants and antifibrinolytic agents. All identified medications should be noted on the nursing care plan
4. Present problem	**4. A.** Active acute blood loss	**4. A.** The normal adult blood volume is 75 cc/kg in males and 67 cc/kg in females. Clinical manifestations of losses approaching 30% are those of hypovolemic shock, with losses of 40–50% being potentially fatal. Laboratory values may be nonreflective of active or acute blood loss. Nursing observation and assessment are more sensitive indicators
	B. Chronic blood loss	**B.** Chronic blood loss, compensated or undiagnosed, may become threatening when the patient is stressed by critical illness or injury. Identification of the patient at risk may avert potential complications through early intervention
	C. Sickle cell crisis	**C.** Patients with known sickle cell disease or positive sickle cell trait may experience a crisis in any situation resulting in hypoxia or decreased oxygenation to the erythrocytes. Careful planning of nursing care activities will avoid undue and unnecessary patient exertion
	D. Infection	**D.** Systemic infections, such as bacteremia and septicemia, may trigger the disseminated intravascular coagulation (DIC) syndrome. Nursing care activities should be performed

(continued)

PARAMETERS	FINDINGS	IMPLICATIONS FOR NURSING CARE
5. Review of systems	**E.** Impaired immunologic defense **5. A.** Hematological system **B.** Cardiovascular system **C.** Pulmonary system **D.** Gastrointestinal system	with special attention to maintenance of aseptic techniques and decreasing potential for cross-contamination between patients **E.** Patients who are iatrogenically immunosuppressed or those with acquired immune deficiencies may require special isolative precautions to avoid contracting concurrent infections **5. A.** Fluid volume, deficit, actual Tissue perfusion, alteration in: all systems Injury, potential for Comfort, alteration in Nutrition, alteration in: less than body requirements **B.** Cardiac output, decreased **C.** Gas exchange, impaired **D.** Hemorrhage, potential for

Assessment of the Hematological System by Inspection

RATIONALE

Evidence for dysfunction of the complex cellular interactions among structures in the hematological system is reflected diffusely throughout body systems (Fig. 6–1). Data are obtained by inspection, with limited use of palpation. For signs and symptoms of hematological dysfunction not reasonably linked to the medical or surgical reason for admission, further validation of suspected etiology is obtained from laboratory data.

PARAMETERS	FINDINGS	POSSIBLE ETIOLOGIES	DOCUMENTATION
1. Central nervous system	1. A. Depressed level of consciousness, initially transient, then sustained B. Confusion, disorientation, inappropriateness C. Restlessness, purposelessness, agitation D. Focal neurological deficits: Dysphasia, aphasia, weakness, hemiparesis, sudden decrease in level of consciousness	1. Impaired cerebral blood flow; subsequent decrease in cerebral perfusion pressure with alteration in cerebral cellular metabolism	• Any decline in level of consciousness Appropriateness of responses • Respiratory rate Alterations in pattern or observations of increased inspiratory effort
2. Pulmonary system	2. A. Tachypnea B. Gasping, struggling, air hunger	2. Hypoxia related to decreased hemoglobin or RBC disorders may result in tachypnea	• Blood pressure and pulse rate Presence and quality of peripheral pulses Time in seconds required for capillary refill (Fig. 6–2)
3. Cardiovascular system	3. A. Poor filling of distal veins (hands, arms, feet) B. Thready pulse, tachycardia C. Prolonged capillary refill	3. Hypovolemia resulting in decreased intravascular volume	
4. Gastrointestinal system	4. A. Abdominal distention B. Upper gastrointestinal bleeding C. Guaiac-positive emesis D. Melena E. Guaiac-positive stool	4. Active or chronic blood loss	• Baseline abdominal girth measurement Rebound Episodes and characteristics of emesis Quantity (if possible) of emesis
5. Renal system	5. A. Decreased urine output B. Hematuria C. Urinary tract infections D. Flank bruising	5. A. Hemolysis of acute transfusion reactions or hypovolemia B. Active or chronic loss may be reflected as gross or microhematuria C. Hemorrhagic cystitis D. Retroperitoneal bleeding	• Urine output and color Location of bruise, size in centimeters, color, any associated pain and tenderness
6. Hepatic system	6. Jaundice (Fig. 6–3)	6. Impaired liver function resulting in inadequate bilirubin excretion	
7. Lymphatic system	7. Lymph adenopathy	7. Immune response (functional) as a response to infection Immune response (dysfunctional) as a result of impaired function or disseminated neoplastic disease	• Body area involved and intensity of color
8. Integumentary system	8. A. Pallor, cyanosis B. Hematomas C. Ecchymosis D. Petechiae	8. Hypoxia or hypovolemia with resultant decreased circulating hemoglobin Alteration in coagulation or bleeding mechanism	• Location palpated, fixed or movable, any associated pain or tenderness (Fig. 6–4)

9. Drainage	9. Quantity, quality, and origin	9. Alteration in coagulation mechanism or alteration in bleeding mechanism indicating impaired hemostasis	• Pallor, cyanosis, dusky or ashen cast Time noted, number, location, and size in centimeters Anatomical distribution
10. Head and neck	10. A. Epistaxsis B. Flushing, pallor, cyanosis C. Lesions D. Gingival bleeding	10. A. Alteration in coagulation or bleeding mechanism B. Hypoxia or hypovolemia resulting in decreased circulating hemoglobin C. Alteration in immunological mechanism or response D. Alteration in coagulation mechanism Alteration in bleeding mechanism	• Cubic centimeters (if possible) (alternative qualifiers may be necessary) Bright red bleeding (BRB), serosanguineous, serous, and presence or absence of clots Anatomical location of drainage if a wound or orifice: Nasogastric tube, surgical drain, urethral catheter, IV insertion site (Fig. 6–5), or others as applicable • Precipitating event, if known, or "spontaneous" if appropriate Quantity in cubic centimeters (if possible) (alternative descriptors may be necessary) Membranes examined Location and number of lesions Presence or absence of gingival bleeding

POSSIBLE NURSING DIAGNOSES

- Cardiac output, alteration in: decreased
- Fluid volume, deficit, actual
- Fluid volume, deficit, potential
- Gas exchange, impaired
- Hemorrhage, potential for
- Injury, potential for
- Oral mucous membranes, alteration in
- Sensory perceptual alteration
- Skin integrity, impairment of: actual
- Tissue perfusion, alteration in

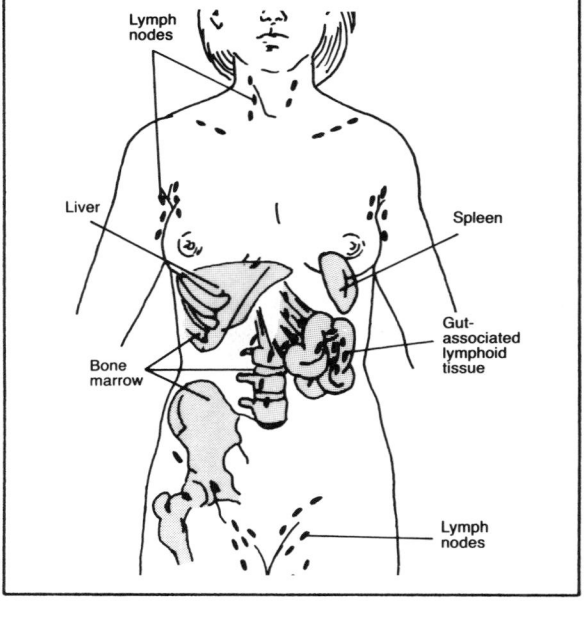

Figure 6–1. Organs of the hematological system.

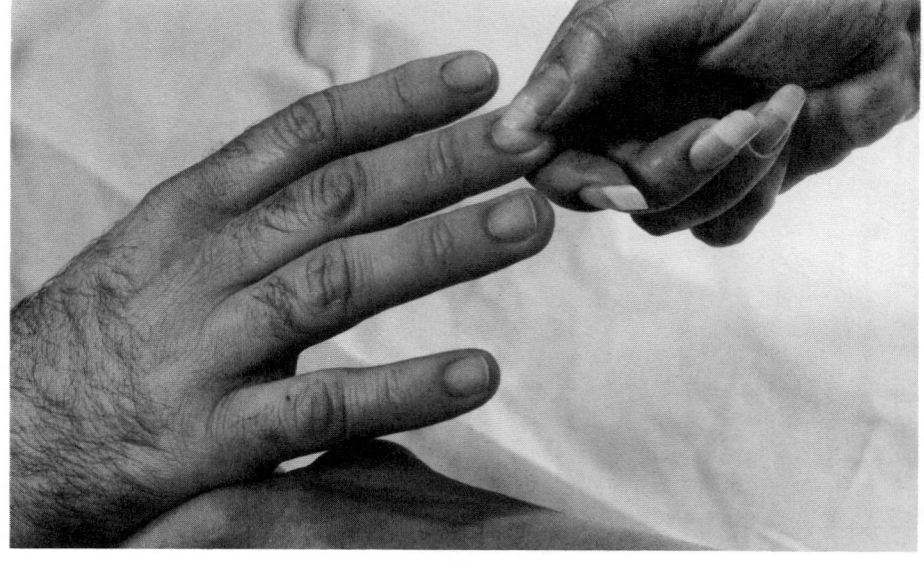

Figure 6–2. Fingertip blanching for capillary refill.

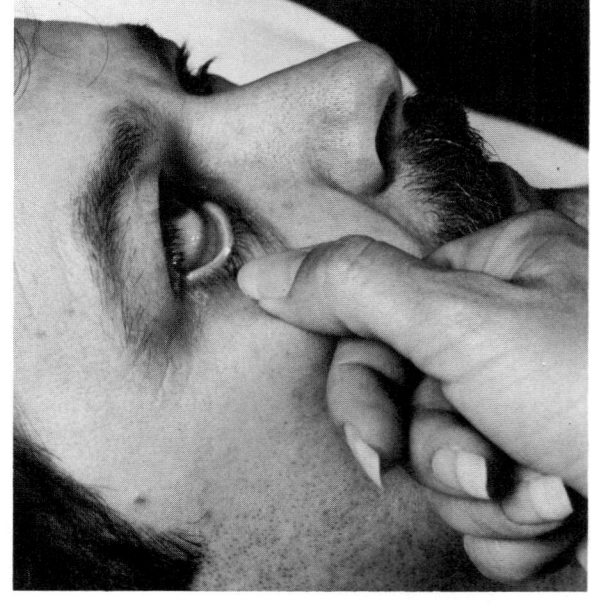

Figure 6–3. Examination of sclera for icterus.

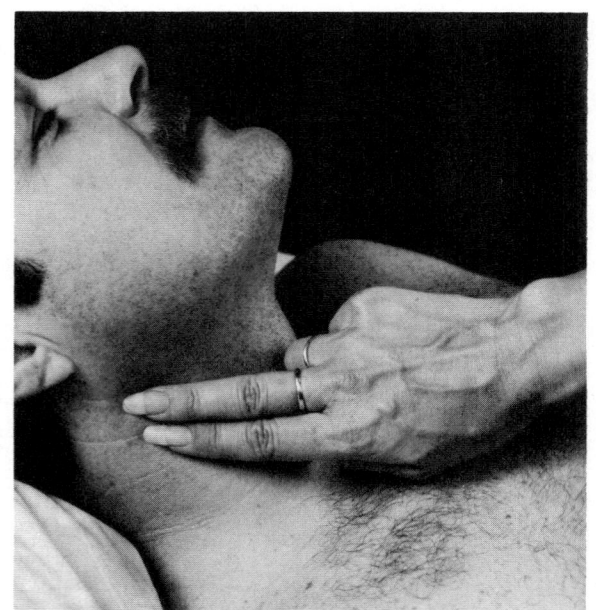

Figure 6–4. Palpation of cervical lymph nodes.

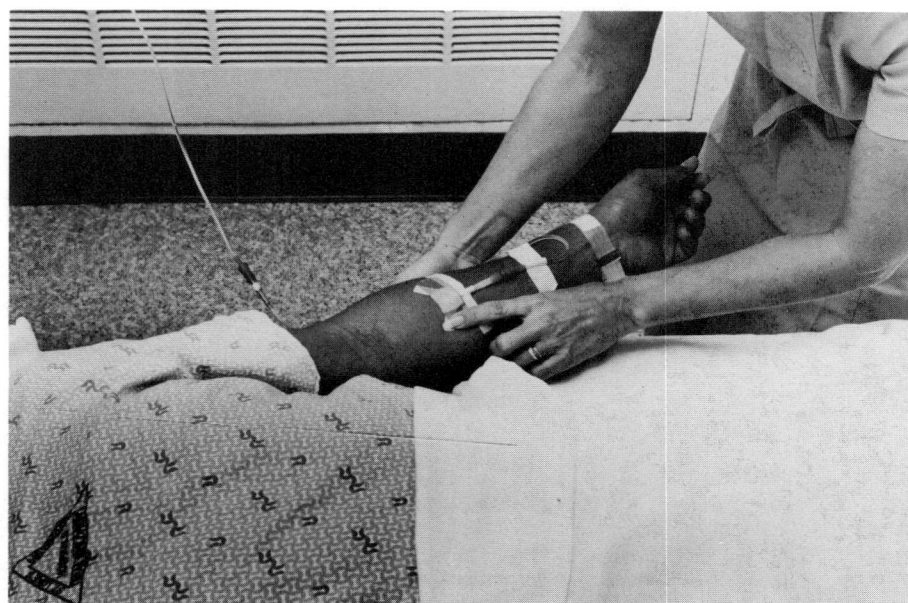

Figure 6–5. Careful inspection of IV insertion sites may detect early signs and symptoms of hematological dysfunction.

Assessment of Pertinent Laboratory Data

RATIONALE The interdependency that exists between the various mechanisms of the hematological system may be reflected only grossly by physical and historical assessment. The most accurate tools available, except in acute, extreme blood loss, are the numerous laboratory tests performed on blood and serum.

PARAMETERS	FINDINGS	POSSIBLE ETIOLOGIES	DOCUMENTATION
	Values listed are normal ranges for each specific test.		The volume of laboratory data generated in any critical care unit may be handled by various systems. To be most useful for patient care, data should be
1. Complete blood count (CBC) A. Hemoglobin (Hgb)	1. A. Male, 16.0 ± 2.0 (g/100 ml); female, 14.0 ± 2.0 (g/100 ml)	1. A. Markedly increased with rapid intravascular hemolysis Moderately increased in sickle cell anemia, thalassemia major, and hemolytic anemias Slightly increased with sickle cell thalassemia	• Reported in a timely fashion • Transcribed accurately • Filed sequentially • Readily available for retrieval
B. Hematocrit (Hct)	B. Male, 30 ml/kg of body weight; female, 24 ml/kg of body weight	B. Decreased with active or chronic blood loss	
C. Red blood cells (RBCs)	C. Male, 5.4 ± 0.8 million/mm^3; female, 4.8 ± 0.6 million/mm^3	C. Increased with polycythemia Decreased with deficient precursor supply, dysfunction in organ of production, hemolytic process, or active or chronic blood loss	
D. White blood cells (WBCs)	D. 5000–10,000/mm^3	D. Increased in presence of acute infection, acute hemolytic processes, acute myocardial infarction, among others Decreased in bacterial infections, septicemia, anaphylactic shock, hematopoietic diseases, among others	
a. Neutrophils	a. 3800/mm^3 (segmented) 620/mm^3 (banded)	a. Elevated in some lymphoma patients during immunosuppression May be decreased in glucose-6-phosphate dehydrogenase (G6PD) deficiency	
b. Lymphocytes	b. 2500/mm^3	b. Abnormal cells are produced in lymphatic leukemia Leukocytosis is noted in acute hemorrhage and acute RBC hemolysis Leukopenia is manifest in pernicious or aplastic anemia, with radiation therapy exposure, or bone marrow depressants	
c. Monocytes	c. 300/mm^3	c. Increased with leukemic diseases, Hodgkin's disease, and malignant lymphomas	
d. Eosinophils	d. 200/mm^3	d. Altered in pernicious anemia, Hodgkin's disease, and polycythemia	

e. Basophils	**e.** 40/mm³	**e.** Increased in polycythemia and Hodgkin's disease Decreased after exposure to radiation, chemotherapy, or immunosuppression
E. Platelets	**E.** 140,000–340,000/mm³	**E.** May be increased in inoperable malignancies that are widely metastasized or in diseases of myeloproliferation Decreased in hereditary factor deficiencies, acquired factor deficiencies, and active blood loss
2. Coagulation studies **A.** Prothrombin time (PT)	**2. A.** Same as control (11–16 seconds)	**2. A.** Increased in factor defects, poor dietary intake, malabsorption, anticoagulant therapy, hepatic impairment, and salicylate abuse
B. Partial thromboplastin time (PTT)	**B.** 22–37 seconds	**B.** Increased in factor defects. Normal in platelet dysfunction If test is properly performed, abnormal in 90% of all patients with coagulation disorders
C. Thrombin time (TT)	**C.** Within 5 seconds of control	**C.** Increased in coagulation defects
D. Bleeding time	**D.** 1–4 minutes (Duke scale)	**D.** Increased in coagulation defects
E. Activated clotting time (ACT)	**E.** 4–12 minutes	**E.** Markedly prolonged with Hageman trait; related to level of severity in hemophilia
F. Fibrinogen	**F.** 200–440 mm/100 ml	**F.** Decreased in neoplastic disease, depletion of other clotting factors, presence of anticoagulants, severe burns, and cirrhosis
G. Fibrin split products	**G.** Positive at a greater than 1:8 dilution	**G.** Positive in DIC
3. Miscellaneous **A.** Erythrocyte sedimentation rate (ESR)	**3. A.** Male, 0–13 mm in 1 hour; female, 0–20 mm in 1 hour	**3. A.** Increased in acute hemorrhage, malignant lymphomas, acute hepatitis, among others Decreased in sickle cell disease and polycythemia
B. Reticulocyte count	**B.** 0.5–1.5% of all erythrocytes	**B.** Increased after blood loss associated with destruction of RBCs Decreased with decreased RBC production
C. Serum iron (SFe)	**C.** Male, 80–160 µg/100 ml; female, 50–150 µg/100 ml	**C.** Increased with hemolytic anemias and decreased RBC production Decreased in iron deficiency anemia and anemias associated with neoplastic disease
D. Total iron binding capacity (TIBC)	**D.** 250–410 µg/100 ml	**D.** Increased in iron deficiency anemia and in acute blood loss. Decreased in anemias associated with chronic diseases
E. Direct Coombs test	**E.** Negative	**E.** Positive in collagen diseases, malignant lymphomas, and various leukemias, among others
F. Indirect Coombs test	**F.** Negative	**F.** Positive in previous transfusion isoimmunization with resultant formation of a specific antibody

POSSIBLE NURSING DIAGNOSES

- Gas exchange, impaired
- Fluid volume, deficit, actual
- Injury, potential for
- Hemorrhage, potential for

SPECIAL NOTE

Frequent Blood Sampling

The frequency of blood tests required for the ICU patient often may result in the unappreciated loss of a significant volume of blood. Replacement of this loss may exceed the capacity of the compromised hematological system's reserves

Quality Control

Since medical intervention is often based on the results of the various laboratory tests, all who obtain blood for sampling should exercise care to:
- Select a peripheral site below the insertion site of peripherally administered solutions (Fig. 6–6)
- Ensure proper identification of all specimens
- Ensure prompt transport of the specimens to the analysis site

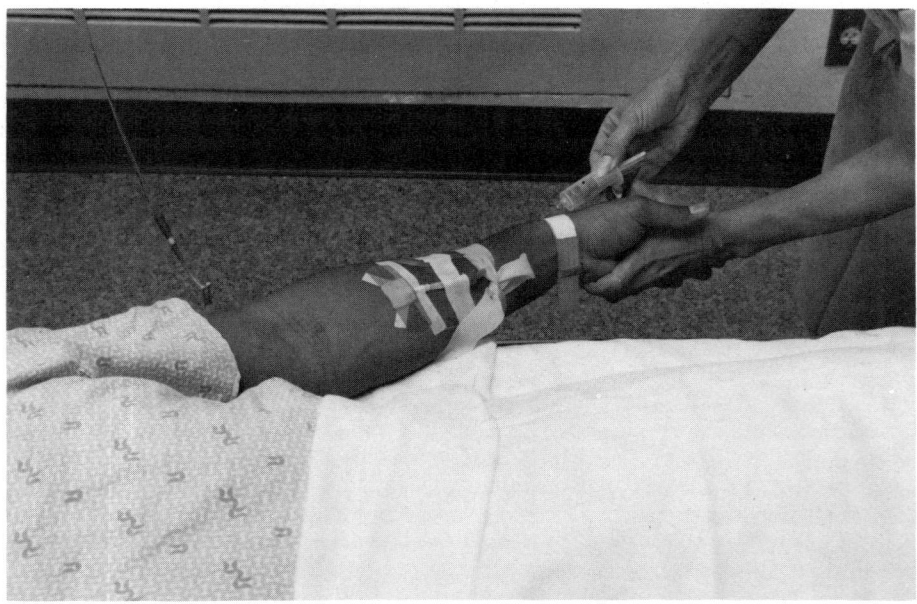

Figure 6–6. To ensure accurate laboratory results, draw blood from below existing IV sites.

Assessment of the Patient Experiencing a Transfusion Reaction

RATIONALE Current estimates for administration of blood components in the United States exceed 12 million units annually. Attention to detail and accurate clinical assessment ensure prompt intervention should one of the seven major transfusion reactions occur.

PARAMETERS	FINDINGS	POSSIBLE ETIOLOGIES	DOCUMENTATION
1. Hemolytic reaction	1. Anxiety, restlessness Localized burning at insertion site Tachycardia Tachypnea, shortness of breath, dyspnea Hypotension Nausea, vomiting Hemoglobinuria Hemoglobinemia	1. In the most acute cases, this reaction occurs during the first 15 minutes of the transfusion due to an incompatibility between recipient plasma antibodies and donor RBC antigens. Capillary obstruction results from agglutination. Massive release of hemoglobin from hemolysis results in hemoglobinemia, hemoglobinuria, and acute renal failure (ARF)	For all administration of blood components, documentation should include: • Baseline vital signs prior to administration • Strict adherence to the identification procedure of patient and component as outlined in your institution policy • Physical assessment findings and subjective reports of discomfort by the patient
2. Allergic reaction	2. Severe vomiting, cramping Severe diarrhea Wheezing Severe dyspnea Abrupt hypotension No temperature elevation	2. Previous sensitization or a congenital IgA deficiency may produce anaphylaxis and death within minutes. Massive release of histamine as cells degranulate results in binding at H_2 receptor sites, increased vascular permeability with fluid migration, vascular collapse, and death	
3. Bacterial reaction	3. Abrupt vomiting Severe abdominal cramping Abrupt hyperthermia Shaking chills Hypotension Blood cultures positive for citrate-metabolizing gram-negative bacilli	3. Although rare, this reaction may occur with the release of endotoxins, resulting in toxic shock. Immunosuppressed patients are at a high risk	Intratransfusion documentation should include: • A continuation of the vital sign documentation • Documentation of any changes in the patient's condition or subjective reports of change
4. Febrile reaction	4. Tachycardia Palpitations Flushing Fever Muscle aches Absent leukoagglutinins Absent RBC hemolysis	4. Considered by some clinical experts to be the most commonly occurring transfusion reaction, it is most likely a result of alloimmunization. Pregnancy or transfusion of 5 or more units should be criteria for recipient antibody screening at least q48h	In the event of an actual or suspected transfusion reaction, documentation should include: • Time symptoms were first noted • Time transfusion was stopped • Maintenance of IV line
5. Circulatory overload	5. Reports of tightness in the chest Dry cough (initially) Base rales on auscultation Dyspnea Restlessness	5. Circulatory overload results with administration of excessive volume or with rapid fluid shift resulting from administration of albumin. Patients with predictable susceptibility include those with preexisting cardiovascular compro-	

	Cyanosis Jugular venous distention (JVD) May deteriorate to congestive heart failure (CHF)	mise or chronic anemia with a decreased hematocrit	• Notification of physician • Institution of emergency life-support measures as necessary
6. Air embolism	6. Shortness of breath Hypotension Reports of chest pain Cough May deteriorate rapidly to arrest	6. Improper maintenance of a closed administration system may result in instillation of air into the patient's vascular system	• Initiation of corrective interventions as necessary • Return of the component and administration set to the blood bank
7. Transmission of infection	7. Delayed symptom onset Malaise Myalgia Nausea, anorexia Joint pain Rash, pruritis Elevated liver function tests (laboratory values)	7. Hepatitis is the infection most commonly transmitted and occurs in 5–10% of transfused patients. Screening with HB_sAg may detect the majority of hepatitis B cases. For hepatitis non-A, non-B, there are no screening tests for detection Infections transmissible by blood transfusion include malaria, seronegative syphilis, Epstein–Barr virus, cytomegalovirus (CMV), Colorado tick fever, infectious mononucleosis, and toxoplasmosis	• Notification of the pathology department (as per your institution policy) • Laboratory studies obtained and sent for analysis • Patient's response to therapeutic interventions

POSSIBLE NURSING DIAGNOSES

Dependent upon the reaction:

• Breathing pattern, ineffective
• Cardiac output, alteration in: decreased
• Comfort level, alteration in
• Gas exchange, impaired
• Injury, potential for

SPECIAL NOTE

Metabolic Complications

Metabolic complications can occur in addition to those reactions already mentioned:
Dilutional coagulopathies
Hypothermia
Citrate toxicity (with pre-existing severe hepatic impairment)
Transient acidosis and subsequent alkalosis

Care of the Patient Receiving Whole Blood

NURSING DIAGNOSIS	RATIONALE	DEFINING CHARACTERISTICS	EXPECTED OUTCOME
Fluid volume, deficit, actual	Whole blood performs the following functions: (1) supplies oxygen and nutrients for tissue maintenance, growth, and repair, (2) transports cellular waste for elimination, (3) transports antibodies, (4) assists regulation and equilization of body temperature, (5) assists regulation of tissue acid-base balance, and (6) assists fluid and electrolyte balance. The average adult circulating blood volume is 5 L. A sudden loss of 1.5 L (30%) requires immediate correction. A loss of 2.5 L (40%) is almost always fatal in the absence of volume replacement.	Severe hypotension Rapid thready pulse rate Decreased pulse volume and pressure Cold, clammy skin	An adequate circulating blood volume will be restored

NURSING INTERVENTIONS

Assure complication-free administration of whole blood (Fig. 6–7).

1. Obtain the patient's transfusion history and report any incidence of adverse reaction during or after a previous blood transfusion
2. Select a large-gauge needle or catheter; an 18 or 19 gauge is recommended for adults. Whole blood should be administered by straight-line, (Fig. 6–8) Y-set, (Fig. 6–9), or tubing that contains an inline microaggregate filter with pore sizes of 40–20 μ. Change administration sets with each unit to avoid clogging the filter and tubing
3. Follow protocol to obtain the blood product. Universal rule: A blood product is not to be returned to the blood bank if it has been out for longer than 30 minutes because of the risks of decreased RBC survival and the greater chance of bacterial comtamination. Do not obtain the blood until you are ready to transfuse it (Fig. 6–10)
4. Identify the blood product and the patient carefully. Verify the following with another licensed person (Fig. 6–11)
   A. Compatibility tag attached to the blood bag and the information printed on the bag itself: ABO group, Rh type, and unit number match. Crossmatching is necessary
   B. Compare the ABO group, Rh type, and physician's order on the patient's chart
   C. Check the expiration date on the blood bag
   D. Inspect the blood product for clots and look for a purplish tinge or excessive bubbling, which may indicate bacterial contamination
   E. Identify the patient by his or her full name and the hospital number on the identification wristband. This information *must* be the same as that found on the blood bag
5. Obtain baseline vital signs: Temperature, pulse, respirations, and blood pressure

6. Use *only* 0.9% (normal) sodium chloride for the starter solution. Any percentage of dextrose could cause intravascular hemolysis, and lactated Ringer's solution causes clot formation due to its high calcium levels. *Never* add medications to the blood bag
7. Start the transfusion *slowly,* no more than 2 ml/min. Even a few drops of incompatible blood can be harmful. Remain with the patient for the first 15 minutes of the transfusion, since the most serious complications occur during this time. Instruct the patient to report or observe closely for any reaction symptoms, including but not limited to chills, headache, low back pain, elevated temperature, dizziness, or nausea
8. Maintain the prescribed transfusion rate. A unit of whole blood should transfuse within 2 hours and should hang no longer than 4 hours. This eliminates the possibility of bacterial proliferation and RBC hemolysis
9. Take and record vital signs frequently during transfusion therapy, watching for any adverse reactions

OUTCOME CRITERIA

1. Previous transfusion reactions will be noted and prophylaxisis initiated
2. Transfusion will be accomplished through intravenous catheter of appropriate gauge
3. Blood will be obtained and transfused in a timely manner
4. Errors in administration due to improper identification procedure will be absent
5. Data base will be obtained
6. Administration with incompatible solutions will be avoided
7. Reactions will be promptly recognized and interventions initiated
8. Transfusion will be completed in a timely fashion
9. Response to transfusion will be closely monitored

DOCUMENTATION

- Patient's pretransfusion vital signs
- Time transfusion was started
- Type of blood product and identification number
- Signature of the person starting transfusion and name of the other licensed person verifying the correct product
- Total volume of fluid transfused (blood and saline)
- Time transfusion was completed
- Patient's response to transfusion, especially any symptoms of adverse reaction
- Any nursing actions taken in response to symptoms of adverse reaction

SPECIAL NOTE

Autotransfusion

The process of autotransfusion was first used in the United States before 1920. Today this method of retrieval for reinfusion is employed in several settings. Emergently it is used for traumatic hemothorax. For selected surgical procedures it is used perioperatively, intraoperatively, and postoperatively. Institutions with large blood bank facilities may offer patients the opportunity to predeposit blood several days before a scheduled surgery, thus assuring themselves of an autologous transfusion should the need arise.

Several manufacturers produce equipment for this procedure, which continues to be evaluated for its therapeutic value and cost effectiveness (Figs. 6–12 and 6–13).

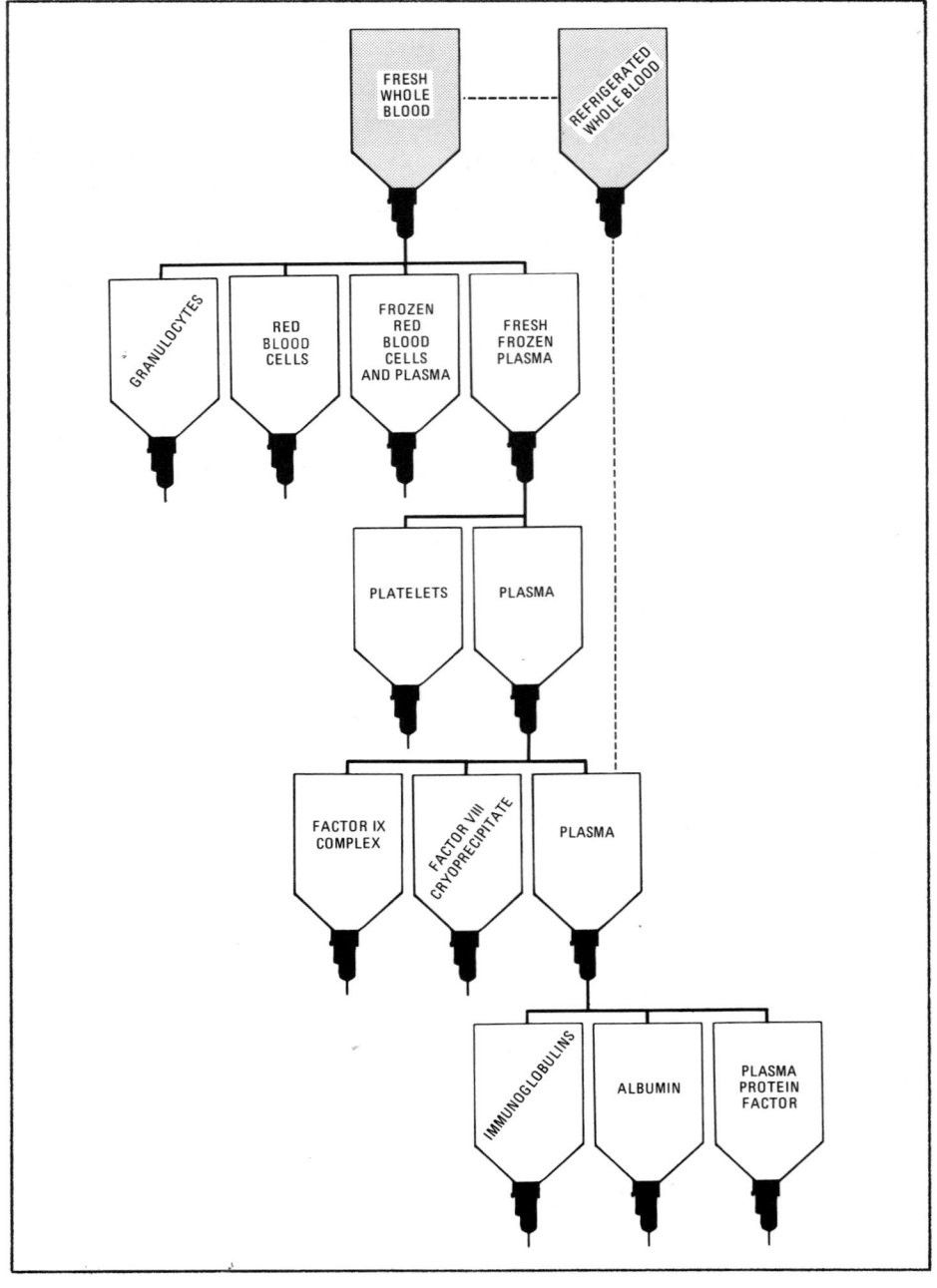

Figure 6–7. Current technology allows various components to be harvested from a unit of whole blood. *(Adapted from Scarlato, M. Blood transfusions today. Nursing 78, 1978, 8(2), 70, copyright 1978, Springhouse Corporation, with permission.)*

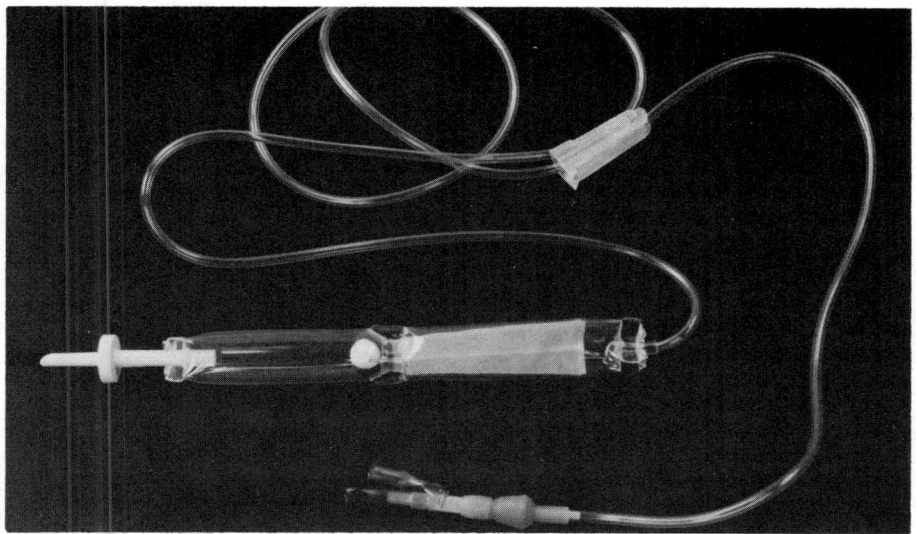

Figure 6–8. Straight-line IV set.

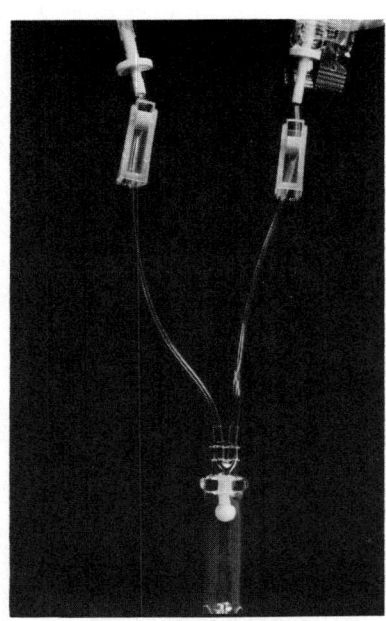

Figure 6–9. Y administration set.

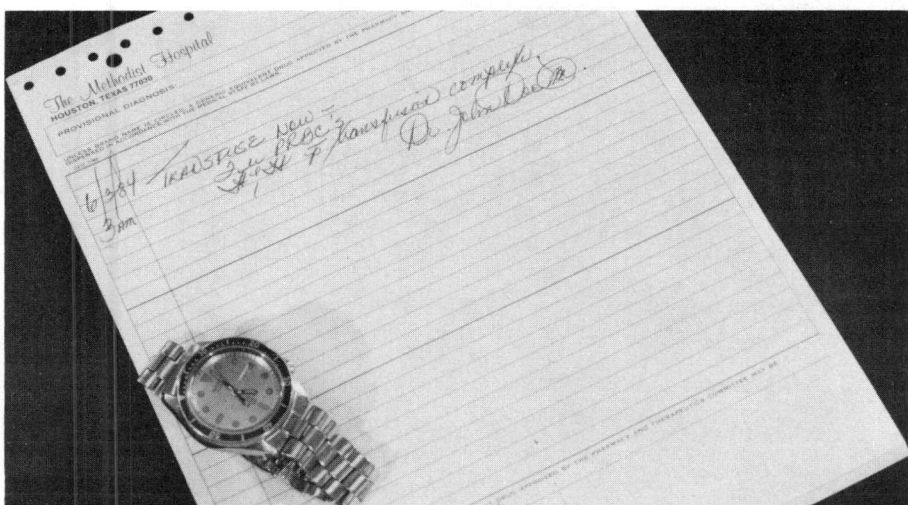

Figure 6–10. Blood may not be returned to the blood bank if it has been out for more than 30 minutes. Do not obtain until you are ready to transfuse.

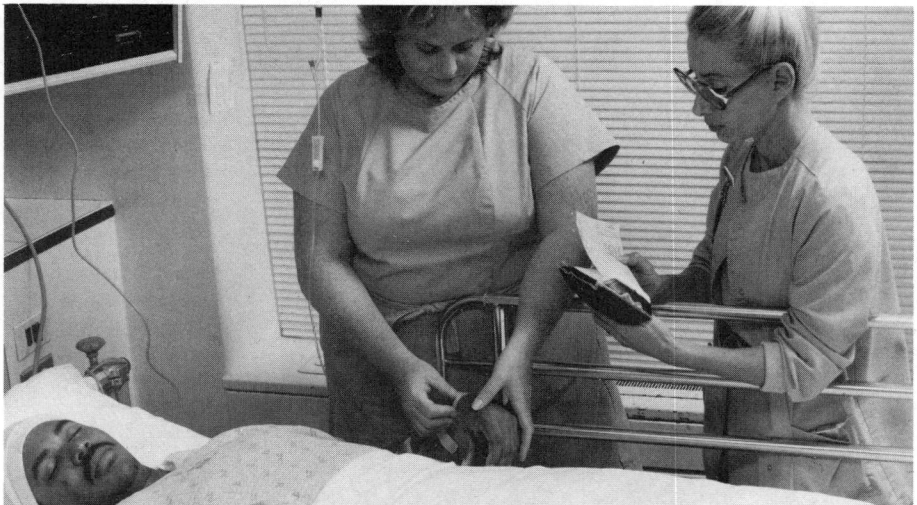

Figure 6–11. To avoid serious patient injury, *always* follow the exact procedure for identification of blood products and recipient.

(continued)

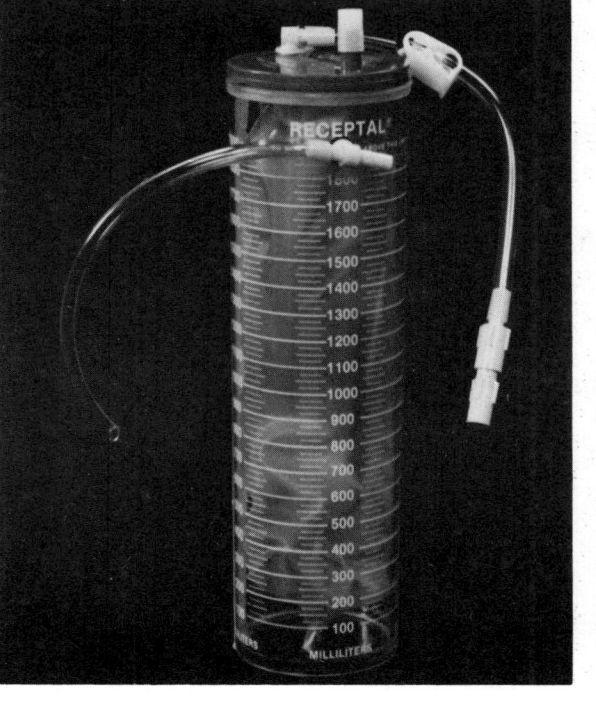

Figure 6–12. Autotransfusion cannister.

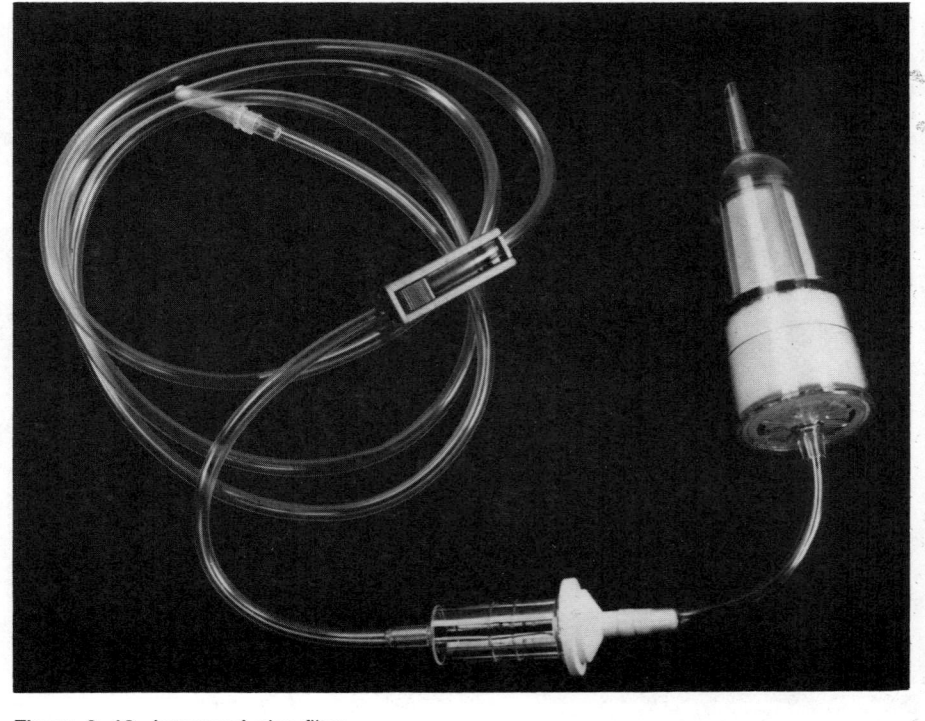

Figure 6–13. Autotransfusion filter.

Care of the Patient Receiving Red Blood Cells

NURSING DIAGNOSIS	RATIONALE	DEFINING CHARACTERISTICS	EXPECTED OUTCOME
Gas exchange, impaired	Altered oxygen-carrying capacity of blood, associated with (1) decreased RBCs from loss, (2) destruction of RBCs from hemolysis, sickle cell anemia, drug poisoning, or thalassemia, (3) decreased production of RBCs from bone marrow suppression, or (4) reduced erythropoietin in chronic renal failure. RBCs have the same oxygen-carrying capacity as whole blood without the hazards of fluid or volume overload. Their use avoids the buildup of potassium and ammonia that sometimes occurs in the plasma of stored blood. The usual volume of 1 unit of RBCs (250–300 ml) has a HCT of 65–85% and should raise an adult recipient's HCT by 3%.	Hypoxemia Tissue hypoxia Hypercapnea Restlessness Confusion Shortness of breath Pallor Dyspnea Chest pain Fatigue Somnolence	The oxygen-carrying capacity of the blood will be improved

NURSING INTERVENTIONS

Assure complication-free administration of red blood cells (Fig. 6–14).

1. Follow the same precautions as when administering whole blood
2. Use microaggregate filter if patient is a candidate for more than two transfusions or has any type of pulmonary dysfunction
3. Always mix thoroughly by rocking bag from side to side. *Do not shake bag*
4. Fill the filter completely to prime the set. Do not squeeze the filter element itself, as this destroys the integrity of the membrane (Figs. 6–15 and 6–16)
5. For routine transfusions, prewarming is unnecessary. Transfuse slowly rather than letting the blood stand at room temperature before beginning to transfuse
6. During the period when the patient's gas exchange is impaired due to RBC deficiency, concentrate on conserving the patient's energy. Discourage unnecessary physical activities. Keep oxygen ready to be administered as needed

OUTCOME CRITERIA

1. Complications associated with administration will be absent or minimized
2. Complications related to microaggregates will be absent or minimized
3. Damage to cell membranes will be absent
4. Filter element will remain undamaged
5. Tranfusion will be accomplished in a timely fashion
6. Impaired gas exchange will be managed without exacerbation

DOCUMENTATION

- Baseline vital signs prior to the transfusion
- Time transfusion was started
- Type of blood product and identification number
- Signature of the person starting the transfusion and the name of the other licensed person verifying the correct product
- Total volume of fluid transfused (product and saline)
- Time transfusion was completed
- Patient's response to the transfusion, especially any symptoms of an adverse reaction
- Any nursing actions taken in response to symptoms of adverse reaction

SPECIAL NOTE

Washed RBCs

This component is indicated for those patients who have developed antibodies to plasma proteins or have shown a previous transfusion reaction to WBCs. Useful in situations requiring extended transfusion therapy when reduced WBC antibody stimulation is desired Most microaggregates are removed during washing; therefore, a regular blood administration set is suitable for transfusion of the unit.

Frozen RBCs, Thawed, Deglycerolized

Frozen RBCs have been useful in the prevention of tissue antigen sensitization and febrile or anaphylactic IgA reactions, as with organ transplant recipients. It is most advantageous when used for unique blood types, since it may be stored for long periods of time. RBCs are preserved by the addition of glycerol as an endocellular cryoprotective agent. It must be washed off prior to use.

Since the thawing and deglycerolization of the frozen RBCs is time consuming, this component cannot be available as a stat item. Transfusions of thawed RBC's should be scheduled with the blood bank well in advance, preferably 24–48 hours before needed. After preparation, the cells must be transfused within 24 hours.

It is not necessary to add saline to the thawed RBCs. Since they are suspended in normal saline, they flow very well.

Microaggregate filter need not be used, since microaggregates have been purged during the washing procedure.

Therapeutic Considerations

The usual volume of 1 unit of RBCs (250–300 ml) has a Hct of 65–85% and should raise an adult recipient's Hct about 3%.

RBCs have the same oxygen-carrying capacity as whole blood without the hazards of fluid or volume overload. Their use avoids the buildup of potassium and ammonia that sometimes occurs in the plasma of stored blood.

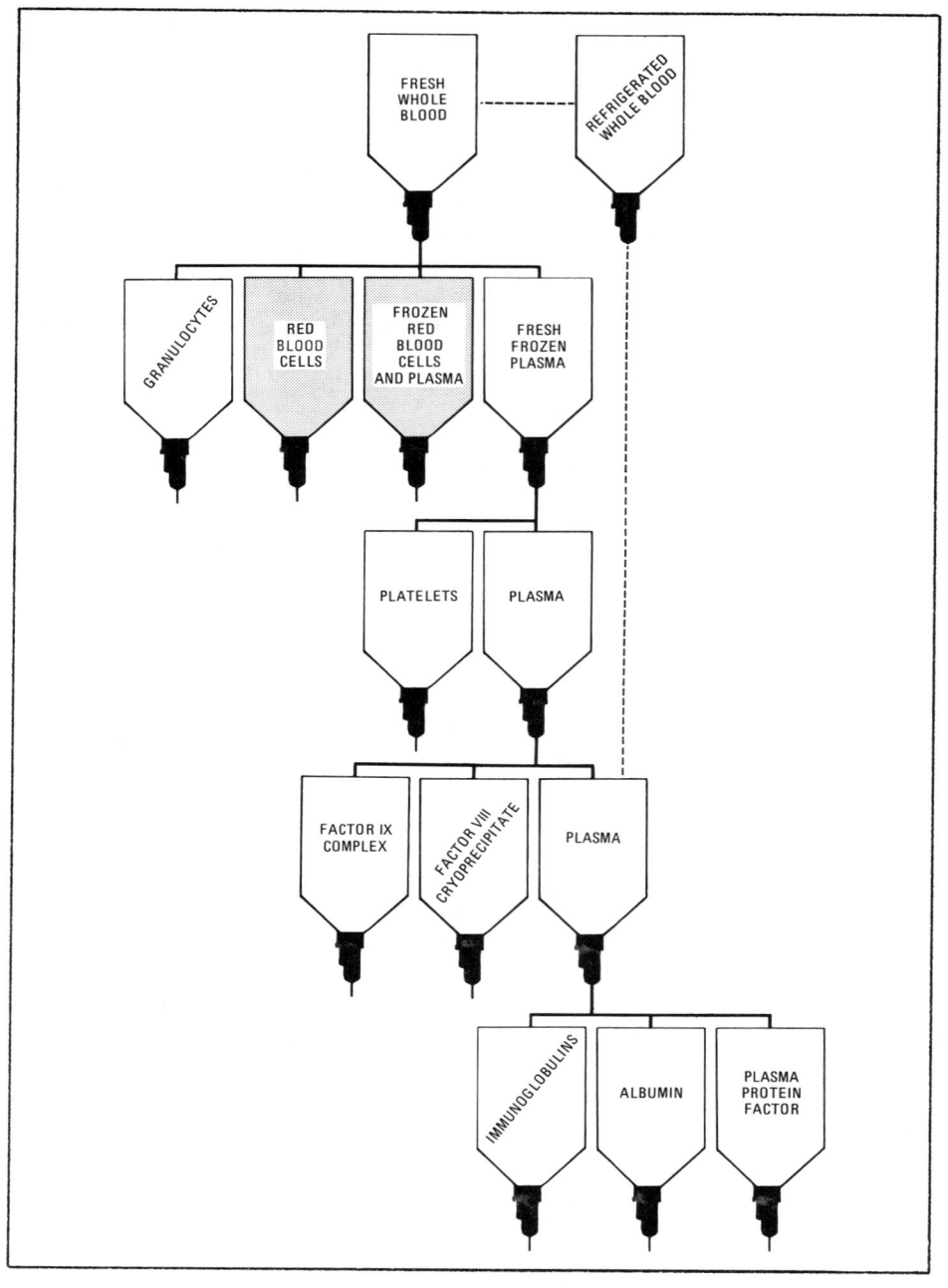

Figure 6–14. RBCs have the same oxygen-carrying capacity as whole blood. *(Adapted from Scarlato, M. Blood transfusions today. Nursing 78, 1978, 8(2), 70, copyright 1978, Springhouse Corporation, with permission.)*

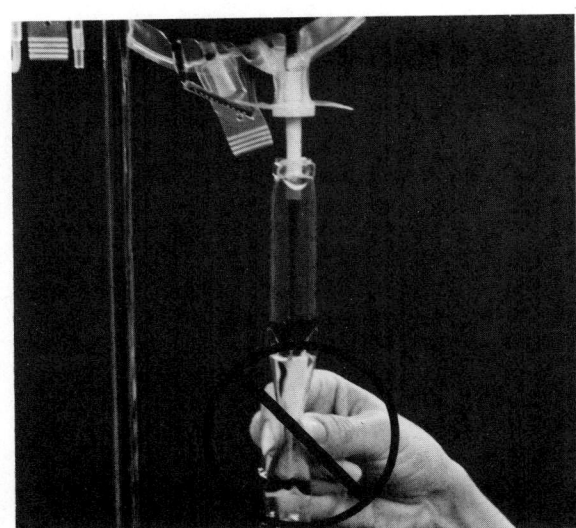

Figure 6–15. When priming the drip chamber, *do not* squeeze the filtering membrane.

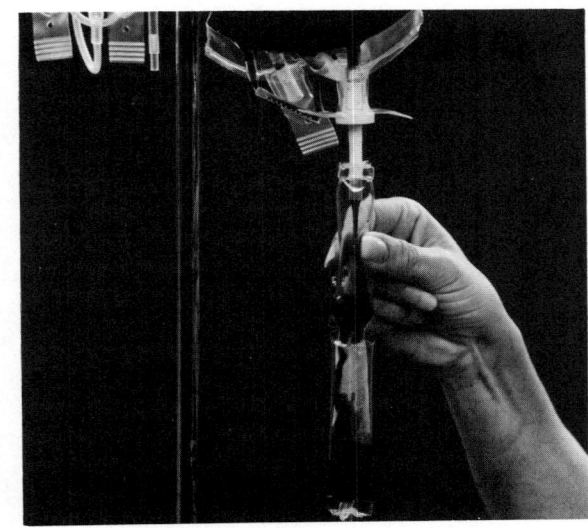

Figure 6–16. Filter being primed correctly.

Care of the Patient Receiving Platelets

NURSING DIAGNOSIS	RATIONALE	DEFINING CHARACTERISTICS	EXPECTED OUTCOME
Hemorrhage, potential for	An altered platelet profile in the host can be associated with (1) decreased platelet production from leukemia or bone marrow depression, (2) increased platelet destruction from immune disorders or drugs, (3) functionally normal platelets in the absence of vitamin B_{12} or folic acid, or (4) dilutional thrombocytopenia after massive blood transfusions. Platelet functions include (1) adherence to injured vessel walls, (2) aggregation, and (3) release of catalytic pre-coagulation factors. Platelet sediment from platelet-rich plasma is resuspended in 30–50 ml of plasma. To raise the platelet count by 5000 mm^3 a usual dosage would be 2 U/kg of patient's weight.	Thrombocytopenia Ecchymoses Petechiae Epistaxis Easily bruised Purpura Bleeding gums Hematuria Guaiac-positive stool	Platelet count will be improved

NURSING INTERVENTIONS

Assure complication-free administration of platelets (Fig. 6–17).

1. ABO compatibility is preferred but not necessary. If not contaminated grossly with RBCs, ABO incompatible platelets may be transfused. When Rh-negative females of child-bearing age receive platelets from Rh-positive donors, Rh_o (D) immune globulin should be administered
2. An order of platelets (4–12 U) must be given through a special filter (Fig. 6–18). A regular blood administration set cannot be used because many of the platelets would be trapped in the filter
3. Gently rotate platelet bag to mix platelets thoroughly prior to transfusion
4. Transfuse platelets over a period of 30–60 minutes for maximum effectiveness. Slower transfusion may be necessary to prevent circulatory overload. The volume of cells is usually 50 ml/U or 200–300 ml total volume
5. For a patient with a history of side effects, administer antihistamines as ordered before beginning the transfusion
6. After platelets have been transfused, flush the line and filter with a small amount of normal saline to assure infusion of all the platelets
7. Make sure that platelets counts, if ordered, are drawn at 1 hour and again at 24 hours following the transfusion. They are usually repeated daily thereafter

OUTCOME CRITERIA

1. Complications associated with ABO incompatibilities will be absent or minimized
2. Component will be transfused through the appropriate filter
3. Damage to cell membranes will be absent
4. Transfusion will be accomplished in a timely fashion

5. Reactions will be absent or minimized
6. Component wastage will be absent or minimized
7. Blood specimens will be obtained in a timely fashion

DOCUMENTATION

- Baseline vital signs prior to transfusion
- Time transfusion was started
- Type of product and identification number
- Signature of person initiating the transfusion
- Total number of units infused and their identification numbers
- Total volume of platelets and saline infused
- Time transfusion was completed
- Patient's response to transfusion, especially any symptoms of an adverse reaction (chills, fever, urticaria, sweating, shortness of breath, or dyspnea)
- All nursing interventions in response to an adverse reaction

SPECIAL NOTE

Platelet Therapy

Platelets can be transfused therapeutically when there is active bleeding, or prophylactically with no symptoms with platelet count below 30,000 mm^3. Spontaneous bleeding can occur with a platelet count below 20,000 mm^3.

Extracorporeal Circulation

More physicians are ordering platelets following extensive cardiovascular surgery, particularly those cases requiring hypothermia or a long period of time on cardiopulmonary bypass (Fig. 6–19). Turbulence of blood flow through the bubble oxygenator may relate to platelet dysfunction postoperatively.

Platelet Survival

Platelet survival is affected by patient's condition. Infection, elevated temperature, and antiplatelet alloantibodies decrease the effectiveness of platelet transfusions.

Plateletpheresis

Plateletpheresis: Platelets are removed from a compatible donor. The platelets are separated from whole blood by a discontinuous blood flow processor. The RBCs and plasma are returned to the donor.

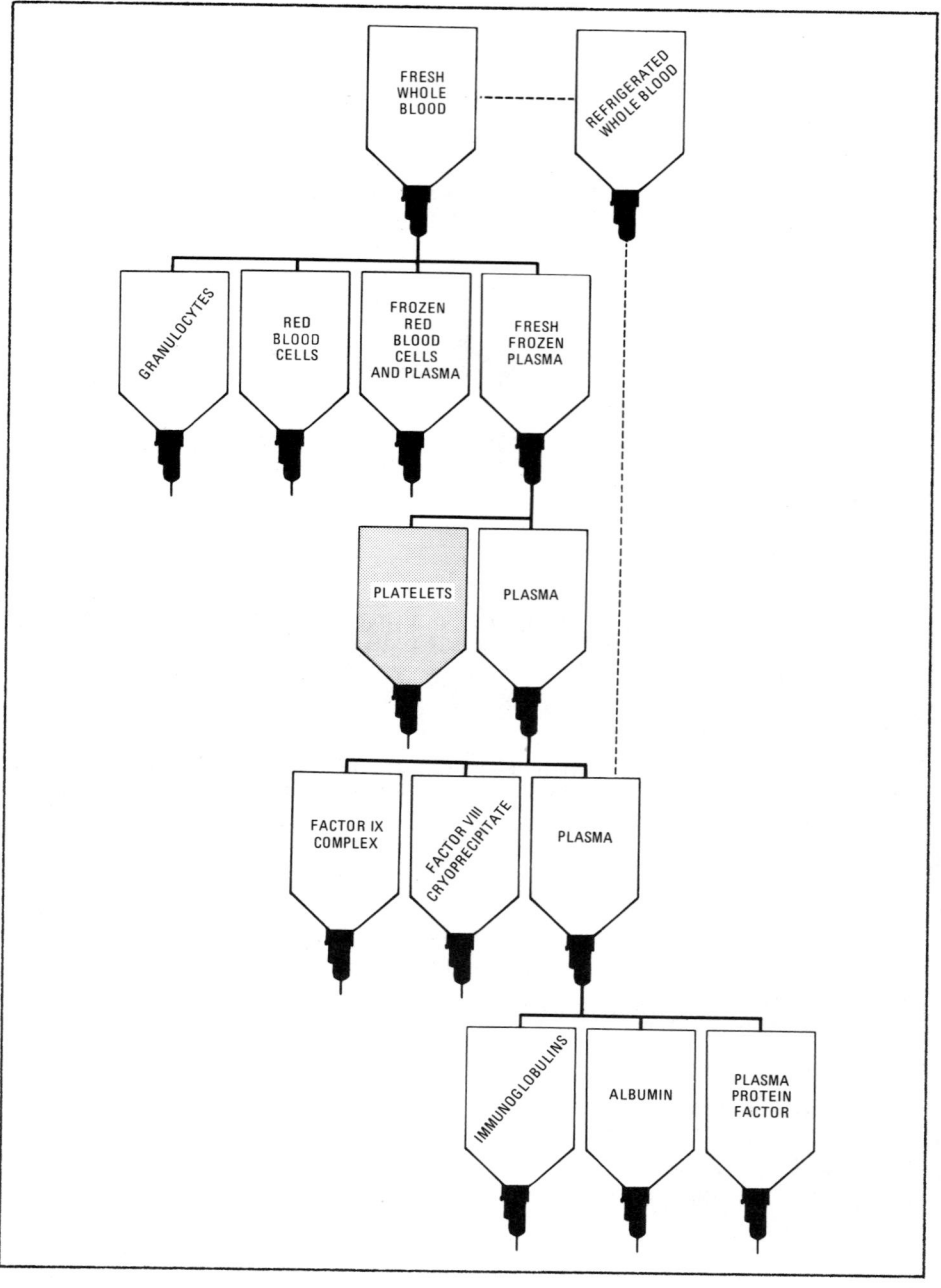

Figure 6–17. Platelets perform 3 critical steps in coagulation of blood. (*Adapted from Scarlato, M. Blood transfusions today. Nursing 78, 1978, 8(2), 70, copyright 1978, Springhouse Corporation, with permission.*)

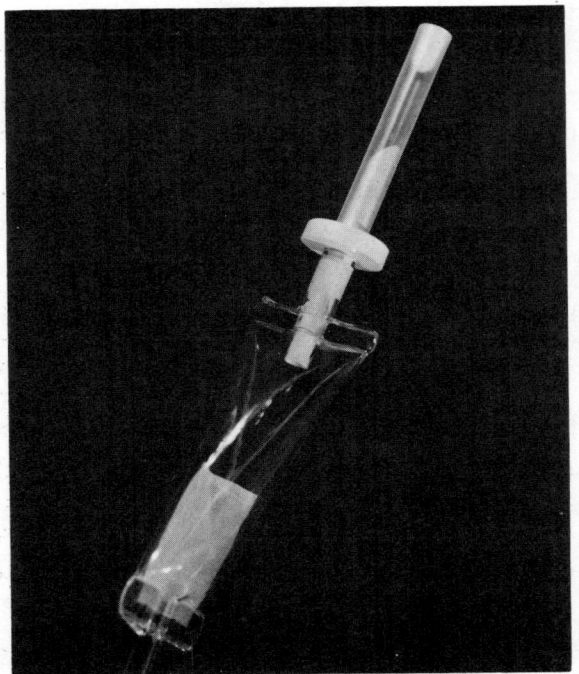

Figure 6–18. Platelet filter.

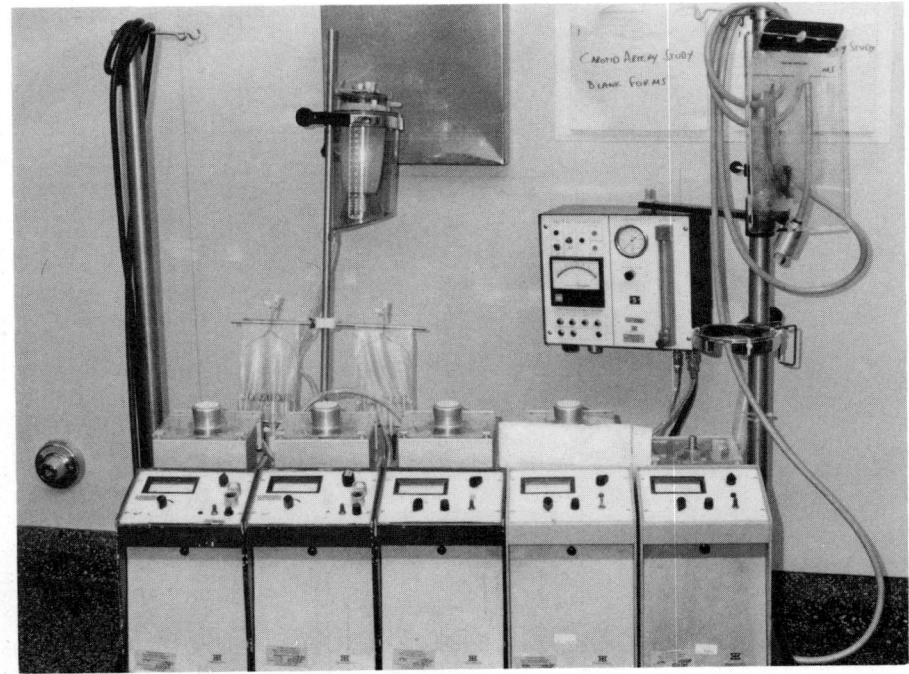

Figure 6–19. Cardiopulmonary bypass pump.

Care of the Patient Receiving Fresh Frozen Plasma

NURSING DIAGNOSES	RATIONALE	DEFINING CHARACTERISTICS	EXPECTED OUTCOME
Hemorrhage, potential for Fluid volume, deficit, actual	An altered clotting profile in the host can be associated with (1) undefined factor deficiency, (2) severe hepatic disease with limited synthesis of plasma coagulation factors, or (3) dilutional hypocoagulability. Hypovolemia resulting from actual loss alters the blood profile and simultaneously impairs perfusion in multiple organ systems. Fresh frozen plasma is prepared from the centrifugation of a unit of whole blood and then by the separation of the plasma from RBCs. Plasma that has been frozen within 6 hours of drawing is known as fresh frozen plasma and can be stored up to 1 year at $-30°F$. One unit of fresh frozen plasma contains all coagulation factors plus 40 mg of fibrinogen (Fig. 6–20).	Altered clotting factors, precise deficiency undefined Hypotension Increased pulse rate Decreased pulse volume Decreased urine output Hemoconcentration Decreased venous filling Increased body temperature Concentrated urine Sudden weight loss Increased serum sodium Change in mental status Poor skin turgor Dry mucous membranes Thirst Weakness Output greater than intake	An adequate circulating blood volume with improved levels of clotting factors will be restored

NURSING INTERVENTIONS

Assure complication-free administration of fresh frozen plasma (Fig. 6–20).

1. Fresh frozen plasma need not be ABO identical but should be compatible with the recipient's RBCs. It can be given regardless of Rh type
2. Fresh frozen plasma should be transfused within 2 hours after thawing to insure that the coagulation factors remain active
3. Plasma used for the replacement of coagulation factor deficiencies should be administered through a filter to remove cell debris and fibrin strands
   Microaggregate (40–20 μ) filters are *contraindicated* because they trap plasma (Fig. 6–21)
4. Smaller needles or catheters, e.g., 21 or 23 gauge, than required for other blood products may be used because plasma is less viscous. Unlike RBCs, the smaller plasma cells will be undamaged by the narrow lumen
5. Administration should be as rapid as possible, but the rate depends upon the patient's ability to tolerate the volume infused. Observe patient for signs of circulatory overload, such as increased heart rate, cough, dyspnea, respiratory distress, restlessness
6. Monitor the patient for adverse reactions, which are usually limited to allergic urticaria or elevated temperature

OUTCOME CRITERIA

1. Complications associated with incompatibilities will be absent or minimized
2. Transfusion will be accomplished in a timely fashion
3. Component will be administered through the appropriate filter
4. Component will be administered through the appropriate gauge needle
5. Complications associated with volume overload will be absent or minimized
6. Reactions will be promptly recognized and interventions initiated

DOCUMENTATION

- Patient's baseline vital signs before the transfusion was started
- Time transfusion was started
- Type of blood product and identification number
- Signature of person initiating the transfusion
- Total number of units infused
- Total volume of fluid infused
- Time transfusion was completed
- Patient's response to the transfusion, especially any symptoms of volume overload
- Any nursing actions taken in response to symptoms of adverse reaction

SPECIAL NOTE

Color Variations

Plasma may appear yellow, cloudy, or greenish, depending on diet, cholesterol levels, and estrogen ingestion (birth control pills) of the donor

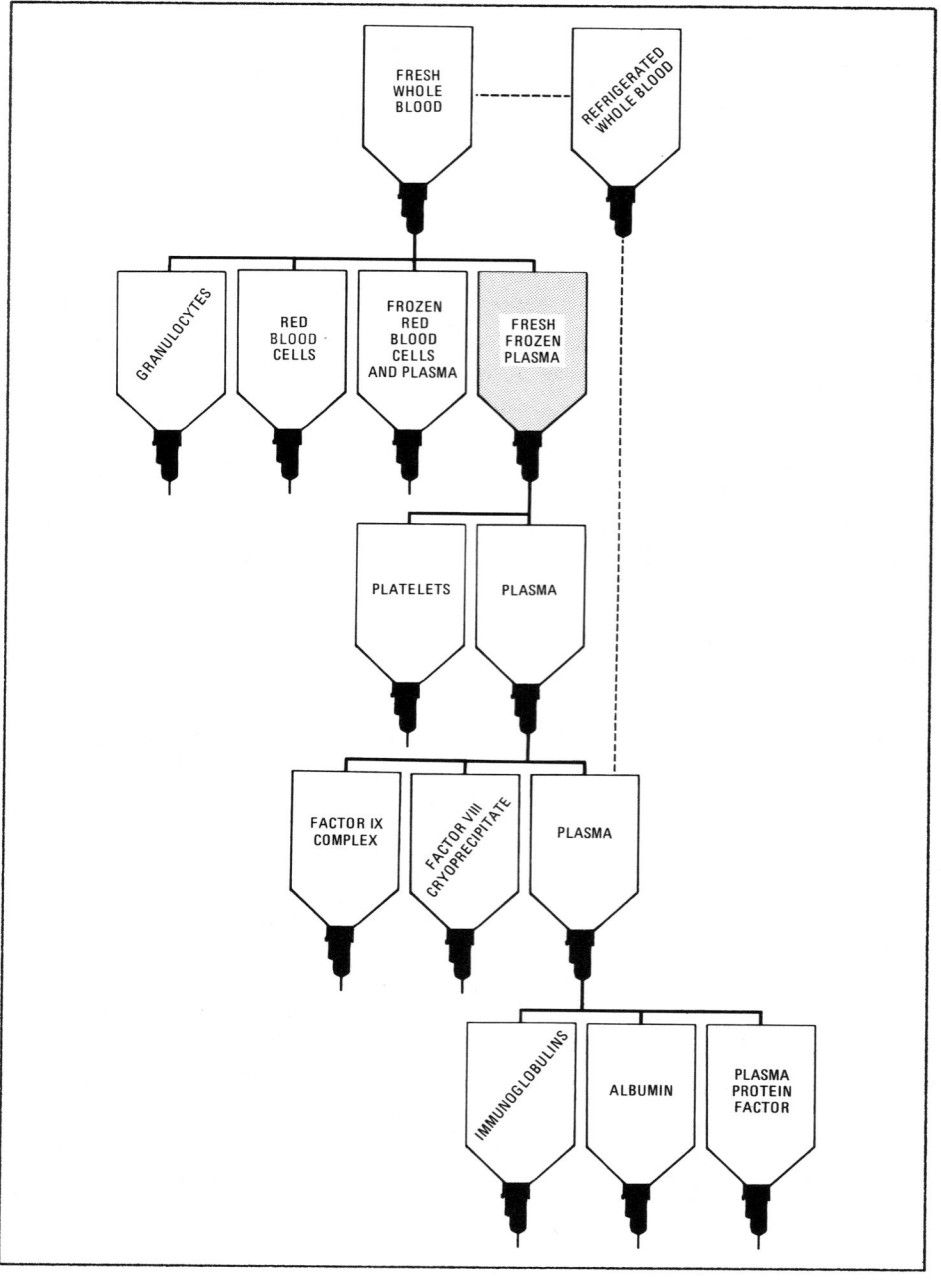

Figure 6–20. Plasma administration restores circulating volume and replaces nonlabile coagulation factors. *(Adapted from Scarlato, M. Blood transfusions today.* Nursing 78, *1978, 8(2), 70, copyright 1978, Springhouse Corporation, with permission.)*

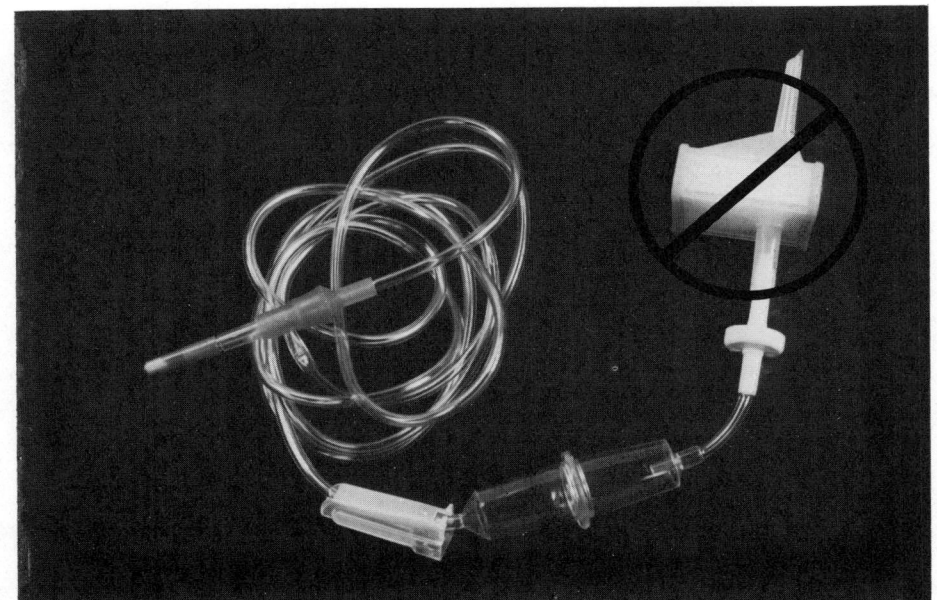

Figure 6–21. Microaggregate filter.

Care of the Patient Receiving Cryoprecipitate

NURSING DIAGNOSIS	RATIONALE	DEFINING CHARACTERISTICS	EXPECTED OUTCOME
Hemorrhage, potential for	An altered clotting profile in the host associated with decreased levels of Factor VIII and fibrinogen may respond to administration of cryoprecipitate, the cold-insoluble portion of plasma recovered from fresh frozen plasma. A unit of cryoprecipitate usually contains 80–120 U of Factor VIII activity in 15 ml. It should be infused as soon as possible after it has been thawed (requires about 20 minutes) in order to avoid loss of activity.	Epistaxis Hematuria Uncontrollable hemorrhage in joints, muscles, or internal organs as a result of minor trauma Hereditary mechanism of altered clotting factors	Problems associated with diminished levels of Factor VIII and fibrinogen will be minimized or resolved

NURSING INTERVENTIONS

Assure complication-free administration of cryoprecipitate (Fig. 6–22).

1. Crossmatching unnecessary. Donor plasma and recipient's RBCs should be ABO compatible
2. Administer as rapidly as possible by syringe or by component drip set only. Rate of administration is 1 U in 5 minutes
3. Initial dose: 1U/6 kg of body weight, follow with 1U/12 kg of body weight at 6–8 hour intervals
4. May be transfused with a 22 or 23 gauge needle, since product is not viscous. Flush the line with saline to insure complete transfusion of all cryoprecipitate
5. Monitor patient for any adverse effects, which include occasional urticaria or vasomotor reaction (chills and tremors not requiring medication). Risk of hepatitis is the same as with transfusing whole blood

OUTCOME CRITERIA

1. Complications associated with ABO incompatibilities will be absent or minimized
2. Transfusion will be accomplished in a timely fashion
3. Adequate amount of component will be administered for patient's body weight
4. Component wastage will be absent or minimized
5. Reactions will be promptly recognized and interventions initiated

DOCUMENTATION

- Time transfusion was started
- Type of blood product infused
- Signature of person initiating the transfusion
- Total volume of cryoprecipitate and saline infused
- Time transfusion was completed

AHF

Factor VIII concentrate anti-hemophilic factor (AHF), is used solely for the prevention and control of bleeding in patients with moderate or severe Factor VIII deficiency due to hemophilia A or acquired Factor VIII deficiency. Unlike cryoprecipitate, it does *not* contain significant fibrinogen.

This product should be reconstituted only with a plastic syringe to prevent binding on the ground glass surfaces. Components should be warmed to room temperature before mixing and administered within 3 hours after reconstitution.

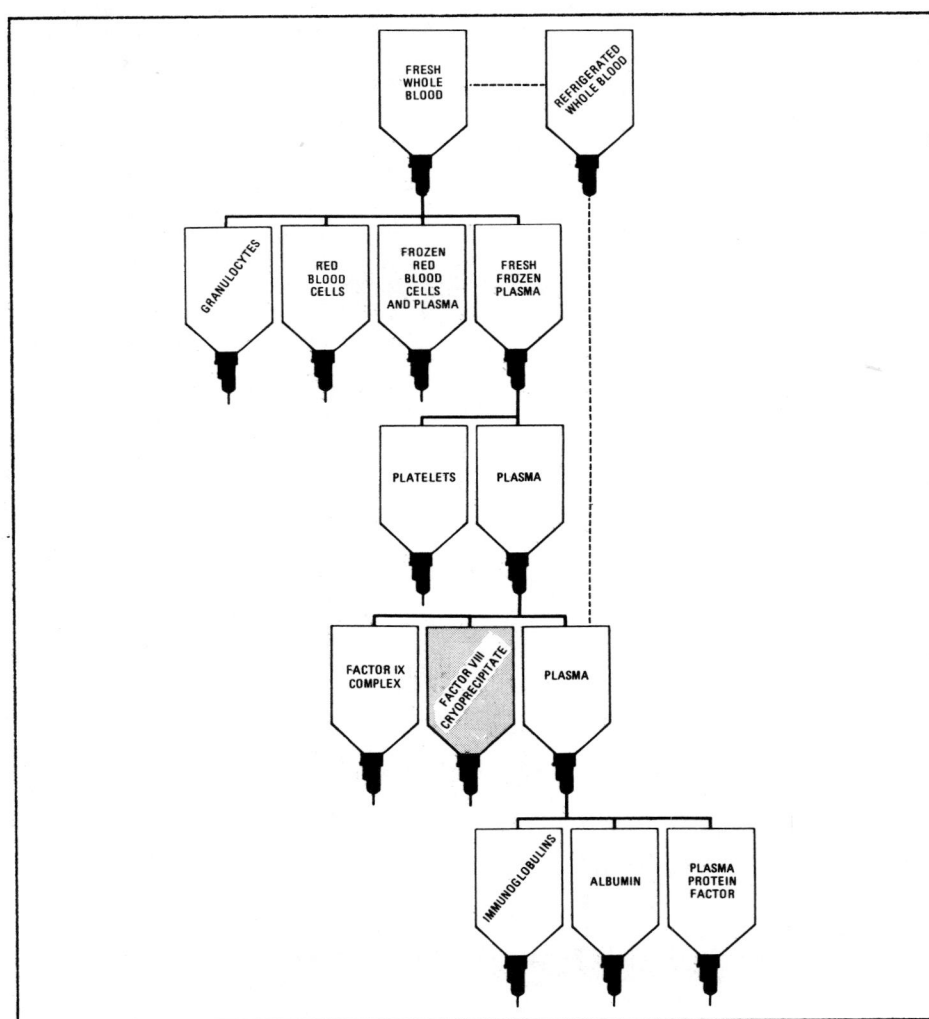

Figure 6–22. Cryoprecipitate is the cold-insoluble portion of fresh frozen plasma. *(Adapted from Scarlato, M. Blood transfusions today. Nursing 78, 1978, 8(2), 70, copyright 1978, Springhouse Corporation, with permission.)*

Care of the Patient Receiving Serum Albumin and Plasma Protein Fraction

NURSING DIAGNOSIS	RATIONALE	DEFINING CHARACTERISTICS	EXPECTED OUTCOME
Active loss, acute	Albumin 5% and albumin 25% (salt-poor) are heat-treated, aqueous, chemically processed fractions of pooled plasma. PPF is a 5% solution of selected proteins from pooled plasma in a buffered, stabilized saline diluent. Both these products are administered when volume expansion is clinically indicated. Mechanism of action involves osmotic pressure principles.	Hypotension Increased pulse rate Decreased pulse volume and pressure Decreased urine output	An adequate volume of circulating blood will be restored

NURSING INTERVENTIONS

Assure complication-free administration of serum albumin and plasma protein fraction (PPF) (Fig. 6–23).

1. Compatibility is not required, since albumin and PPF contain no RBCs or plasma antibodies
2. Administer both products with a straight-line set (supplied) (Fig. 6–24). Do not mix in the same line with protein hydrolysates or alcohol solutions
3. Dosage will vary with individual patient. Normally, an initial infusion of 100 ml of 25% albumin is suggested. In hypovolemic shock, a unit of albumin should be administered as rapidly as necessary to improve the condition of the patient. It may be repeated in 15–30 minutes after initial infusion. When given to patients with normal blood volume, the infusion rate should be slow (1 ml/min) to prevent rapid expansion of plasma volume with consequent circulatory overload. For PPF, 500 ml is suggested initially, with additional amounts used as clinical picture dictates
4. When greater protein concentration is desired or sodium restriction is indicated, it is preferable to use albumin rather than PPF
5. Albumin 5% is osmotically equivalent to blood and draws fluid into the bloodstream from the surrounding spaces equally as well. Albumin is active osmotically, and when injected intravenously, 50 ml of 25% albumin draws approximately 175 ml of additional fluid into the circulation within 15 minutes, except in the presence of marked dehydration. Observe the patient carefully for signs of pulmonary edema and symptoms of fluid overload: dyspnea, venous distention, bounding pulse, and mental changes
6. Rapid infusion of more than 10 ml/min of PPF may produce hypotension. The infusion should be slowed or discontinued if sudden hypotension occurs
7. The rapid rise in blood pressure that may follow the rapid administration of albumin or PPF requires careful observation of the injured patient to detect bleeding points that failed to bleed at lower blood pressure
8. The incidence of untoward reactions to both products is low, although nausea, vomiting, increased salivation, and febrile reactions occasionally occur

OUTCOME CRITERIA

1. Administration will be accomplished without a delay for typing or crossmatching
2. Administration with incompatible solutions will be avoided
3. Rate of administration will be in accordance with clinical indicators
4. Sodium restriction will be maintained
5. Complications associated with fluid overload will be absent or minimized
6. Hypotension will be promptly recognized and interventions initiated
7. Occult bleeding sites will be detected
8. Reactions will be promptly recognized and interventions initiated

DOCUMENTATION

- Baseline vital signs prior to infusion
- Time infusion was started
- Concentration of product
- Total volume of albumin or PPF infused
- Time infusion was completed
- Patient's response to therapy, particularly blood pressure and respiratory status
- Any nursing actions taken in response to adverse reactions

SPECIAL NOTE

Cerebral Vasospasm

In some facilities, volume expansion is the preferred treatment for complications associated with cerebral vasospasm. Specific systolic blood pressure parameters should be obtained from the physician prior to starting the infusion.

Hepatitis

Albumin and PPF are sterilized by pasteurization and carry less risk of hepatitis than whole blood.

Osmotic Pressure

Albumin 25% has five times as much osmotic pressure as an equal volume of blood and is useful in treating hypoproteinemia and renal failure.

Coagulation Factors

All coagulation factors are missing from PPF, and therefore fresh frozen plasma may be required to treat patients needing replacement of labile coagulation factors.

Precautions

PPF must be used cautiously when the patient has CHF from added fluid and salt load or has renal or hepatic failure from added protein load. PPF contains not less than 85% albumin, and the remainder consists of about 17% alpha- and beta-globulins.
Warning for PPF: Do not use if fluid is turbid or more than 4 hours after container has been entered.

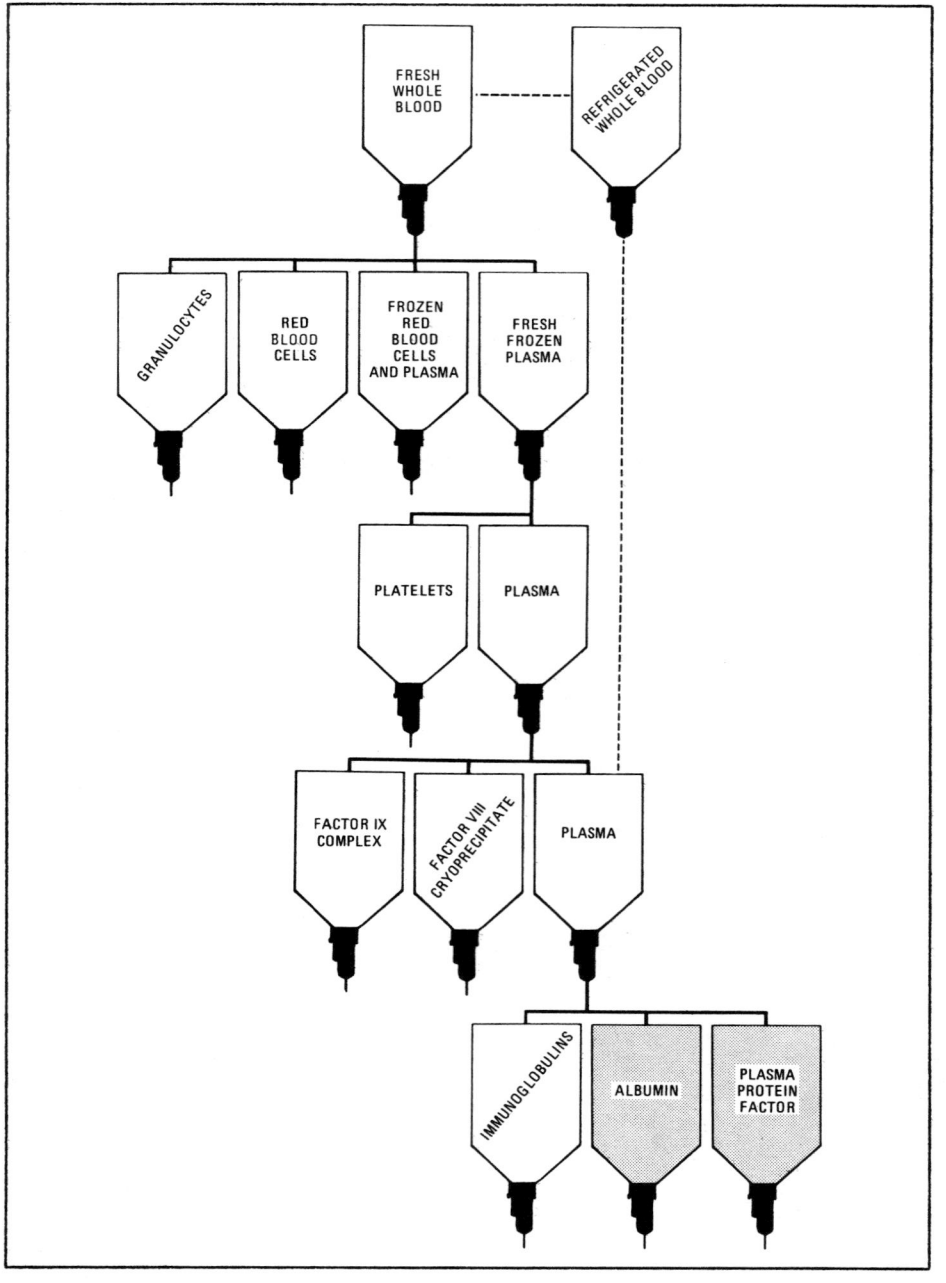

Figure 6–23. Albumin and plasma protein fraction are recovered from pooled plasma. *(Adapted from Scarlato, M. Blood transfusions today. Nursing 78, 1978, 8(2), 70, copyright 1978, Springhouse Corporation, with permission.)*

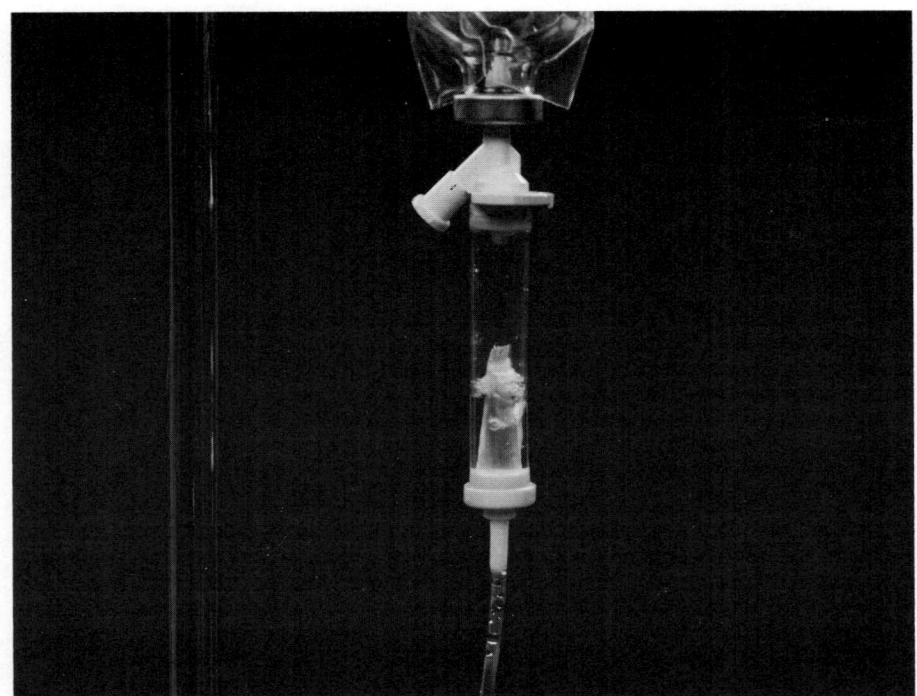

Figure 6–24. Albumin filter.

Care of the Patient Receiving Factor IX Complex

NURSING DIAGNOSIS	RATIONALE	DEFINING CHARACTERISTICS	EXPECTED OUTCOME
Hemorrhage, potential for	Factor IX complex is indicated whenever one or more of the coagulation factors (II, VII, IX, or X) must be elevated to prevent or stop a bleeding episode. Two units per kilogram of body weight will cause an average in vivo increase of about 3% in the level of Factor IX when measured 15 minutes after administration. Factor IX complex is prepared from pooled human plasma and is available from several manufacturers.	Epistaxis Hematuria Uncontrollable hemorrhage in joints, muscles, or internal organs Hereditary mechanism of altered clotting factors	Problems resulting from inadequate levels of Factors II, VII, IX, or X will be minimized or resolved

NURSING INTERVENTIONS

Assure complication-free administration of Factor IX complex (Fig. 6–25).

1. Factor IX complex should be refrigerated until used and should be reconstituted at the time of use with sterile water for injection
2. Give only by IV route. Administer slowly, at a rate of approximately 2–3 ml/min. Infusion should begin within 3 hours after reconstitution
3. Observe patient carefully for symptoms of intravascular coagulation, such as changes in blood pressure and pulse rate, respiratory distress, chest pain, and cough. If these symptoms appear, promptly discontinue the infusion
4. Serial PTTs may be required beginning a few hours after infusion. Results determine any additional need for correction of the deficient factor

OUTCOME CRITERIA

1. Component storage and preparation will be accomplished in an appropriate manner
2. Administration will be accomplished in a timely fashion
3. Complications associated with administration will be promptly recognized and interventions initiated
4. Laboratory specimens will be obtained in a timely fashion

DOCUMENTATION

• Time transfusion was started
• Type of blood product administered
• Signature of person initiating the transfusion
• Total volume of Factor IX complex infused
• Time transfusion was completed

SPECIAL NOTE

Hepatitis

Because of the high hepatitis risk with this product, serious consideration should be given whenever possible to the management of the patient by using fresh frozen plasma.

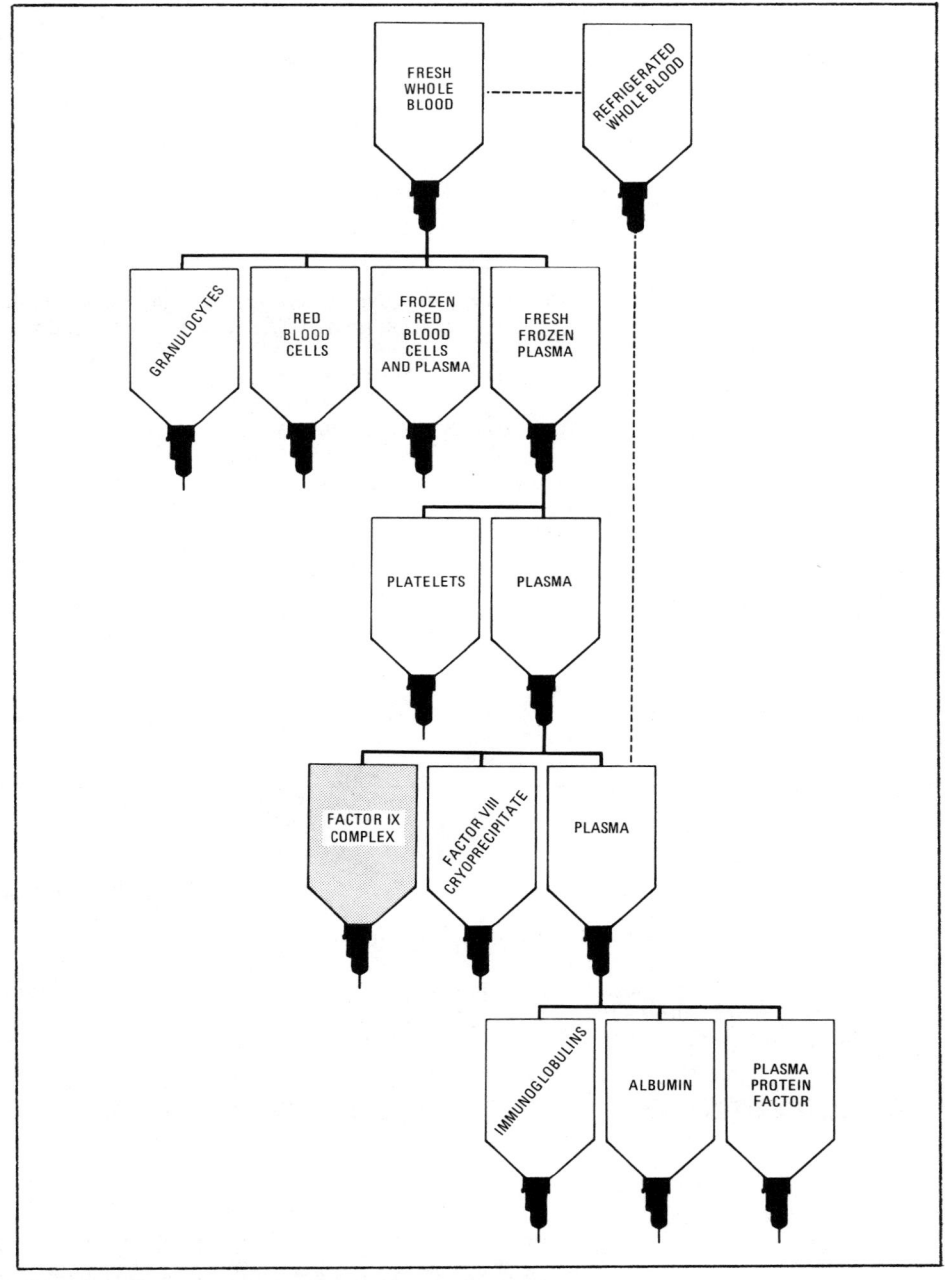

Figure 6–25. Factor IX complex is retrieved from pooled plasma. *(Adapted from Scarlato, M. Blood transfusions today. Nursing 78, 1978, 8(2), 70, copyright 1978, Springhouse Corporation, with permission.)*

Care of the Patient Receiving Granulocytes

NURSING DIAGNOSIS	RATIONALE	DEFINING CHARACTERISTICS	EXPECTED OUTCOME
Infection, potential for	White blood cells (leukocytes) are generally grouped into three major categories: Granulocytes, lymphocytes, and monocytes. Granulocytes are further subdivided into neutrophils, eosinophils, and basophils. As mediator of the body's immune response mechanism, a severely depressed leukocyte count (leukopenia, agranulocytosis, or neutropenia) predisposes the patient to contraction of a concurrent infection	Leukopenia: WBC below 5000/μl Neutropenia: Neutrophil count below 2000/μl Absolute neutropenia: Neutrophil count below 500–1000/μl Impairment of or absence of usual signs of infection Malaise, weakness	The level of circulating granulocytes will be increased

NURSING INTERVENTIONS

To insure complication-free administration of granulocytes (Fig. 6–26):

1. A major crossmatch is required prior to transfusion
2. Donor and recipient must be ABO compatible
3. Microaggregate filter should *not* be used
4. The verification procedure for recipient and component must be documented
5. Administer over a 2–4 hour period
6. Reactions may occur
   A. Fever and shaking chills: Common and may be the desired response as circulating granulocytes begin phagocytosis
   B.* Allergic reactions: May be a reaction to the RBCs contained in the infusion. *Stop the transfusion.* Maintain a patent IV line. Notify the physician.
   C. Graft vs host (GVH) reaction: Occurs in immunosuppressed patients as donor lymphocytes attack recipient's cells. *Stop the transfusion.* Maintain a patent IV line. Notify the physician.
   D.* Hemolysis: Occurs in response to erythrocytes. *Stop the transfusion.* Maintain a patent IV line. Notify the physician
   E. Severe hypotension: *Stop the transfusion.* Maintain a patent IV line. Notify the physician
   F. Respiratory distress: May occur if the lungs are the site of infection. *Stop the transfusion.* Maintain a patent IV line. Notify the physician

OUTCOME CRITERIA

1. Incompatibilities between donor and recipient will be identified
2. Transfusion reactions related to ABO incompatability will be absent or minimized
3. Granulocytes and platelets will not be removed by a microaggregate filter

*Current state of the art does not allow for complete removal of every RBC by pheresis, thus these reactions may occur.

4. Errors in administration due to improper identification procedure will be absent
5. Complications associated with rapid administration will be avoided
   Complications associated with other causes will be promptly identified and remedial measures instituted
6. Complications associated with administration will be absent or minimized

DOCUMENTATION

- Baseline vital signs
- Time transfusion was started
- Type of blood product administered
- Signature of person verifying identification information and signature of second licensed person verifying correct product
- Volume of fluid infused
- Time transfusion was completed
- Any nursing interventions taken in response to an adverse reaction

SPECIAL NOTE

Leukopheresis

Because of the high degree of variability of granulocytes obtainable from a unit of blood, granulocyte pheresis (or leukopheresis) is the preferred method of harvest.
   The procedure involves an ABO- and Rh-compatible donor who can spend 5–6 hours several times weekly in the donation process
   By use of an automated cell separation process, donor blood is filtered for the desired component and then returned to the donor
   Efficiency of the cell separator and the use of steroids to induce elevated donor granulocyte production will affect the number collected

Alternative Interventions

Use of laminar airflow rooms, protected environments, and reverse isolation procedures have all been employed for severely granulocytopenic patients. All methods have been reported as offering varying degrees of success. Administration of granulocytes for prophylaxis remains controversial.

Shift

In some instances, the WBC count with a differential is described as having a "shift to the left" or a "shift to the right." The origin of this description evolves from the display of the various WBC types in a left to right sequence as determined by the maturity of their development. Thus a shift to the left may indicate a predominance of immature WBCs (polymorphonuclear neutrophils), and a shift to the right may indicate a regenerative phase with a predominance of mature WBCs, such as lymphocytes or monocytes.

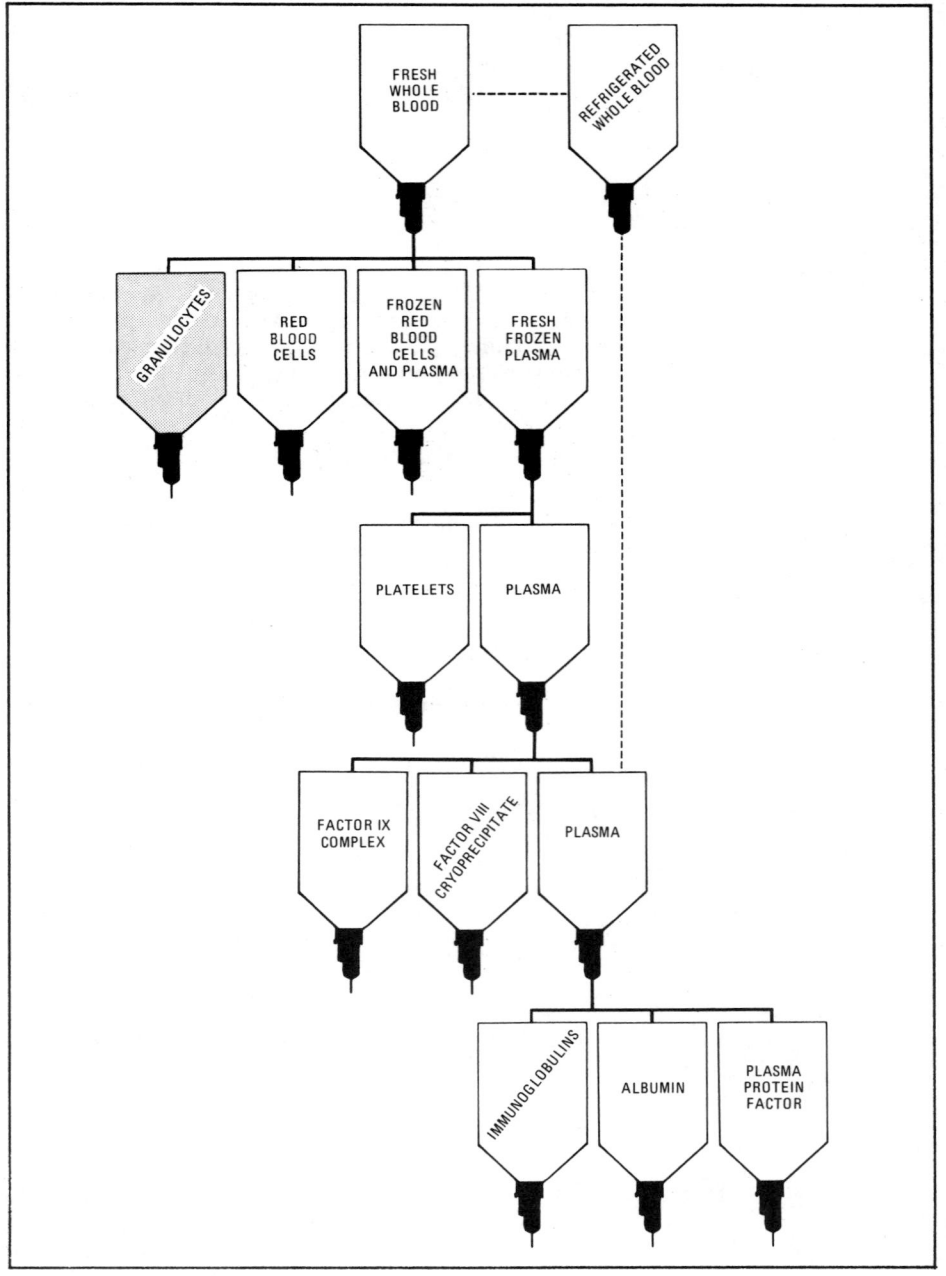

Figure 6–26. Granulocytes are obtained from a donor by the process of leukopheresis. *(Adapted from Scarlato, M. Blood transfusions today. Nursing 78, 1978, 8(2), 70, copyright 1978, Springhouse Corporation, with permission.)*

Care of the Patient with Disseminated Intravascular Coagulation

NURSING DIAGNOSIS	RATIONALE	DEFINING CHARACTERISTICS	EXPECTED OUTCOME
Hemorrhage, potential for	Hemostasis is normally achieved by balanced activity between the body's coagulation and fibrinolytic systems. In the syndrome of DIC, the initial vascular insult stimulates an overproduction of thrombin, resulting in excessive clotting. As the clots begin to lyse, released autologous anticoagulants inhibit any normal clotting activity. As continued circulating clotting depletes the circulating factor levels, stable clot formation is impossible, and uncontrolled bleeding may occur. Since DIC is not, in itself, a disease, the treatment of choice is the treatment of the underlying disease process. An alternative method of therapy is to administer replacement blood components. When treatment of the underlying pathology is not possible, anticoagulant therapy with heparin may be used to prohibit the formation of thrombin and thus attempt to control the clotting process	History of intrinsic system activation (Factor XII) • Extensive trauma or burns • Transplant rejection • Acute hemolysis (transfusion reaction, infection, snake bite) • Extracorporeal circulatory bypass History of extrinsic system activation (thromboplastic substances) • Obstetrical conditions (retained uterine contents, abruptio placentae) • Neoplastic diseases History of • Cirrhosis • Septicemia (acute bacterial infection) • Acute hepatitis • Shock Laboratory values • Fibrin split products (FSP): elevated fibrin degradation products (FDP): present • PT: prolonged • PTT: prolonged • TT: prolonged • Factor assays for V, VII, VIII, X, XIII: reduced • Fibrinogen: reduced (but may be within normal limits) • Platelet count: reduced Evidence of thrombocytopenia	Complications associated with disseminated intravascular coagulation will be promptly identified and minimized

NURSING INTERVENTIONS

1. Vital signs q1h
2. Neurological vital signs and Glasgow coma scale scores q2h
3. Intake and output q1h
4. Inspection of IV insertion sites q1h (Fig. 6–27)
5. Inspection of tube or drain insertion sites q2h
6. Inspection of preexisting wounds (surgical or traumatic) q2h
7. Assessment of skin q4h
8. Assessment of oral mucous membranes and gingiva q4h
9. Guaiac testing of emesis and stool every occurrence
10. Guaiac testing of nasogastric drainage q4h
11. Observation of venipuncture sites q15min × 6 after blood is drawn
12. Cushioning devices on bed
13. Protective padding on bony prominences
14. Extreme care when handling, turning, or transferring patient
15. Administration of blood or blood products as ordered
16. Administration of heparin as ordered
17. Ensure that laboratory specimens are promptly and appropriately obtained

OUTCOME CRITERIA

1. Signs of hypotension will be promptly detected and investigated
2. Changes in neurological status will be promptly recognized and investigated
3. Alteration in quantity of urine output will be promptly noted and investigated. Evidence of hematuria will be promptly recognized and reported
4. Any oozing or bleeding from IV insertion sites will be promptly noted and corrected
5. Any evidence of oozing or bleeding from insertion site will be promptly recognized and investigated
6. Any increase in wound drainage will be promptly noted and investigated
7. Change in or appearance of hematomas, ecchymoses, or petechiae will be promptly noted and reported
8. Any evidence of oral lesions and gingival bleeding will be promptly recognized and reported
9. Guaiac-positive results of emesis and stool will be promptly noted and reported
10. Guaiac-positive results of nasogastric drainage will be promptly noted and reported
11. Abnormal bleeding will be promptly detected, reported, and corrected
12. No injury will occur in bed
13. No injury will occur to bony prominences
14. No injury will occur when handling, turning, or transferring patient
15. Restoration of adequate volume and component levels will be restored
16. Anticoagulation efforts will be reflected by laboratory studies
17. Specimens will be obtained in a safe, timely, and cost-effective manner

DOCUMENTATION

- Blood pressure, heart rate, respiratory rate, and temperature
- Supporting physical assessment findings; notification of appropriate personnel for changes and interventions initiated, if any
- Neurological vital signs
- Glasgow coma scale scores
- Urine output
- Presence or absence of bleeding at IV insertion sites
- Presence or absence of bleeding from insertion site of tubes or drains
- Amount of wound drainage
- Increase in volume or change in quality of drainage
- Notification of appropriate personnel and interventions, if any initiated

(continued)

- Hematomas or evidence of ecchymosis
- Integrity of oral mucosa and presence or absence of gingival bleeding
- Results of guaiac testing
- Presence or absence of oozing or bleeding at venipuncture sites
- Placement of eggcrate mattress, water mattress, foam, or sheepskin; initiation of air-fluidized therapy
- Use of draw sheet for turning, lifting, or transferring and instructions given to paraprofessionals
- Documentation of identification procedure
- Patient's response to therapy
- Administration of medication
- Laboratory values

SPECIAL NOTE

Nomenclature

Other names for disseminated intravascular coagulation:
Consumptive coagulopathy
Defibrination syndrome
Intravascular coagulation–fibrinolysis

Pharmacological Blockade

Heparin and the coumarin derivatives are commonly used anticoagulating agents. Whereas the coumarin derivatives act as vitamin K antagonists, the primary action of heparin is to inactivate thrombin, thus preventing its interaction with fibrinogen. This pharmacological blockade then assists in the management of DIC by reducing the intravascular clotting process and raising the circulating levels of factors, restoring the capacity for normal clotting.

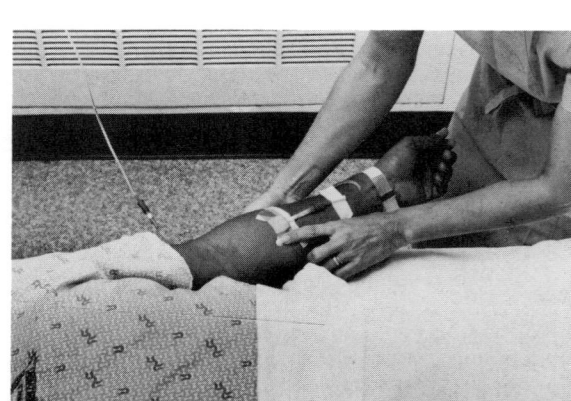

Figure 6–27. Inspection of IV site.

Albumin: A type of simple protein widely distributed throughout the tissues and fluids in plants and animals; found in blood, milk, and muscle.

Anemia: Any condition in which the number of red blood cells/mm^3, the amount of hemoglobin in 100 ml of blood, and the volume of packed red blood cells/100 ml of blood are less than normal. Clinically, generally pertaining to the concentration of oxygen-transporting material in a designated volume of blood.

Basophil: A type of leukocyte that has an affinity to stain specifically with basic dyes under specific pH conditions; constitutes approximately 0.5% of the total white blood cell count.

Bleeding Time: Following a small puncture, the time elapsing between the appearance of the first drop of blood and the removal of the last drop of blood. Normally between 1 and 3 minutes. Normal in hemophilia; prolonged in some liver diseases, thrombocytopenia, and in the presence of decreased prothrombin levels.

Coagulation: Clotting; the process of changing from liquid to solid, especially of blood.

Coagulopathy: Any disease affecting the coagulability of the blood.

Cryoprecipitate: Precipitate that forms when soluble material is cooled, especially with reference to the precipitate that forms in normal blood plasma that has been subjected to cold precipitation and is rich in antihemophilic globulin (Factor VIII).

Direct Coombs' Test: For detecting sensitized erythrocytes in erythroblastosis fetalis and in cases of acquired hemolytic anemia; the agglutination that results during the test indicates the presence of incomplete or univalent antibodies on the surface of the erythrocytes.

Disseminated Intravascular Coagulation: A hemorrhagic syndrome that occurs following the uncontrolled activation of clotting factors and fibrinolytic enzymes throughout small blood vessels. Fibrin is deposited, platelets and clotting factors are consumed, and fibrin degradation products inhibit fibrin polymerization, resulting in tissue necrosis and bleeding.

Eosinophil: A type of leukocyte that stains readily with eosin dye; constitutes approximately 2.5% of the total white blood cell count.

Eosinophilia: Eosinophilic leukocytosis.

Erythrocyte: A mature red blood cell.

Erythrocyte Sedimentation Rate: The degree of rapidity with which the red blood cells sink in a mass of drawn blood.

Fibrin: An elastic filamentous protein derived from fibrinogen by the action of thrombin, which releases fibrinopeptides A and B from fibrinogen.

Fibrinogen: Factor I; a globulin of blood plasma that is converted into the coagulated protein, fibrin, by the action of thrombin in the presence of ionized calcium.

Hematocrit: Percentage of the volume of a blood sample occupied by cells; hematocrit as opposed to plasma component.

Hemoglobin: The red, respiratory protein of erythrocytes, consisting of approximately 6% heme and 94% globin; transports oxygen from the lungs to the tissues; this oxygenated form is termed *oxyhemoglobin*.

Leukocyte: White blood cell; 20 potential descriptors identified.

Leukocytosis: An abnormally large number of leukocytes, as observed in acute infections.

Leukopenia: Any situation in which the total number of leukocytes in the circulating blood is less than normal, the lower limit of which is generally regarded as 5000/mm^3.

Monocyte: A relatively large mononuclear leukocyte.

Neutrophil: A mature white blood cell in the granulocytic series; constitutes approximately 50–75% of the total white blood cell count. Primary function is ingestion of bacteria.

Plasma: The fluid noncellular portion of the circulating blood; distinguished from the serum obtained after coagulation.

Platelet: An irregularly shaped disc found in blood, containing granules in the center and clear protoplasm peripherally; one-third the size of an erythrocyte and contains no hemoglobin. Important in the coagulation process by activation of the surface lipoprotein platelet Factor III.

Prothrombin: Factor II; in the presence of thromboplastin and ionized calcium, prothrombin is converted to thrombin.

Reticulocyte: A yound red blood cell occurring during the process of active regeneration of blood.

Sickle cell disease: Characterized by the presence of crescent- or sickle-shaped erythrocytes in peripheral blood, excessive hemolysis, and active hemopoieses.

Thrombin: An enzyme found in shed blood that converts fibrinogen into fibrin by hydrolyzing peptides; it is formed by the action of prothrombinase.

Thrombocytopenia: A condition in which there is an abnormally small number of platelets in the circulating blood.

Bibliography

Alspach, J. G., & Williams, S. (Eds.). *Core curriculum for critical care nursing* (3rd ed.). American Association of Critical Care Nurses. Philadelphia: Saunders, 1985.

Berk, J. L., & Sampliner, J. E. (Eds.). *Handbook of critical care* (2nd ed.). Boston: Little, Brown, 1976.

Blood component administration manual. The Procedure Committee of the Nursing Service and the Transfusion Service (Pathology) of The Methodist Hospital, Houston, Texas, 1982.

Circular of information for the use of human blood and blood components (Rev.). Washington, D.C.: American Association of Blood Banks and the American Red Cross, 1981.

Hahn, A. B., Backin, R. L., & Oestreich, S. K. J. (Eds.). *Pharmacology in Nursing* (15th ed.). St. Louis, Mo.: Mosby, 1982.

Jennings, J. M. Improving your management of DIC. *Nursing 79,* May 1979, 60–67.

Kazak, A. Processing blood for transfusion. *American Journal of Nursing,* 1979, 931–934.

Kirkis, E. J., & Ettorre, D. M. Seven sticky problems (and their solutions) in blood transfusions. *RN,* April 1983, 59, 62, 94.

Lewis, S. M., & Collier, I. C. *Medical-surgical nursing: Assessment and management of clinical problems.* New York: McGraw-Hill, 1983.

Leser, D. R. Synthetic blood; a future alternative. *American Journal of Nursing,* March 1982, 5432–5455.

Smith, L. B. Reactions to blood transfusions. *American Journal of Nursing,* September 1984, 1096–1101.

Wallack, J. *Interpretation of diagnostic tests: A handbook synopsis of laboratory medicine* (3rd ed.). Boston: Little, Brown, 1978.

7

ENDOCRINE SYSTEM

Carol W. La Croix

Care of the Patient Requiring Therapy
for Hypoglycemic Crisis

NURSING DIAGNOSIS	RATIONALE	DEFINING CHARACTERISTICS	EXPECTED OUTCOME

Metabolism, alteration in: glucose	Hypoglycemic crisis is a medical emergency caused by an alteration in the balance between release of and utilization of glucose in the body. The majority of cases occur in diabetics, but it can occur independently of diabetes. Contributing factors include insulin overdose, liver disease, and end-stage renal dysfunction.
	
	Immediate management of hypoglycemia is necessary to prevent permanent brain damage as a result of cellular glucose deprivation.
		Past medical history
		  Pancreatic or hepatic disease
		  Increase in insulin dosage in type I diabetics
		  Pituitary or adrenal dysfunction
		  Steroid therapy
		Physical assessment
		  Decreased level of consciousness
		  Altered mental status
		  Slow, slurred speech
		  Generalized seizures, coma
		  Visual disturbances: Blurred or double vision, visual halos
		  Tachycardia, elevated blood pressure
		  Diaphoresis
		  Shallow respirations
		Laboratory data
		  Blood glucose less than 60 mg/dl
		  Negative urine ketones
		  Glucose levels below 40 mg/dl can cause loss of consciousness, generalized seizures, and dilated pupils
		  Glucose levels below 20 mg/dl can cause bradycardia, shallow respirations, coma, brain damage, and death if prolonged
			Serum glucose will be restored to normal levels

NURSING INTERVENTIONS

1. Administer IV glucose as ordered: 1–2 ampules 50% dextrose IV push over 5–10 minutes, followed by infusion of D_5W until glucose levels return to normal range. During IV administration of 50% dextrose, assess needle placement every 5–10 ml as this solution is very irritating to body tissues and can cause tissue necrosis if infiltrated. A 50 ml vial of 50% dextrose contains 25 g of glucose and can raise blood glucose levels as much as 200 mg/dl
2. Administer glucagon as ordered. Glucagon is a potent hormone produced by the pancreas that stimulates glycogen release from the liver, thereby raising blood glucose levels. A dose of 1 mg intramuscularly (IM) or subcutaneously (SC) should alleviate symptoms in about 15 minutes. If there is no response, a second dose can be given, but in elderly or debilitated patients with depleted glycogen stores, this may not be helpful, and administration of 50% dextrose IV push may be required
3. Seizure precautions until glucose returns to normal range

4. Glasgow coma scale and pupil checks q1h until alert and oriented, then q4h for 24 hours
5. Vital signs q15min until stable, then q2h for 24 hours
6. Obtain glucose levels as ordered q15min until glucose reaches 60 mg/dl, then q1h for 24 hours or until stable and within normal range
7. Administer oral carbohydrate when patient is alert and able to swallow

OUTCOME CRITERIA

1. Blood glucose will be greater than 60 mg/dl within 10 minutes
2. Blood glucose will be maintained between 70 and 120 mg/dl
3. Sequelae from seizure activity will be prevented or minimized
4. Glasgow coma scale scores will improve or return to normal level
5. Vital signs will be within normal range
6. Serum glucose levels will reflect improvement of hypoglycemic status. Directional trends will be promptly identified

DOCUMENTATION

- Administration of IV dextrose as ordered, including route and dosage
- Glucagon administration as ordered, including dosage, route, and location of administration
- Seizure precautions taken, presence or absence of seizures, characteristics of seizures, interventions initiated, and any sequelae sustained as a result of seizures
- Glasgow coma scale scores q1h or as ordered
- Vital signs as ordered
- Serum glucose levels drawn, with results
- Oral carbohydrate administration, including type and amount given and any intolerance of oral intake

Documentation of directional trends, abnormalities, and other changes will include notification of physician, any interventions taken, and patient's response to therapy. The use of a laboratory flowsheet for recording of sequential laboratory data is invaluable for assessing trends and determining progress of therapy.

SPECIAL NOTE

Somogyi Effect

Somogyi effect is the rebound hyperglycemia that results when a very low blood glucose causes release of epinephrine, adrenal corticosteroids, and growth hormone. This rebound effect can cause very erratic shifts in blood glucose values. Somogyi effect may be seen following an acute hypoglycemic episode; however, if the patient has had *very* low glucose levels (less than 30 mg/dl), this effect may not occur.

Medic-Alert

It is highly recommended that patients prone to hypoglycemic reactions carry a Medic-Alert card or bracelet, since hypoglycemic symptoms often mimic alcohol intoxication or cerebral vascular accident (CVA).

Reagent Strips

There are two types of reagent strips used for blood glucose determinations that can be read visually, without the use of a glucometer. These are ChemStrip bG by BioDynamics and Visidex by Ames. Although these strips may be slightly less accurate than those used with a glucometer, they can be very useful tools for rapid assessment of a patient's current glucose level.

Autonomic Neuropathy

Patients with significant autonomic neuropathy, a long-term complication of diabetes, or those receiving beta-blockers, such as propranolol (Inderal), may not exhibit the adrenergic warning symptoms of hypoglycemia, such as tachycardia, diaphoresis and anxiety. Neurological signs and symptoms, such as decreased level of consciousness, slurred speech, or visual disturbances, may be the first clues to hypoglycemia. Blood glucose monitoring is especially important for these patients.

Care of the Patient Requiring Therapy
for Diabetic Ketoacidosis

NURSING DIAGNOSES	RATIONALE	DEFINING CHARACTERISTICS	EXPECTED OUTCOME

Metabolism, alteration in: glucose
 	
Fluid volume, alteration in, deficit, actual
	Diabetic ketoacidosis (DKA) is one of the most prevalent endocrine emergencies. It occurs when there is an insulin deficiency associated with some form of physical or emotional stress. Serum glucose levels rise, and fat stores are converted into free fatty acids, causing hyperglycemia and ketonuria. These two conditions lead to osmotic diuresis, significant volume depletion of up to 15% total body fluid, and dehydration. Precipitating factors include inadequate secretion of insulin, infection, pregnancy, and omission of insulin.
	
	    Death as a result of DKA is often due to shock but can be caused by underlying illness or infection, myocardial infarction, or complications of therapeutic management. Mortality rates approach 10%, but prompt recognition and aggressive therapy can reduce this rate to less than 2%. Complications, if not detected and managed expediently, can lead to and include
	  Shock, cardiac dysrhythmias
	  Acute renal failure
	  Pulmonary edema
	  Cerebral edema and seizures
	  Hypoglycemia, hypokalemia, hypophosphatemia
	  Aspiration
	  Coma, death
		Past medical history
		  Hyperthyroidism
		  Type I diabetes mellitus, uncontrolled
		  Infection
		  Recent stress or surgery
		Physical assessment
		  Polyuria, polydipsia
		  Flushed, dry skin with poor turgor
		  Elevated temperature
		  Tachypnea or Kussmaul respirations
		  Acetone breath
		  Nausea, vomiting, abdominal tenderness
		  Decreased level of consciousness: Lethargy and confusion
		  Hypotension
		  Tachycardia
		  Cardiac dysrhythmias
		Laboratory data
		  Plasma glucose greater than 300 mg/dl
		  Plasma ketones to 4+
		  Elevated plasma lipids: Cholesterol greater than 300 mg/dl; triglycerides greater than 190 mg/dl
		  BUN equal to or greater than 24 mg/dl
		  Positive urine glucose and ketones
		  Arterial blood gases (ABGs) consistent with metabolic acidosis; arterial pH less than 7.35
		  Serum bicarbonate less than 22 mEq/L
		  Serum potassium (K^+) normal to high; greater than 5.0 mEq/L (initial serum K^+ may be normal to low or elevated but becomes rapidly depleted once therapy has been started)
			Optimal glucose levels will be restored, and fluid balance will be returned to normal

NURSING INTERVENTIONS

1. Vital signs q1h
2. Glasgow coma scale q2h until patient is alert
3. Continuous ECG monitoring for rhythm changes related to K^+ shifts, with rhythm strip q1–2h
4. Intake and output q1h
5. Administer IV fluid therapy as ordered. Fluid replacement usually consists of isotonic saline (0.9% NS) for hypotensive patients or 0.45% normal saline. Infusion rates are rapid and may be up to 1 L in the first 30 minutes, 1 L over the next hour, then 300–500 ml/hr over 24 hours. The actual rate depends on blood pressure, urine output, and overall patient response to a rapid increase in circulatory volume. When blood glucose is less than 240 mg/dl, IV fluid is changed to a solution containing dextrose
6. Administer insulin therapy as ordered. Methods include IV bolus, continuous IV infusion, and frequent SC injections. Low-dose IV insulin therapy has been shown to produce fewer complications (hypokalemia and hypoglycemia) while returning blood sugar to normal levels. Regular insulin IV bolus (5–10 U) is usually given, followed by a continuous infusion of regular insulin (6–12 U/hr). Amount of insulin given decreases as blood glucose decreases but is not discontinued until patient is able to tolerate oral fluids and food and receive SC insulin. Since insulin may bind to plastic IV tubing, it is advisable to flush 50 cc of the mixed IV insulin solution or albumin through the tubing before starting the continuous infusion. An infusion pump is mandatory to accurately regulate the amount of insulin administered (Fig. 7–1)
7. Central venous pressure (CVP) or pulmonary capillary wedge pressure (PCWP) q1h. Pulmonary artery catheter placement can be invaluable in monitoring fluid volume status during replacement therapy
8. Obtain blood glucose q1h until stable (Fig. 7–2)
9. Urine specific gravity, glucose, and ketones q1h (urethral catheter necessary)
10. Monitor serum sodium (Na) and potassium (K^+) levels q2h
11. Administer potassium replacement as ordered: Potassium replacement is usually required, since serum potassium levels decrease once fluid and insulin therapy are initiated due to rapid fluid replacement. Potassium chloride, 40–80 mEq/L of IV fluid, is sufficient to maintain potassium levels necessary to reduce the occurrence of cardiac dysrhythmias. Potassium phosphate can also be administered as an IV additive. It is useful in maintaining serum phosphate levels, which are often depleted in patients with DKA
12. Monitor skin condition every shift: Color, temperature, turgor
13. Daily weights
14. Nasogastric tube to low suction to decrease possibility of aspiration. Position patient on side

OUTCOME CRITERIA

1. Vital signs will be optimal for the patient
2. Glasgow coma scale scores will remain stable or improve
3. Any dysrhythmias will be promptly identified
4. Urine output will be greater than 30 cc/hr
5. Patient will be rehydrated
6. Blood glucose will be restored to less than 150 mg/dl
7. CVP will be maintained between 5 and 10 cm H_2O
8. Directional trends in blood glucose will be promptly identified
9. Urine specific gravity will be maintained between 1.010 and 1.030
10. Serum sodium will be maintained between 135 and 145 mEq/L, and directional trends will be promptly identified
11. Serum potassium will be maintained between 3.5 and 5.0 mEq/L, and directional trends will be promptly identified
12. Changes in skin condition will be promptly identified
13. Weight will be optimal for the patient
14. Risk of aspiration will be minimized

(continued)

DOCUMENTATION

- Vital signs as ordered
- Glasgow coma scale q2h
- ECG rhythm with rhythm strip q1–2h
- Intake and output q1h
- IV fluid therapy as ordered, including type, amount, and rate of solution infused
- Insulin therapy as ordered, including type, route, amount, and rate of insulin administered
- Central pressure readings q1h. Type of reading taken (CVP vs PCWP) should be noted
- Blood glucose levels drawn, with result
- Urine specific gravity, glucose, ketones q1h
- Electrolyte values drawn, with results
- Potassium replacement therapy as ordered. Type, route, dosage, and rate of potassium administered should be documented
- Skin condition on admission, then every shift
- Weight on admission, then daily
- Presence of nasogastric tube, with degree of suction, character and amount of drainage noted

Documentation of directional trends, abnormalities, and other changes will include notification of physician, any interventions taken, and patient's response to therapy.

SPECIAL NOTE

Glucometer

The use of glucometers for bedside determination of blood glucose levels has increased the rapidity of assessment and treatment. There are, however, some legal implications of which the critical care nurse *must* be aware. Nurses using a bedside glucometer should be proficiency-verified, and some form of quality control must be initiated. Laboratory verification of results at random intervals has been suggested. It is conceivable that an initiated treatment, based on an erroneous glucose determination, could have serious consequences not only for the patient but also for the nurse.

Glycohemoglobin

Assessment of glycohemoglobin can be done via a blood sample drawn on the patient's arrival to the ICU. The results of the test, however, may not be available for several days and will not influence the *immediate* management of DKA. Glycohemoglobin results will provide the clinician with useful information regarding the patient's previous state of metabolic control. Results suggesting poor control may alert the nurse to an existing knowledge deficit. Reassessment of patient teaching–learning needs may be indicated.

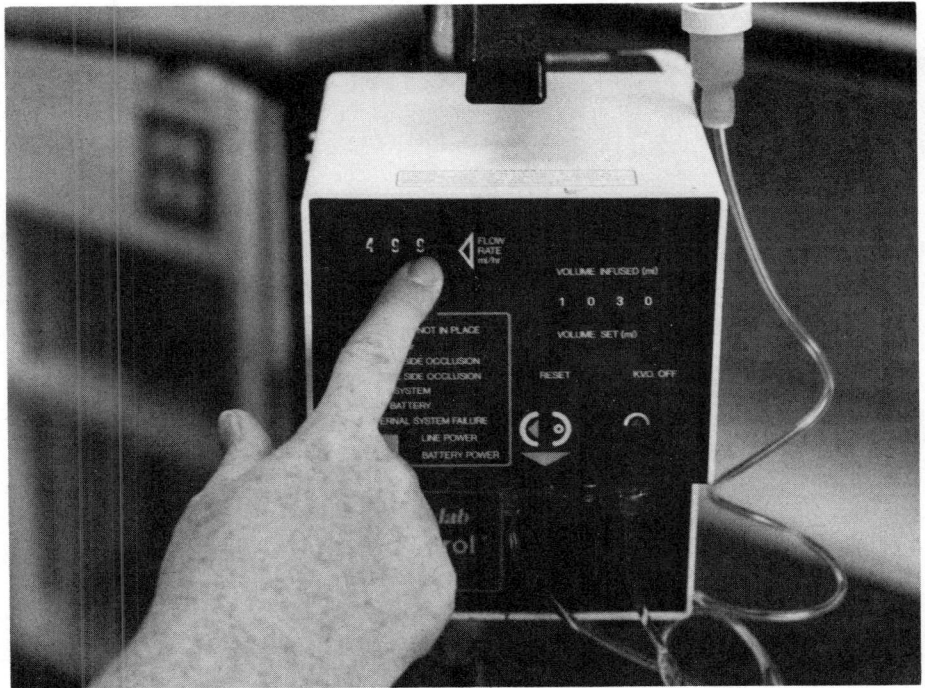

Figure 7–1. A volume control infusion pump is mandatory for accurate administration of IV insulin.

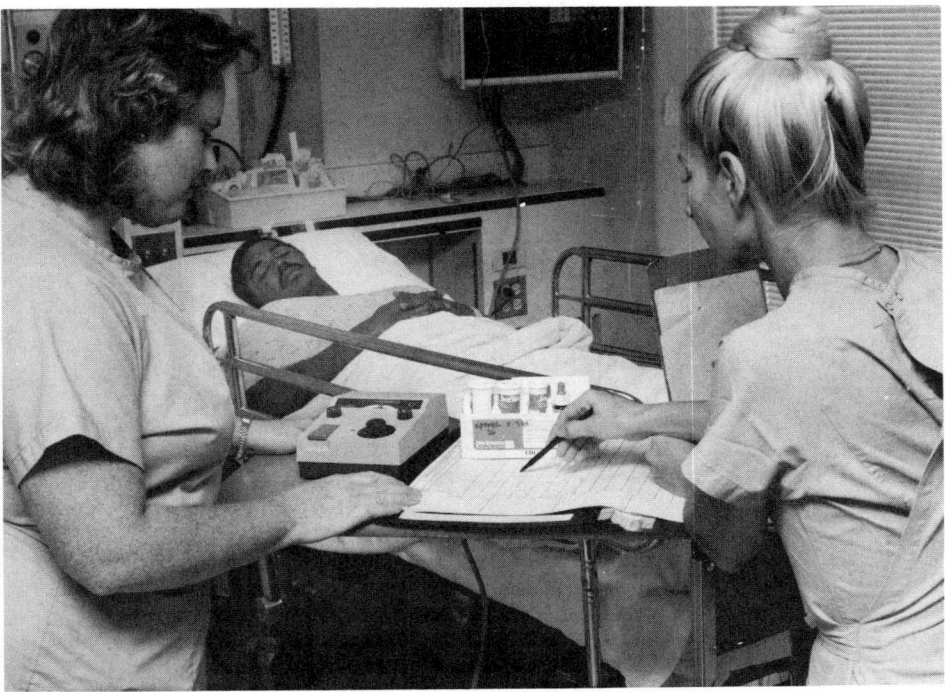

Figure 7–2. Blood glucose levels can be rapidly obtained through the use of a bedside glucometer.

Care of the Patient Requiring Therapy for Hyperosmolar Hyperglycemic Nonketotic Coma

NURSING DIAGNOSIS	RATIONALE	DEFINING CHARACTERISTICS	EXPECTED OUTCOME
Fluid volume, alteration in, deficit, actual	Hyperosmolar hyperglycemic nonketotic coma (HHNK) is usually seen in type II (non-insulin dependent) diabetics but may occur in any individual receiving large amounts of glucose for a sustained time period, such as with total parenteral nutrition. Glucose intolerance occurs, causing a rise in blood glucose, which produces an osmotic diuresis. Continued diuresis leads to dehydration, a shift in electrolyte balance, and if uncorrected, eventual coma and death. Precipitating factors include major stress, infections, malnutrition, and diabetes mellitus. Certain drugs are also thought to precipitate HHNK, including diuretics, steroids, and immunosuppressive drugs. Patients receiving peripheral amino acid solutions may also be at risk for development of HHNK due to the gluconeogenic properties of some of the amino acids. The reason these patients do not become ketotic is not clear. One theory suggests that the patient's insulin level is sufficient to prevent ketosis but not to reduce the blood sugar. Another theory states that the hyperosmolar state may have an inhibitory effect on lipolysis, preventing ketosis by reducing the flow of free fatty acids to the liver. Death occurs in approximately one third of these patients *within the first 24 hours* and is usually a result of shock, electrolyte imbalance, underlying disease, or cerebral edema	Past medical history 　Type II diabetes mellitus 　Total parenteral nutrition 　Chronic steroid therapy 　Recent stress: Burns, infections Physical assessment This condition can produce significant dehydration, resulting in a 25% loss of total fluid volume. Symptoms may include 　Decreased level of consciousness progressing to coma 　Muscular weakness 　Possible seizures 　Decreased urinary output 　Dry, flushed skin with very poor turgor 　Elevated temperature 　Tachycardia 　Hypotension and shock 　Tachypnea Laboratory data 　Plasma glucose greater than 600 mg/dl 　Serum osmolality greater than 320 mOsm/kg 　BUN greater than 60 mg/dl 　Very high urine glucose, 2% or greater 　Negative urine ketones 　Serum sodium less than 135 mEq/L	Fluid balance will be restored and life-threatening complications associated with a hyperosmolar state will be prevented or minimized

NURSING INTERVENTIONS

1. Vital signs q1h
2. Glasgow coma scale q1h
3. Seizure precautions
4. Administer IV fluids as ordered. IV therapy consists of rapid fluid replacement of up to 10 L in the first 24 hours (Fig. 7–3). If the patient is normotensive, 0.45% normal saline will probably be infused, whereas 0.9% normal saline will be used in hypotensive patients. Because many HHNK patients are elderly with underlying cardiac or renal impairment, close monitoring during fluid replacement is *imperative*. PCWPs

are recommended over CVP readings to more accurately monitor tolerance of the fluid load (normal PCWP is 6–12 cm H_2O; normal CVP is 5–10 cm H_2O). Patients should be carefully watched for signs of fluid overload: Pulmonary rales, edema, elevated blood pressure, and bounding pulse

5. Administer insulin therapy as ordered. Insulin therapy is initiated with caution, as a too rapid decrease in blood glucose can produce a fluid shift, resulting in cerebral edema. HHNK patients tend to be very sensitive to the effects of insulin and should be closely monitored during therapy. Insulin is usually administered IV but may be given SC if circulation is adequate. Small doses of 10–20 U/hr are used until the patient's response to insulin can be assessed
6. Administer potassium replacement therapy as ordered
7. CVP readings or pulmonary artery catheter readings q1h
8. Obtain serum glucose levels q1h
9. Intake and output q1h (urethral catheter necessary)
10. Urine specific gravity q1h
11. Monitor electrolytes: Sodium, potassium, and chloride
12. Assess skin condition every shift: Color, temperature, and turgor (Fig. 7–4)
13. Daily weights

OUTCOME CRITERIA

1. Vital signs will be optimal for the patient
2. Glasgow coma scale scores will be stable or improve
3. Patient will experience no injury or complications as a result of seizures
4. Adequate hydration status will be restored
5. Plasma glucose will be restored and maintained between 70 and 150 mg/dl
6. Potassium will be maintained between 3.5 and 5.0 mEq/L
7. CVP will be restored to 5–10 cm H_2O; PCWP will be restored to 6–12 cm H_2O
8. Urine output will be greater than 30 cc/hr
9. Urine specific gravity will be restored to a range of 1.010 to 1.030
10. Directional trends in sodium and potassium levels will be promptly identified
11. Changes in skin condition will be promptly identified
12. Weight will be optimal for the patient

DOCUMENTATION

- Vital signs q1h
- Glasgow coma scale scores q1h
- Seizure precautions taken, presence or absence of seizures, including type, duration, and residual impairment
- IV fluid therapy as ordered, including type, volume, and rate of solutions infused
- Insulin therapy as ordered. Type, dosage, and route of insulin administered should be noted
- Potassium replacement therapy as ordered, including dosage and route of administration
- CVP or PCWP readings q1h. Type of reading taken (CVP or PCWP) should be noted
- Serum glucose levels drawn, with results
- Intake and output q1h
- Urine specific gravity q1h
- Electrolyte values drawn, with results
- Skin condition on arrival to unit, then every shift
- Weight on admission, then daily

Documentation of directional trends, abnormalities, and other changes will include notification of physician, any interventions taken, and patient's response to therapy.

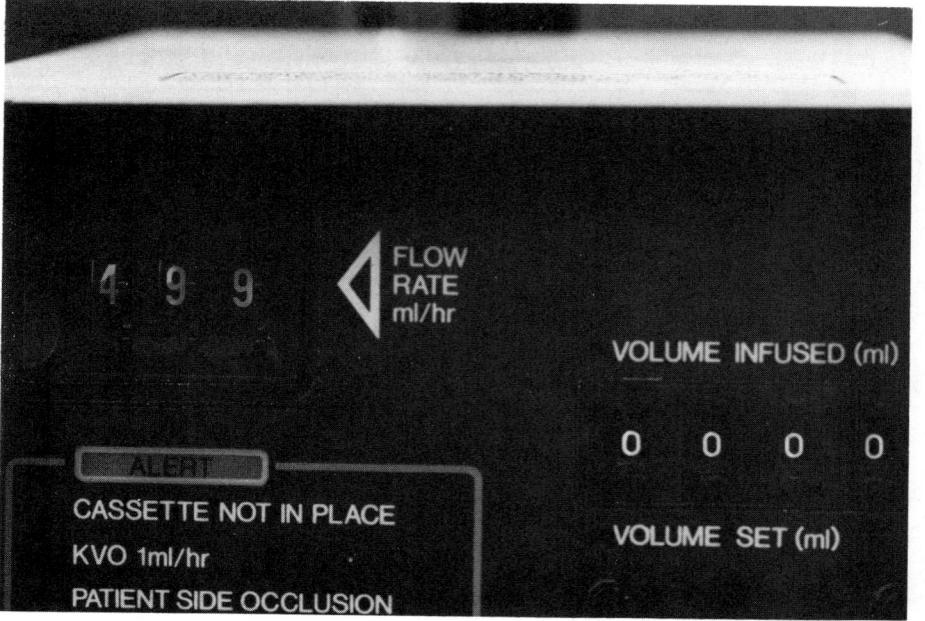

Figure 7–3. Use of a volume control infusion pump is necessary for accurate and rapid administration of large fluid volumes.

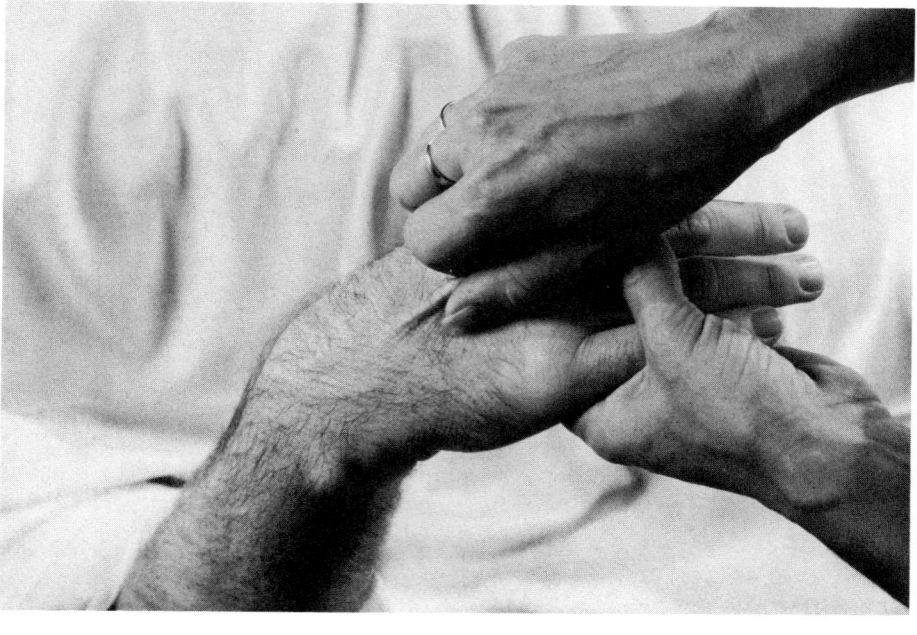

Figure 7–4. Skin turgor can provide valuable information regarding current hydration status.

Care of the Patient Requiring Therapy for Diabetes Insipidus

NURSING DIAGNOSIS	RATIONALE	DEFINING CHARACTERISTICS	EXPECTED OUTCOME

Fluid volume, alteration in, deficit, actual	Diabetes insipidus (DI) is a disorder resulting either from insufficient secretion of antidiuretic hormone (ADH) or from the inability of the renal tubules to respond to circulating ADH (nephrogenic DI). This condition is characterized by severe polyuria, sometimes exceeding 10 L/day, and polydipsia. Precipitating causes are surgical procedures involving the pituitary or hypothalamus, pituitary or hypothalamic lesions, and severe head injuries
	
	Uncontrolled diabetes insipidus can rapidly lead to dehydration, significant weight loss, hypovolemia, and a hyperosmolar state despite fluid intake. Recognition and prompt treatment are essential to prevent these life-threatening complications.
		Past medical history
		  Hypophysectomy
		  Head trauma
		  Surgical manipulation of pituitary or hypothalamus glands
		  Cerebral edema, postoperative or posttraumatic
		Physical assessment
		  Dramatically increased urine output (up to 15 L/day) (Fig. 7–5)
		  Extreme thirst
		  Dry skin with poor turgor
		  Weight loss (up to 5 pounds/day)
		  Hypotension
		Laboratory data*
		  Urine specific gravity less than 1.005
		  Elevated plasma osmolality, greater than 287 mOsm/kg
		  Elevated serum sodium, greater than 145 mEq/L
		
		*Water deprivation tests are often used to differentiate between diabetes insipidus and other types of polyuria. In diabetes insipidus, urine osmolality remains the same despite dehydration.
			Circulating levels of ADH and fluid volume will be restored to normal

NURSING INTERVENTIONS

1. Vital signs q1h
2. Intake and output q1h (urethral catheter as indicated)
3. Urine specific gravity q1h (Fig. 7–6)
4. Administer vasopressin therapy as ordered
   A. Available preparations
      Aqueous vasopressin: SC or IM routes; duration of action is 3–6 hours with onset in 30–60 minutes
      Vasopressin tannate in oil: IM route; duration of action is 24–72 hours. Critical that the active ingredient be properly suspended through warming and gentle agitation of vial—roll between palms, do *not* shake
      Lysine vasopressin spray: Intranasal route; duration of action is 4 hours. Poorly absorbed through inflamed nasal mucosa, can cause rise in blood pressure and upper respiratory infections
      Deamino-D-arginine vasopressin spray (DDAVP): Intranasal route; duration of action is 8–24 hours.

Absorption can occur through inflamed nasal mucosa; very few side effects

Aqueous vasopressin is preferred in the critical care setting due to short duration of action that allows for recognition of returning posterior pituitary function and prevention of water intoxication in patients receiving IV fluids. Vasopressin IV drip is also being used in some institutions to provide better control of DI in patients with head trauma

   B. Guidelines for administration (by physician order only)

      Urine output greater than 200 ml/hr for 2 or more hours

      Urine specific gravity less than 1.005

      Serum sodium greater than 145 mEq/L

      Excessive thirst

5. Monitor for adverse reactions to vasopressin therapy

   A. The primary side effect of vasopressin therapy is water intoxication, which is evidenced by weight gain, weakness, decreased level of consciousness, headache, bounding pulse, elevated blood pressure, generalized seizures, or coma

   B. Nausea and abdominal cramping may also occur and can be minimized by oral intake of one to two glasses of water at the time of vasopressin administration

   C. Nephrogenic DI is not always responsive to vasopressin therapy and can be treated with thiazides and other diuretics

6. Monitor serum sodium levels (usually q2h)

7. Administer IV fluid therapy as ordered (critical care patients are often unable to tolerate oral intake)

8. Balance output with comparable intake, every shift (as ordered by physician)

9. Assess for presence of thirst mechanism

10. Assess and monitor skin condition every shift

11. Daily weights

OUTCOME CRITERIA

1. Vital signs will be optimal for the patient
2. Urine output will be less than 200 cc/hr
3. Urine specific gravity will be maintained between 1.010 and 1.030
4. Vasopressin will be administered correctly
5. Side effects of vasopressin therapy will be promptly recognized and controlled or eliminated
6. Directional trends in serum sodium values will be promptly identified
7. Hydration status will remain optimal for the patient
8. Intake will be equal to urinary output for each shift
9. Presence or absence of thirst will be identified
10. Skin condition changes will be promptly identified
11. Directional weight changes will be identified

DOCUMENTATION

- Vital signs q1h
- Intake and output q1h. If patient has a urethral catheter, this should be noted
- Urine specific gravity q1h, with results
- Vasopressin therapy as ordered, including type, dosage, and route of administration
- Any adverse reactions to vasopressin therapy
- Serum sodium levels drawn, with results

(continued)

- IV fluid therapy as ordered, including type, volume, and rate of solutions infused
- Compensatory intake as ordered, with type and volume of fluid given
- Presence or absence of thirst mechanism to be assessed every shift
- Skin condition on arrival to unit, then every shift
- Weight on admission, then daily

Documentation of directional trends, abnormalities, and other changes will include notification of physician, any interventions taken, and patient's response to therapy.

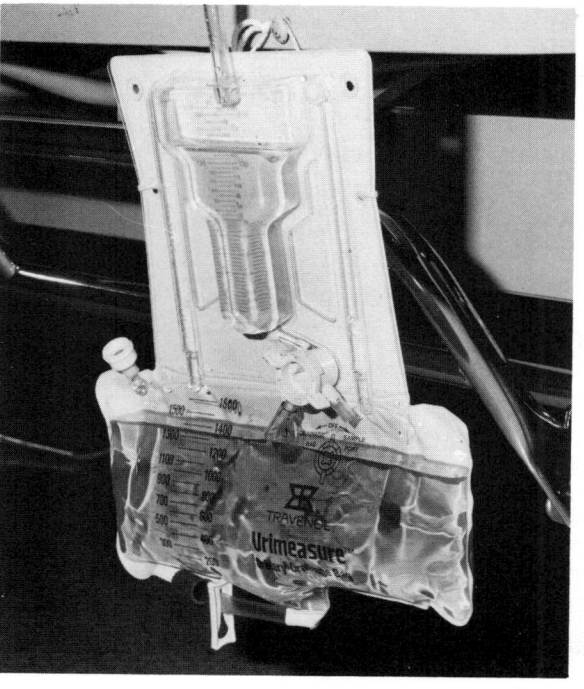

Figure 7–5. Dramatically increased urine output is a hallmark of diabetes insipidus.

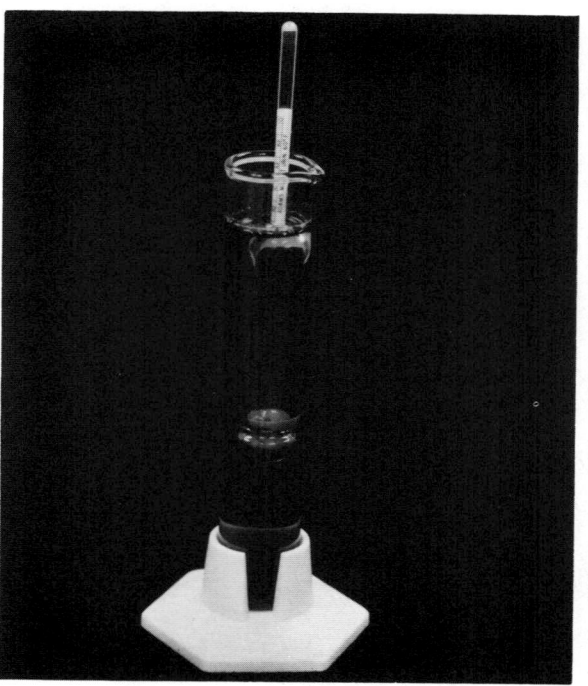

Figure 7–6. Urimeters can be used at the bedside to determine urine specific gravity.

Care of the Patient Requiring Therapy for Syndrome of Inappropriate Antidiuretic Hormone

NURSING DIAGNOSIS	RATIONALE	DEFINING CHARACTERISTICS	EXPECTED OUTCOME

Fluid volume, alteration in, overload, actual	Antidiuretic hormone is responsible for regulating the delicate water balance necessary for the maintenance of adequate fluid volume. Whenever body fluids become volume depleted, as in dehydration, or concentrated, as in elevated serum glucose or sodium, the pituitary gland responds by releasing ADH. This increase in ADH signals the kidneys to reabsorb more fluid through increased renal tubule permeability. Volume expansion occurs and is detected by pressor receptors in the major vessels, and ADH production decreases. Syndrome of inappropriate ADH secretion (SIADH) is the continuous secretion of ADH unrelated to fluid volume, which leads to water intoxication and serum sodium dilution. Precipitating factors may include hemorrhage, head trauma, surgical procedures, and certain types of tumors. Complications of severe water intoxication and hyponatremia include seizures, coma, and death. Prompt recognition and intervention are necessary to prevent the occurrence of these complications.	Past medical history
		  CNS disorders (subdural hematoma, brain tumors, cerebral vascular thrombosis) or head trauma
		  Ectopic ADH production (lung malignancies)
		  Drug therapy (morphine, barbiturates, thiazide diuretics)
		  Intermittent positive pressure breathing (IPPB) therapy (stimulates ADH secretion)
		Physical assessment
		  Decreased level of consciousness
		  Seizures
		  Lethargy
		  Diminished reflexes
		  Hyperventilation
		  Headache, nausea, and cramps
		  Decreased urine output to less than 600 ml/24 hr
		  Dry skin with poor turgor
		  Unusual thirst
		  Weight gain
		Laboratory data
		  Serum sodium less than 130 mEq/L
		  Urine sodium greater than 20 mEq/L
		  Serum chloride less than 95 mEq/L
		  Serum osmolality less than 280 mOsm/kg
		  Urine specific gravity greater than 1.030
			Electrolyte balance will be restored to optimal level

NURSING INTERVENTIONS

1. Vital signs q1h (potential for cardiovascular overload)
2. Glasgow coma scale q2h
3. Intake and output q1h (urethral catheter as indicated)
4. Restrict oral fluid intake to 800–1000 ml/day
5. Urine specific gravity q1h
6. Monitor serum osmolality daily
7. Monitor serum sodium daily
8. Administer diuretics as ordered: Furosemide (Lasix) or mannitol IV bolus
9. With furosemide administration, monitor for potassium depletion (ECG monitoring)

10. Administer sodium replacements as ordered: Oral (high-sodium liquids) and IV fluids (hypertonic saline infused over several hours). Infusion of 3–5% hypertonic saline solution over 2–4 hours is often the method of choice to correct serious hyponatremia. Patients receiving rapid saline infusions must be monitored carefully for signs of volume overload, especially when they are elderly or have a history of CHF. Simultaneous administration of diuretics will decrease chance of fluid overload
11. Monitor CVP and PCWP q1h
12. Monitor skin condition every shift: Color, turgor, edema
13. Daily weights

OUTCOME CRITERIA

1. Vital signs will be optimal for the patient
2. Glasgow coma scale scores will be stable or improve
3. Urine output will be greater than 30 cc/hr
4. Oral intake will be limited to less than 1000 ml/24 hr
5. Urine specific gravity will be restored to range of 1.010 to 1.030, and directional trends will be promptly identified
6. Serum osmolality will be restored to range of 280 to 295 mOsm/kg, and directional trends will be promptly identified
7. Directional trends in serum sodium will be promptly identified
8. Decrease in fluid volume will be accomplished
9. Serum potassium will remain at greater than 3.5 mEq/L, and directional trends will be promptly identified
10. Serum sodium will be restored to range of 135 to 145 mEq/L
11. Complications associated with pulmonary edema will be absent or minimized
12. Skin condition changes will be promptly identified
13. Directional weight changes will be promptly identified

DOCUMENTATION

- Vital signs q1h
- Glasgow coma scale scores q2h
- Intake and output q1h. Presence of urethral catheter should be noted, if applicable
- Oral fluid restrictions, indicating amount of restriction for 24 hours and for each shift
- Urine specific gravity q1h
- Serum osmolality drawn, with results
- Serum sodium levels drawn, with results (Fig. 7–7)
- Diuretic therapy as ordered, including drug, dosage, and route given
- Serum potassium levels drawn, with results
- Sodium replacement therapy
   Oral: Type, volume of fluid administered
   IV: Type, rate, volume of solution given
- Bilateral breath sounds q4h; presence or absence of rales or rhonchi, location of rales, presence or absence of decreased breath sounds should be noted
- Skin condition on arrival at unit, then every shift
- Weight on arrival, then daily

Documentation of directional trends, abnormalities, and other changes will include notification of physician, any interventions taken, and patient's response to therapy.

(continued)

SPECIAL NOTE

Serum Osmolality

Serum osmolality can be calculated at the bedside using the following formula:

$$2(Na + K) + \frac{BUN}{2.7} + \frac{Glucose}{18}$$

The values obtained by using this formula are approximately 5% greater than those obtained through conventional laboratory methods.

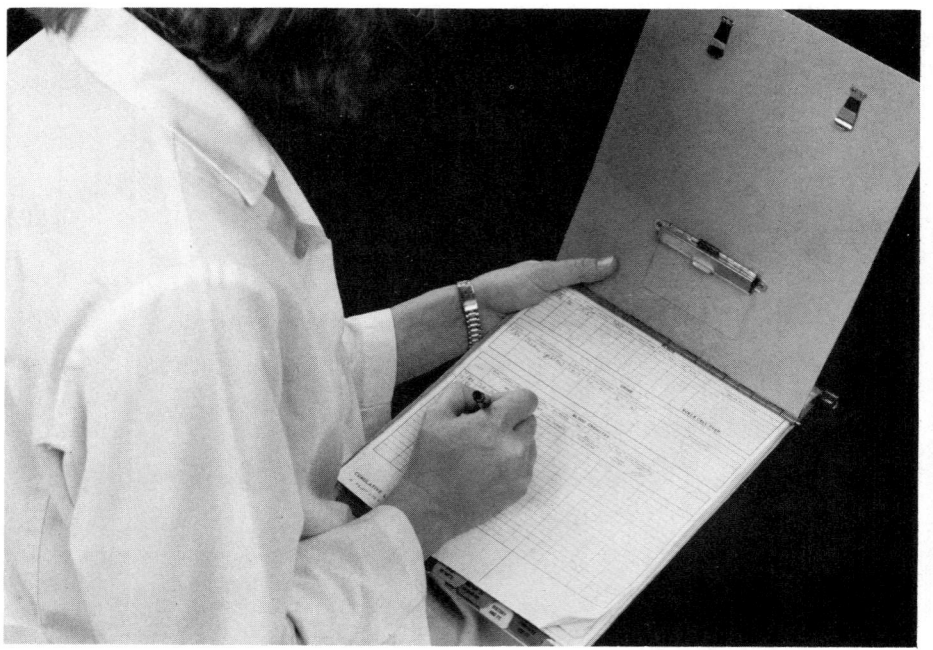

Figure 7–7. Charting laboratory results on flowsheets can assist the nurse in determining trends and current status.

Care of the Patient Requiring Therapy for Myxedema Coma

NURSING DIAGNOSIS	RATIONALE	DEFINING CHARACTERISTICS	EXPECTED OUTCOME

Metabolism, alteration in: decreased	Thyroid hormone functions regulate the metabolic activities of the body and affect all body systems. Myxedema coma is the serious and extreme end result of hypothyroidism, with a mortality rate approaching 70%. Respiratory failure remains the major cause of death. A frequent finding is previously undetected, chronic hypothyroidism, which after a precipitating event, such as infection, surgery, or exposure to cold, results in a state of coma. Severely hypothyroid patients are unable to metabolize drugs properly and are very susceptible to overdoses and toxicity reactions, further increasing the risk of coma	Past medical history
		  Thyroidectomy or thyroid irradiation
		  Head injury
		  Iodine deficiency
		  Pituitary or hypothalamic disease or ablation
		Physical assessment
		  Mental depression
		  Hypothermia, less than 90°F, cold intolerance
		  Hypotension
		  Bradycardia
		  ECG changes: Flat T-wave, prolonged PR interval
		  Hypoventilation
		  Decreased urine output
		  Diminished reflexes with delayed relaxation phase in deep tendon reflexes
		  Weakness
		  Dry, rough skin with nonpitting facial edema
		Laboratory data
		  Decreased T_3 resin uptake; less than 25% (depends on resin used)
		  Increased thyroid-stimulating hormone (TSH); greater than 0.2 μ/ml
		  Decreased T_4 (normal range varies)
		  Decreased glucose; less than 110 mg/dl
		  Hyponatremia; less than 130 mEq/dl
			Metabolic function will be restored to normal level

NURSING INTERVENTIONS

1. Vital signs q1h
2. Glasgow coma scale q2h
3. Continuous ECG monitoring
4. Ventilatory assistance as required to maintain adequate respiration (Fig. 7–8)
5. Administer IV fluids as ordered. Administration of IV solutions, such as 5% dextrose in saline, will usually correct any glucose deficits that exist. IV therapy should be instituted with care, especially in elderly patients, to avoid the development of CHF. Use of an infusion pump is recommended
6. Administer pressor agents, such as dopamine, as ordered to maintain blood pressure
7. Administer thyroid medications as ordered. Prompt thyroid hormone replacement is essential and usually accomplished through IV administration of L-thyroxine or T_4. Usual dosage is 500 μg IV bolus, with subsequent maintenance doses of 50–100 μg IV bolus daily until patient is able to tolerate oral forms of

thyroid replacement. The potential risk of rapid increase in metabolic rate, which can stress cardiac reserves and precipitate CHF, dysrhythmias, or angina, must be weighed against the high mortality rate associated with lack of treatment. Signs and symptoms of thyroid hormone overdose include tachycardia, diaphoresis, anxiety, nervousness, insomnia or inability to maintain sleep states

8. Administer cortisol as ordered. Administration of a soluble hydrocortisone (Solu-Cortef) is recommended to cover the patient until cortisol levels can be established. Institution of rapid thyroid replacement and subsequent rise in metabolic rate in patients with underlying hypothalamic or pituitary hypothyroidism can promote adrenal crisis. Usual dosage is hydrocortisone 100 mg q6h IV
9. CVP readings q2h
10. Strict intake and output q1h (urethral catheter as indicated)
11. Auscultate heart sounds q4h (potential for cardiac tamponade)
12. Keep patient warm (gradual passive measures, such as blankets)
13. Monitor for drug toxicity related to hypometabolism of drugs. Hypometabolism can potentiate the action of many drugs, especially analgesics, sedatives, and anesthetics. In addition, drug dosage requirements are usually decreased for such drugs as digoxin and insulin. Patients should be constantly monitored for symptoms of overdose and toxicity for any drugs administered. Also, remember that drug requirements will change as the patient returns to a euthyroid state
14. Assess skin condition every shift: Color, temperature, edema, texture
15. Monitor electrolytes
16. Monitor blood glucose levels

OUTCOME CRITERIA

1. Vital signs will be optimal for the patient
2. Glasgow coma scale scores will be stable or improved
3. Cardiac rhythm disturbances will be promptly identified
4. Respiratory rate will be maintained at greater than 12/min with a volume of 6 L/min
5. Blood glucose will be maintained between 70 and 110 mg/dl, and adequate hydration will be restored
6. Blood pressure will be maintained greater than 100/70
7. Thyroid hormone levels will return to normal range, and side effects of thyroid medications will be promptly identified
8. Cortisol levels will return to range of 2 to 27 μg/100 ml
9. CVP will be maintained between 5 and 10 cm H_2O, and directional trends will be promptly identified
10. Urine output will be greater than 30 cc/hr
11. Indications of cardiac tamponade will be promptly identified
12. Symptoms of drug toxicity will be promptly identified
13. Skin condition changes will be recognized
14. Directional trends in electrolytes will be identified
15. Directional trends in blood glucose levels will be promptly identified

DOCUMENTATION

- Vital signs q1h
- Glasgow coma scale scores q2h
- ECG q2h, with rhythm strips to document abnormalities
- Ventilatory assistance, with time initiated, initial respiratory assessment, type, volume, rate of respirator, and any changes in settings
- IV fluid therapy as ordered, including type, volume, and rate of fluid administered
- Administration of pressor agents as ordered, including drug, dosage, and route of administration
- Administration of thyroid medications as ordered, including drug, dosage, and route of administration
- Cortisol administration as ordered, including drug, dosage, and route of administration
- Initial CVP reading, then q2h

(continued)

- Intake and output q1h, noting presence of urethral catheter if applicable
- Cardiac auscultation with initial heart sounds, then q4h
- Any warming measures taken, including type of passive warming device used and temperature setting of room
- Any signs or symptoms of drug toxicity as they occur
- Skin condition on arrival to unit, then every shift
- Electrolyte values drawn, with results
- Blood glucose levels drawn, with results

Documentation of directional trends, abnormalities, and other changes will include notification of physician, any interventions taken, and patient's response to therapy.

SPECIAL NOTE

Thyroid Function Results

Thyroid function studies can be distorted by the following factors:

- Hemolysis of the blood sample
- Drugs, such as steroids, propranolol, estrogen or oral contraceptives, and large doses of aspirin
- Pregnancy
- Topical iodine solutions
- IV contrast media (iodine dyes)
- High dietary iodine intake

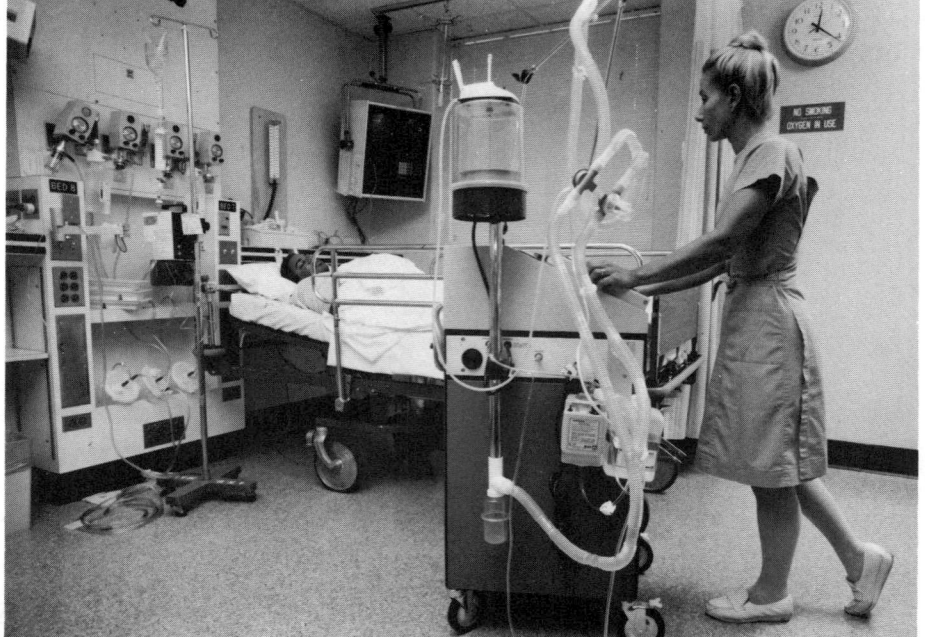

Figure 7–8. Ventilatory assistance is frequently required for patients with myxedema coma to maintain adequate respiratory function.

Care of the Patient Requiring Therapy
for Thyrotoxic Crisis

NURSING DIAGNOSIS	RATIONALE	DEFINING CHARACTERISTICS	EXPECTED OUTCOME

Metabolism, alteration in: increased	Thyrotoxic crisis or thyroid storm, is a medical emergency characterized by multi-system decompensation secondary to severe hyperthyroidism. Metabolic functions are accelerated and central nervous system, cardiovascular and gastrointestinal abnormalities are frequently present.
	
	Thyrotoxic crisis occurs most often in undiagnosed hyperthyroid patients who are experiencing a major stress, such as infection, trauma, or surgery, but may develop spontaneously.
	
	Prompt treatment of this syndrome is essential to prevent development of coma, shock, and death. Therapeutic intervention should be initiated immediately, even if thyroid levels have not been confirmed.
		Past medical history
		  Recent major stress: Physiological or psychological
		  Thyroid replacement therapy
		  Manipulation and palpation of thyroid gland
		  Premature or abrupt cessation of antithyroid medications
		Physical assessment
		  Hyperthermia greater than 100°F, with diaphoretic, flushed skin
		  Hypertension
		  Tachycardia, palpitations, S_3
		  Cardiac dysrhythmias
		  Extreme agitation, anxiety
		  Quick, jerky movements, tremors
		  Altered mental status: Delirium or psychosis
		  Increased gastric motility with nausea, vomiting, diarrhea, and cramps
		  Goiter
		  Recent significant weight loss
		Laboratory data
		  Increased serum T_3
		  Normal to increased T_4
		  Increased thyroid I-131 uptake
		  Decreased plasma cortisol: Less than 5 μg/100 ml in the morning; less than 2 μg/100 ml in the evening
		  Increased blood glucose: Greater than 150 mg/dl
		  Abnormal liver function studies
		
		Since thyroid hormone values are similar, if not identical, in both thyrotoxic crisis and hyperthyroidism, it is important to note that diagnosis of thyrotoxic crisis is based primarily on clinical signs and symptoms, which will be dramatically increased over those of hyperthyroidism.
			Metabolic function will be stabilized

1. Vital signs q1h. Rectal temperatures q1h or by continuous probe monitoring
2. Glasgow coma scale q4h
3. Continuous ECG monitoring
4. Administer antithyroid medications as ordered
   A. Sodium iodide: Given PO or IM, inhibits thyroid hormone release, lowers basal metabolic rate and decreases heart rate. Is not used in cases of acute thyroid hormone poisoning. Drug dosages may vary depending on the patient's metabolic state
   B. Lithium; Given PO, is the drug of choice for patients with iodine sensitivity. Inhibits thyroid hormone release. Potential for toxicity is great due to the narrow dosage safety margin. Dosage is 300–600 mg PO up to 4 times daily depending on serum lithium levels. Symptoms of toxicity include diarrhea, vomiting, weakness, lethargy, and incoordination
   C. Propylthiouracil (PTU): Given PO or by lavage, blocks the synthesis of thyroid hormone within approximately 1 hour of administration and, therefore, should be given 1 hour before iodine therapy is initiated. Also aids in inhibiting conversion of T_4 to T_3. Sudden withdrawal of PTU can cause thyroid storm. Dosage is 300–400 mg q8h and is decreased as necessary as patient improves
   Beta-blocking drugs, such as propranolol, are used as supportive therapy to prevent cardiac failure but also inhibit conversion of T_4 to T_3
5. Decrease temperature through use of cooling devices or antipyretics as ordered. (*Note:* Aspirin should *not* be used, since it prevents binding of thyroid hormones. Also note that shivering increases metabolic rate and body temperature; muscle-relaxing drugs can be prescribed to decrease incidence of shivering)
6. Administer insulin therapy as ordered. Increased metabolic rate accelerates glycogenolysis and may cause insulin resistance and impaired secretion. Treatment may not be used for mild hyperglycemia; IV or SC regular insulin can be used to control significant glucose elevations. Dosage will vary with degree of hyperglycemia
7. Administer IV fluids as ordered. Patients in thyrotoxic crisis can develop either fluid deficit or fluid overload due to rapid metabolic rates and subsequent therapy. IV infusion rates should therefore be controlled by infusion pumps and closely monitored, especially in elderly patients and those with renal or cardiac disease. IV solutions of 5% dextrose in saline are normally infused at a rate of 100–150 cc/hr
8. CVP readings q1h
9. Strict intake and output
10. Obtain and monitor serum glucose levels q1h
11. Urine glucose and ketones q2h
12. Urine specific gravity every shift
13. Assess and monitor skin condition every shift
14. Daily weights

1. Vital signs will be optimal for the patient
2. Glasgow coma scale scores will be stable or improved
3. Cardiac rhythm will be normal
4. Thyroid hormone levels will be stable
5. Temperature will be reduced to normal range
6. Blood glucose will be maintained between 70 and 100 mg/dl
7. Adequate hydration will be maintained
8. CVP will be maintained between 5 and 10 cm H_2O, and changes will be promptly identified
9. Urine output will be greater than 30 cc/hr
10. Directional trends in blood glucose levels will be promptly identified
11. Urine glucose and ketones will return to negative state
12. Specific gravity will be restored to a range of 1.010 to 1.030
13. Skin condition changes will be recognized
14. Directional weight changes will be promptly identified

(continued)

DOCUMENTATION

- Vital signs q1h. Use of a continuous probe monitor should be included, if applicable
- Glasgow coma scale scores q2h
- ECG every shift, with initial rhythm and any changes in rhythm supported by rhythm strips
- Administration of antithyroid medications as ordered. Drug, dosage, and route used should be included
- Measures to decrease temperature, including type of cooling devices used, date and time initiated, and presence or absence of shivering
- Insulin therapy as ordered. Should include type, dosage, and route of insulin given
- IV fluid therapy as ordered, with type, volume, and rate of solution infused
- Initial CVP reading, then q1h
- Intake and output q1h
- Serum glucose levels drawn, with results
- Urine testing done, with results
- Urine specific gravity done, with results
- Skin condition on admission, then every shift
- Weight on arrival, then daily

Documentation of directional trends, abnormalities, and other changes will include notification of physician, any interventions taken, and patient's response to therapy.

Care of the Patient Requiring Therapy for Adrenal Crisis

NURSING DIAGNOSIS	RATIONALE	DEFINING CHARACTERISTICS	EXPECTED OUTCOME
Tissue perfusion, alteration in: decreased	Adrenal crisis occurs when there is a severe shortage of glucocorticoids and mineralocorticoids in the body. Decreased cortisol levels lead to alterations in water and sodium balance, glucose metabolism, and production of digestive enzymes. Risk of vascular collapse and shock in these patients is high, with volume depletion often approaching 20% of total body fluid volume. Precipitating factors include surgery, trauma, infection, or other forms of stress	Past medical history Addison's disease (chronic adrenal insufficiency) Change in chronic steroid therapy Recent stress: Physiological or psychological Surgical removal of pituitary or adrenal glands Physical assessment Hypotension or shock Tachycardia Weak, rapid pulse Cardiac dysrhythmias or ECG changes: Peaked T-waves, widened QRS complex, diminished P-wave, lengthening PR interval Elevated temperature Dry skin with poor turgor Oliguria, anuria Anorexia Nausea, vomiting, diarrhea, and cramps Muscle weakness, lethargy Diminished reflexes Constant headache Depression, irritability, anxiety Hyperpigmentation of the skin creases, joints, lips, gums, or buccal mucosa Laboratory data Decreased plasma cortisol: Less than 5 µg/100 ml in the morning; less than 2 µg/100 ml in the evening Decreased blood glucose: Less than 65 mg/dl Decreased serum sodium: Less than 130 mEq/L Elevated serum potassium: Greater than 5.0 mEq/L Increased BUN: Greater than 24 mg/dl Increased serum calcium: Greater than 10.5 mg/dl	Restoration of cortisol level and fluid balance to normal

1. Obtain blood for cortisol, ACTH levels immediately, then as ordered by physician
2. Vital signs q15min until stable, then q1h until crisis resolved
3. Continuous ECG monitoring for dysrhythmias
4. CVP or PCWP readings q1h
5. Administer fluid replacement as ordered. Usual fluid replacement therapy consists of 5% dextrose in saline at rapid infusion rates, with the patient receiving as much as 1–2 L over the first 2 hours. Infusion rates depend largely upon the patient's response to rapid volume expansion. Fluid replacement therapy will be regulated according to patient's volume status, hemodynamic response, and restoration of sodium and glucose levels
6. Administer glucocorticoid therapy as ordered. Administration of glucocorticoids usually begins with hydrocortisone (Solu-Cortef) 100–200 mg IV push. In addition, IV fluids will usually contain 100 mg hydrocortisone/L. Physicians may order an IM injection of cortisone acetate 100 mg to provide additional coverage in the event of erratic IV absorption or infiltration. Supplemental mineralocorticoids, such as deoxycorticosterone, are usually unnecessary, since large doses of steroids will provide adequate mineralocorticoid effects. Glucocorticoid therapy will be tapered on a daily basis depending on response to therapy and the presence or absence of infection or other stressors. Steroid therapy can cause the following side effects: Amenorrhea, edema, headache, gastrointestinal distress, alopecia, and mood swings. The physician should be alerted to these signs so that steroid dosage can be adjusted.
7. Intake and output q1h (urethral catheter as indicated)
8. Place patient in standard shock position (unless contraindicated, as in patients with increased intracranial pressure)
9. Glasgow coma scale q2h
10. Monitor electrolytes, especially potassium
11. Monitor ABGs for acidosis (pH less than 7.35, bicarbonate less than 15)
12. Assess and monitor skin condition every shift
13. Daily weights

OUTCOME CRITERIA

1. Abnormal cortisol levels will be promptly identified and interventions initiated
2. Vital sign changes will be promptly identified and reported to physician
3. Cardiac rhythm disturbances will be promptly identified and interventions taken for correction
4. CVP readings will be restored to a range of 5 to 10 ml H_2O, and changes will be promptly identified
5. Glucose will be maintained between 70 and 100 mg/dl
   Adequate hydration will be restored
6. Cortisol levels will be restored to range of 2 to 27 µg/100 ml
7. Urine output will be greater than 30 cc/hr
8. Adequate perfusion of major organs will be maintained
9. Glasgow coma scale scores will remain stable or improve
10. Directional trends in electrolytes will be promptly identified
11. Arterial pH will remain above 7.35, and changes will be promptly identified
12. Changes in skin condition will be identified
13. Weight changes will be promptly noted

DOCUMENTATION

- Plasma cortisol and ACTH levels drawn on arrival, with results, then as ordered
- Vital signs as ordered
- ECG every shift, with initial rhythm and any changes in rhythm supported by rhythm strips
- Initial CVP or PCWP reading, then readings q1h. Type of reading (CVP vs PCWP) should be included
- IV fluid therapy as ordered, with type, rate, and volume of solution infused
- Glucocorticoid therapy as ordered. Drug, dosage, and route of administration should be noted

(continued)

- Intake and output q1h, with notation of urethral catheter, if applicable
- Use of shock position, with time initiated. Any complicating factors that negate shock position should be noted
- Glasgow coma scale scores q2h
- Electrolyte values drawn, with results
- ABGs drawn, with results
- Skin condition on arrival, then every shift
- Weight on admission, then daily

Documentation of directional trends, abnormalities, and other changes will include notification of physician, any interventions taken, and patient's response to therapy.

SPECIAL NOTE

Oral Contraception

Patients receiving oral contraceptives also may have many of the side effects produced by steroid overdose.

Long-term Steroid Therapy

All patients on long-term steroid therapy should carry emergency medical identification (such as Medic-Alert tag or card), stating disease, drug, and physician to notify.

Care of the Patient Requiring Therapy for Hypocalcemic Crisis

NURSING DIAGNOSIS	RATIONALE	DEFINING CHARCTERISTICS	EXPECTED OUTCOME

Injury, potential for: tetany	Hypocalcemic crisis is a medical emergency seen with increasing frequency in the critical care setting.
	
	A decrease in serum calcium causes neuromuscular irritability that correlates directly with the degree of hypocalcemia. This deficiency usually presents as tetany, and the cause may be apparent, as in parathyroid or thyroid surgery, or obscure, such as with malabsorption syndromes or hypoparathyroidism.
	
	Prompt recognition and therapy are essential to prevent the development of hypotension, seizures, laryngeal spasms, and cardiac arrythmias.
		Past medical history
		  Recent neck surgery (thyroid, parathyroid, laryngeal cancer)
		  Multiple blood transfusions (caused by precipitation of serum ionized calcium)
		  Nephrotic syndrome
		  Drug therapy
		  Hepatic disease
		Physical assessment
		  ECG changes: Prolonged QT interval (correct for heart rate, age, and sex), inverted T-wave
		  Central and peripheral nervous system changes: Seizures, hyperactive reflexes, paresthesias of the hands and feet
		  Carpopedal spasms
		  Muscular weakness, cramps
		  Circumoral numbness or tingling
		  Decreased level of consciousness or changes in mental status
		Laboratory data
		  Decreased ionized calcium: Less than 4.6 mEq/L (or 3.2 mg/dl)*
		  Decreased total serum calcium: Less than 9 mg/dl
		  Elevated serum phosphorus: Greater than 2.6 mEq/L (or 4.5 mg/dl)*
		Drugs, such as heparin, insulin, and magnesium salts, can cause difficulty in obtaining a correct measurement of serum calcium.
		
		*Since several assays are available, more than one value may be shown.
			Symptoms of tetany will be alleviated through restoration and maintenance of normal calcium level

NURSING INTERVENTIONS

1. Vital signs q1h
2. Obtain baseline serum calcium level, then monitor calcium levels q4–6h for duration of calcium therapy
3. Continuous ECG monitoring for dysrhythmias
4. Administer IV calcium replacement as ordered. Two forms of parenteral calcium are currently used: calcium chloride and calcium gluconate. Calcium can be administered either as a slow IV bolus of 1–2 amps

10% calcium gluconate or as an IV infusion of 2 amps 10% calcium gluconate in 100 ml D_5W infused over 15 minutes. In either case, the patient should be carefully monitored for signs and symptoms of hypercalcemia, since the calcium level will rise quickly and tend to fluctuate. IV sites should be checked frequently, since infiltration of calcium salts can produce necrosis and sloughing of tissues (Fig. 7–9). Special attention should be given to patients receiving digitalis and calcium salts concurrently, since these drugs are synergistic and will produce increased inotropic and toxic effects

5. Glasgow coma scale q1h
6. Assess reflexes every shift
7. Assess for Trousseau's and Chvostek's sign every shift. Trousseau's sign is the presence of carpopedal spasms related to decreased blood flow to the extremities. It can be elicited by placing a tourniquet on the upper arm for several minutes. The presence of spasm is indicative of a positive sign (Fig. 7–10). Chvostek's sign is a reflex produced by neuromuscular irritability and may be an early indication of hypocalcemia. To elicit this sign, gently tap the area in front of the ear just over the facial nerve and observe for twitching of the facial muscles (Fig. 7–11). Twitching is indicative of a positive reflex
8. Monitor electrolytes

OUTCOME CRITERIA

1. Vital signs will be optimal for the patient
2. Baseline calcium level will be obtained within 15 minutes of admission
   Directional trends in calcium levels will be identified
3. Cardiac dysrhythmias will be promptly recognized and interventions initiated
4. Serum calcium will be restored to a range of 9 to 11 mg/100 ml
5. Glasgow coma scale scores will be optimal for the patient
6. Changes in reflexes will be promptly identified
7. Presence or absence of Trousseau's and Chvostek's signs will be recognized and changes will be promptly detected
8. Directional trends in electrolytes will be identified

DOCUMENTATION

- Vital signs q1h
- Baseline calcium level drawn, with results, then calcium levels drawn as ordered, with results
- ECG q2h, with baseline rhythm and any dysrhythmias supported by rhythm strips
- IV calcium therapy as ordered, with drug, dosage, and method of administration (bolus vs infusion)
- Glasgow coma scale scores q1h
- Reflexes assessed on admission, then every shift
- Trousseau's and Chvostek's sign assessed on arrival, then every shift
- Electrolyte values drawn, with results

Documentation of directional trends, abnormalities, and other changes will include notification of physician, any interventions taken, and patient's response to therapy. The use of laboratory flowsheets for recording of sequential laboratory data is invaluable in assessing trends and interpreting success of therapy.

SPECIAL NOTE

Tetany and Tetanus

The spasms of hypocalcemic tetany, occurring in the extremities, can be distinguished from spasms caused by *Clostridium tetani* infection, or tetanus, which produces spasm in the head and neck.

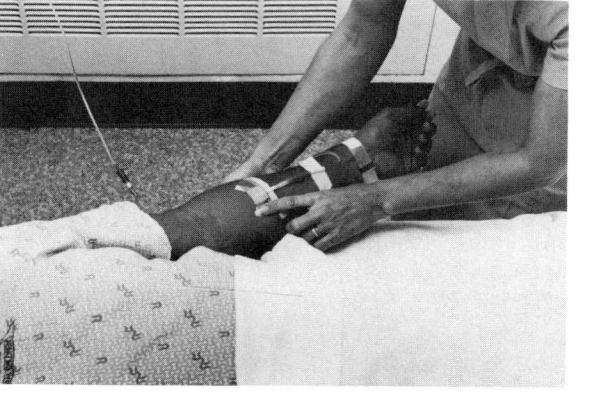

Figure 7–9. IV sites should be closely monitored during infusion of IV calcium to prevent tissue damage related to infiltration of calcium salts.

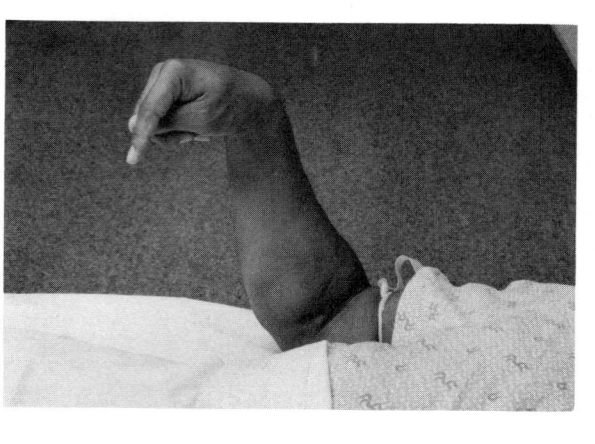

Figure 7–10. Trousseau's sign or carpopedal spasms can be elicited in patients with hypocalcemia by placing a tourniquet on the arm for several minutes.

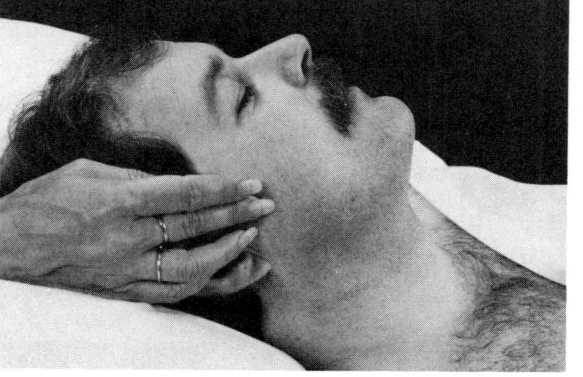

Figure 7–11. Chvostek's sign or twitching of the facial muscles, is an early sign of hypocalcemia.

Care of the Patient Requiring Therapy for Hypercalcemic Crisis

NURSING DIAGNOSIS	RATIONALE	DEFINING CHARACTERISTICS	EXPECTED OUTCOME

Fluid volume, alteration in, potential	Hypercalcemia most commonly occurs in patients with hyperparathyroidism but can occur as a result of malignancies, vitamin D excess, and sensitivity to calcium. Elevated serum calcium levels cause polyuria as the kidneys attempt to rid the body of excess calcium. Dehydration occurs as the renal tubules lose responsiveness to ADH as a result of elevated parathyroid hormone levels, further increasing serum calcium concentrations	Past medical history
		  Hyperparathyroidism
		  Malignancies
		  Hyperthyroidism
		  Increased gastrointestinal absorption of calcium, as in sarcoidosis
		  Excess of vitamin D
		Physical assessment
		  Nausea, vomiting, diarrhea
		  Anorexia
		  Mental confusion, lethargy
		  Muscle atrophy, weakness, or paralysis
		  Coma
		  ECG changes: Shortened QT complex, ventricular dysrhythmias
		  Hypertension
		  Tachycardia
		  Skin condition indicative of dehydration: Warm, dry, poor turgor and mobility
		  Polyuria
		Laboratory data
		  Serum calcium* greater than 12 mg/dl
		  Serum phosphate less than 2.5 mg/dl
		  Urine specific gravity less than 1.005
		  Potassium greater than 3.5 mEq/L
		
		*When decisions to treat are based on laboratory results, it is important to note that since half of the calcium ions are free or ionized and half are bound to plasma proteins, albumin levels and arterial pH must also be evaluated. As arterial pH increases, more calcium binds to protein; as pH decreases, the opposite occurs, with an increase in ionized calcium.
			Calcium levels will be within normal range

NURSING INTERVENTIONS

1. Vital signs q1h
2. Glasgow coma scale q2h
3. Continuous ECG monitoring
4. Administer IV fluids as ordered. IV solution of choice is normal saline (0.9%) infused rapidly, with up to 1 L during the first hour and 4–5 L daily. Patients should be observed closely for signs of fluid overload: Elevated blood pressure, polyuria, bounding pulse

5. Administer diuretics as ordered. IV furosemide (Lasix), given with saline infusion, enhances reduction of serum calcium levels; thiazides should *not* be used, as these enhance hypercalcemia
6. Administer calcium-reducing medications as ordered*
   A. Mithramycin: The most effective for lowering serum calcium through decreased bone resorption. Given in dosages calculated by weight (25 μg/kg IV over 8 hours), will reduce calcium levels within 24–48 hours and maintain reduction for up to 2 weeks. Major side effect is thrombocytopenia, but its incidence is infrequent. Primarily used for hypercalcemia caused by malignancy
   B. Calcitonin: Given SC q12h in dosages of 2–8 SI U/kg, will decrease calcium levels for up to 72 hours. Very effective for hypercalcemia caused by excessive PTH secretion
   C. Other drugs known to lower serum calcium levels include glucocorticoids, salicylates, indomethacin
7. Monitor calcium levels
8. Monitor potassium levels. Patients receiving digitalis should be observed for digitalis toxicity, which may occur with hypokalemia
9. Monitor CVP q1h
10. Intake and output q1h (urethral catheter as indicated)
11. Assess skin condition every shift

OUTCOME CRITERIA

1. Vital signs will be optimal for the patient
2. Glasgow coma scale scores will remain stable or improve
3. Cardiac dysrhythmias will be recognized and interventions initiated
4. IV therapy complications will be detected and controlled
5. Diuretics will be correctly administered
6. Side effects of calcium-reducing medications will be promptly detected and controlled or eliminated. Calcium levels will be restored to a range of 8.5 to 11 mg/dl
7. Directional trends in serum calcium levels will be identified
8. Potassium will be maintained in a range of 3.5 to 5.0 mEq/L. Changes will be promptly recognized
9. CVP will be maintained between 5 and 10 cm H_2O. Changes will be promptly identified
10. Urinary output will be greater than 30 cc/hr
11. Changes in skin condition will be recognized

DOCUMENTATION

- Vital signs q1h
- Glasgow coma scale scores q2h
- ECG every shift and as necessary, with initial rhythm and rhythm changes supported by rhythm strips
- IV fluid therapy as ordered, including type, volume, and rate of solutions infused
- Diuretic therapy as ordered, with time administered, drug, dosage, and route
- Calcium-reducing medications as ordered, with time administered, drug, dosage, and route
- Calcium levels drawn, with results
- Potassium levels drawn, with results
- Initial CVP reading, then readings q1h
- Intake and output q1h, with urethral catheter noted, if applicable
- Skin condition on admission, then every shift

Documentation of directional trends, abnormalities, and other changes will include notification of physician, any interventions taken, and patient's response to therapy.

Patients should be carefully monitored during the calcium-reduction phase, since serum calcium levels can decrease by as much as 25%, resulting in hypocalcemia

Glossary

Azotemia: Increased nitrogen wastes, especially urea, in the blood; also called uremia.

Carpopedal spasms: Spasms of the hands and feet caused by hypocalcemia; can be elicited through use of a tourniquet on extremity for 3–5 minutes.

Chvostek's sign: A hyperactive reflex related to decreased calcium levels; unilateral facial spasm elicited by a slight tap over the facial nerve.

Euthyroid: State of normal thyroid function.

Exophthalmia: Abnormal protrusion of the eyeball, associated with hyperthyroidism.

Gluconeogenesis: The formation of glucose in the liver from proteins and possibly fats; occurs with decreased carbohydrate intake or starvation.

Ionized calcium: Free (or unbound) serum calcium ion, most important calcium fraction to physiological function; measurement tends to be unreliable.

Osmolality: Osmotic concentration that is determined by the number of ions in solution.

Osmolarity: A measure of water concentration; increased osmolarity indicates decreased water concentration.

Paresthesias: Abnormal sensations, such as numbness, tingling, prickling, or a heightened sensitivity.

Polydipsia: Excessive thirst usually resulting in excessive fluid consumption.

Polyphagia: Eating unusually large amounts of food at a meal.

Polyuria: Excessive volume of urine; urine produced is pale in color with a low specific gravity.

Reagent: Any substance possessing a particular chemical action used to measure another substance.

T_3: Triiodothyronine; an amino acid hormone containing iodine secreted by the thyroid.

T_4: Thyroxine; an amino acid hormone containing iodine secreted by the thyroid.

Trousseau's sign: A hyperactive reflex related to decreased calcium levels and manifested as carpopedal spasms.

Bibliography

Adams, C. E. Pulling your patient through an adrenal crisis. *RN*, 1983, *10*, 36–38.

Alspach, J. G., & Williams, S. (Eds.), *Care curriculum for critical care nursing* (3rd ed.). Philadelphia: Saunders, 1985.

Anderson, B. J. Antidiuretic hormone: Balance and imbalance. *Journal of Neurosurgical Nursing*, 1979, *11*(2), 71–73.

Burch, W. M. *Endocrinology for the house officer.* Baltimore: Waverly Press, 1984.

Cavalier, J. P. Crucial decisions in diabetic emergencies. *RN*, 1980, *11*, 32–37.

Coleman, P. Antidiuretic hormone: Physiology and pathophysiology—A review. *Journal of Neurosurgical Nursing*, 1979, *11*(4), 199–203.

Doenges, M. E., Jeffries, M. F., & Moorhouse, M. F. *Nursing care plans,* Philadelphia: F. A. Davis, 1984.

Evangelisti, J. T., & Thorpe, C. J. Thyroid storm—A nursing crisis. *Heart and Lung,* 1983, *12*(23), 184–193.

Freitag, J. L., & Miller, L. W. (Eds.). *Manual of medical therapeutics* (23rd ed.). Boston: Little, Brown, 1980.

Hennessy, K. HHN dehydration. *American Journal of Nursing*, 1983, *10*, 1425–1426.

Hershman, J. M. *Practical endocrinology.* New York: Wiley, 1981.

Honigman, R. E. Thyroid function tests. *Nursing*, 1982, *82*(4), 68–71.

Lane, J., & Pierce, A. G. When persistence pays off. *Nursing*, 1982, *82*(4), 44–47.

McFadden, E. A., Zaloza, G., & Chernow, B. Hypocalcemia: A medical emergency. *American Journal of Nursing*, 1983, *2*, 227–230.

Quinlan, M. Solving the mysteries of calcium imbalance: An action guide. *RN*, 1982, *45*(11), 50–54, 100.

Smith, J. Nursing management of diabetes insipidus. *Journal of Neurosurgical Nursing*, 1979, *11*, 71–73.

Soloman, B. L. The hypothalamus and the pituitary gland. *Nursing Clinics of North America*, 1980, 9, 446–450.

Stock-Barkman, P. Confusing concepts. *Nursing*, 1983, *6*, 33–41.

Wake, M. M., & Bresinger, J. F. The nurse's role in hypothyroidism. *Nursing Clinics of North America*, 1980, *15*(3), 453–467.

8

PSYCHOSOCIAL FACTORS

Kemba D. DeGroot

Assessment of the Pertinent Psychosocial History

RATIONALE

Developing the skill of critically analyzing the patient's psychosocial history will provide the ICU nurse with information essential to gaining a broader perspective on the patient as a whole, to mobilizing strengths and resources, and to anticipating maladaptive coping mechanisms. Often a psychological history on the chart will not be adequate to assess the psychosocial needs of the patient. The ICU nurse may, therefore, need to obtain information through observation of the interactions between visitors, discussions with family members, and conversations with the patient (Fig. 8–1).

PARAMETERS	FINDINGS	IMPLICATIONS FOR NURSING CARE
1. Family history	1. **A.** Family members: Immediate and extended	1. **A.** Patient's relationship with family members (likes and dislikes, dependencies, rivalries, conflicts) affects the level of stress during visiting periods and during discharge planning; indicates to whom the patient may turn for support Patient may use family member who has some similar medical problem as a role model, suggesting the outcome of his or her current condition. The effect depends upon the patient's view of this family member, as well as how others responded to the affected person The patient's reaction to a suicide or mental illness in the family is of more significance than the isolated fact itself
	B. Home environment: Economic class of neighborhood, living arrangements crowded, individual leads a solitary, reclusive existence	**B.** Inadequate privacy or isolation may affect the patient's desire to return home. The patient's need for privacy, if he or she is used to living alone, may be invaded by the ICU setting
	C. Economic considerations: Patient's responsibility for the economic well-being of the family	**C.** Stress over the sacrifice the family may need to make to pay for medical or surgical services can affect the emotional stability of the patient. Patients may be prone to refuse services offered for fear of cost to their loved ones
	D. Ethnic, cultural, and religious traditions: Related to physical and mental illness	**D.** How the family views and responds to illness, such as with superstition or shame, can significantly affect the patient's desire to recover, level of anxiety, self-esteem, and compliance
2. Past health history	2. **A.** Previous illness and operations: Complications, outcomes, and patient's reactions to hospitalization	2. **A.** A positive outcome of previous health problems provides a basis for hope in the patient, whereas a negative outcome may result in despair The time of life of the previous hospitalization, as well as the outcome, and any chronic condition resulting from that incident will have an impact on how the patient perceives the current condition Reactions of the patient indicate how he or she may tend to cope with the current situation
	B. Mental disorders: Particularly those with anxiety as a precipitating factor	**B.** The ICU environment may seriously stress the patient and cause reemergence of symptomatology, particularly anxiety-precipitated disorders, such as the more severe neuroses (phobias, obsessions and compulsions, conversion reactions, such as hysterical blindness or paralysis), psychosomatic disorders, and at the panic level of anxiety, psychotic episodes

3. Patient profile	**3. A.** Age, sex	It is not uncommon for patients with no previous psychological problems to experience high levels of anxiety and fear upon awakening in the ICU, particularly when complications were unanticipated and the patient is not prepared for a stay in this environment. The ICU nurse should be prepared to calm this patient when the person becomes aware of the strangeness of the surroundings
		3. A. Age and sex of the patient should be considered in relation to developmental stages and tasks. These functions are put at risk as a result of the illness, trauma, or surgery. Consequential limitations of hospitalization can also affect subsequent developmental stages of this individual
	B. Socioeconomic status	**B.** Socioeconomic status of the patient influences compliance and cooperation with physicians and nurses, as well as with hospital requests and requirements. In very general terms, working class people tend to view their lives to a greater extent as externally controlled. Family structure is more authoritarian. They are more likely to conform to the external authority of hospital staff. Middle class people and those with advanced educational preparation feel that control of their lives is more internally directed. Family structure is usually more democratic. They are more likely to resist at authoritarian approaches that do not include recognition of their desire to have input
	C. Ethnic, cultural, and religious beliefs	**C.** Ethnic practices, culture, and religious beliefs hold important restrictions and customs pertaining to diet, medication, transfusions, and other medical and psychological aspects of care
	D. Role identity	**D.** Roles that the patient has or expects to have and the physical limitations now imposed on the ability to resume or assume them can be a source of serious conflict. Self-esteem and values are tied to these roles, and when roles are threatened, will induce levels of anxiety concomitant with their perceived importance to the patient
	E. Coping style	**E.** Methods of coping used by the patient during previous stressful events will be mobilized first. Should they be perceived to be ineffective by the patient, regression to forms of coping found functional in earlier stages of life will emerge. If the stress is overwhelming to the patient, psychological defense mechanisms that enable the patient to deny the problem will be activated. If this fails to return the anxiety to a manageable level, there exists a high potential for the development of neurosis and, at the panic level, psychotic episodes
4. Present problem	**4. A.** Surgical intervention	**4. A.** Surgical intervention results in alteration or removal of a body part. Diminished capacity, temporary or permanent, will require adjustment of the patient's self-concept, including body image, self-esteem, role performance, and personal identity ICU syndrome may be precipitated by sleep deprivation, sensory overload or deprivation, and forced immobilization. The nurse should implement preventive measures to minimize the effects of this syndrome
	B. Exacerbation of chronic illness	**B.** Significant levels of anxiety and fear may be manifested as the patient becomes aware of the ICU environment Should the prognosis be poor, the nurse will assist the family to prepare for the impending loss
	C. Life-threatening or terminal illness	**C.** As the patient and family begin to grieve an immediate or potential loss, the nurse should be ready to provide assistance as necessary to support the patient and family during this process Spiritual distress may require the nurse to respond by alerting the chaplain or patient's

(continued)

PARAMETERS	FINDINGS	IMPLICATIONS FOR NURSING CARE
	D. Trauma	spiritual counselor. Assistance may be necessary to provide the privacy of other accommodations for varying rituals of final rites **D.** Generally, the patient and family are unprepared to cope with unexpected physical trauma and will require special care and orientation to the events that are taking place around them Self-inflicted trauma should alert the ICU nurse to be aware of signs of self-destructive behavior so that precautions can be instituted
5. Review of systems	**5.** Response to past or present stressors	**5.** Anxiety Coping, family: potential for growth Coping, ineffective family: compromised Coping, ineffective family: disabling Coping, ineffective individual Family process, alteration in Fear Grieving, anticipatory Grieving, dysfunctional Powerlessness Self-concept, disturbance in: body image, self-esteem, role performance, personal identity Sensory–perceptual alteration: visual, auditory, kinesthetic, gustatory, tactile, olfactory Sleep pattern disturbance Social isolation Spiritual distress Thought processes, alteration in Violence, potential for: self-directed or directed at others

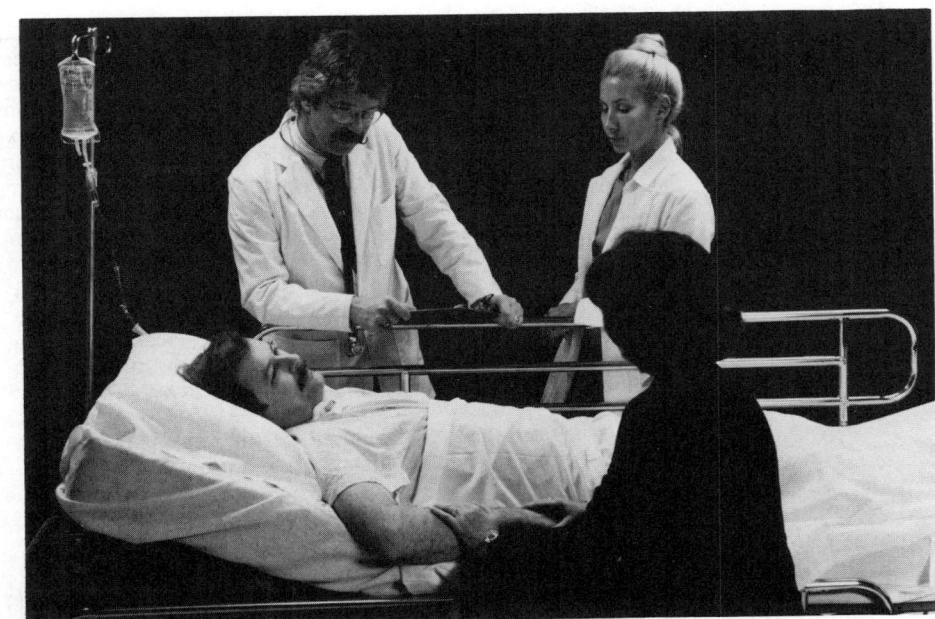

Figure 8–1. Astute observation of interactions among the patient, family members, and medical staff will often provide the ICU nurse with insight into the psychosocial history of the patient.

Care of the Patient with ICU Syndrome

NURSING DIAGNOSES	RATIONALE	DEFINING CHARACTERISTICS	EXPECTED OUTCOME
1. Sleep pattern, disturbance in 2. Sensory–perceptual alteration 3. Social isolation 4. Powerlessness	The syndrome of ICU psychosis is manifested by a gradual alteration in the accuracy of reality perception (Fig. 8–2). The following stressors combine to contribute to the development of this syndrome. 1. Sleep deprivation: May be demonstrated after 2–5 days in ICU. This is the most frequently mentioned cause of ICU syndrome and involves not only the number of hours needed for sleep but also the quality and duration of sleep. Routine external interruptions include monitoring vital signs, suctioning, and positioning 2. Sensory overload: This begins with the initial exposure to the unfamiliar ICU environment. The noise of multiple alarm systems and electronic equipment combined with constant light and activity are 24-hour stressors for the patient. Also, there are a large number of people coming and going at the bedside, few of whom the patient recognizes 3. Sensory deprivation: Constant low-level noise from many electrically powered machines results in drone auditory input. The patient is unable to distinguish timeframes or understand the technical language spoken around the bedside. Personnel tend to talk about the patient without including him or her in the conversation. In addition to being socially isolated from their families except for short periods, strict hospital routines tend to dehumanize individual patient care 4. Restraint: Forced immobilization resulting from tubings, catheters, ECG leads, protective restraints, endotracheal tubes, casts, and machines contribute to a patient's feeling of powerlessness. Emotional equilibrium is further challenged by physical dependence and compromised psychological resilience	Disorientation may be displayed in deteriorating stages • Clouding of consciousness: Reduction in awareness of environment and actions • Inability to concentrate: Lack of capacity to focus intellectual energies on a definite task, easily distracted • Impaired orientation for time: Does not know year, month, season, day, or time of day, under conditions where patient could reasonably be expected to know • Impaired orientation to place: Does not know where he or she is or the geographic relationship to surrounding places, under conditions where the patient could reasonably be expected to know • Impaired orientation to person: Does not know or cannot identify others, such as family members, who he or she is usually expected to remember or recognize • Impaired orientation of self: Does not know his or her name or occupation Visual and auditory hallucinations may be characterized by • Visual perception for which there is no external stimulus, such as "seeing visions" that no one else sees • Auditory perception for which there is no external stimulus, such as "hearing voices" that no one else hears. The patient responds to environmental cues of which the observer is unaware or unable to perceive Perceptual distortion may be characterized by illusions, a false perception or misinterpretation of an actual sensory stimulus Paranoia may be displayed as delusions of persecution despite lack of evidence: Patient firmly and fixedly believes others are planning to interfere and harm his or her physical and psychological well-being; unrealistic belief that others are "against me" or "out to get me"	Accurate perception of reality will be maintained or reestablished

1. Schedule medication, procedure, and treatment routines to permit uninterrupted periods of sleep, especially on the night shift
   Lower lighting during specified sleep periods to reestablish diurnal rhythms
   Monitor the patient's sleep patterns to assess the degree of sleep deprivation
2. Verbalize orienting information to include time, date, place, and person q2h while the patient is awake
   Thoroughly explain equipment sounds and alarms to the patient
   Inform the patient of his or her condition and progress during periods of reality orientation
3. Provide properly functioning eyeglasses and hearing aids
   Recognize cultural variables that affect patient's response to stimulus and accommodate insofar as possible
   Encourage visits from family members and friends as allowed by the patient's condition
4. Demonstrate range of limb movement with lines and equipment in place
   Allow patient control over as many aspects of the environment as possible
   Encourage verbal and nonverbal expression

OUTCOME CRITERIA

1. Patient is provided with periods of uninterrupted sleep, as close to his or her normal sleep patterns as possible
2. Patient maintains reality orientation to person, place, and time
3. Patient will be provided with meaningful social interaction and stimulation
4. Patient will understand the need for monitoring lines, ECG leads, and catheter tubing and will be encouraged to move with assistance while these are in place

DOCUMENTATION

In order to more accurately assess the patient's perception of reality and to assure continuity of care, precise documentation should be encouraged for each of the following parameters.

- The patient has experienced _____ hours of uninterrupted sleep this shift
- The patient is oriented to person, place, and time q2h
- The patient's eyeglasses and hearing aids are in place during waking hours, and are functioning properly
- Relationship of visitors, i.e., spouse, sister, friend, and so on
- Range of motion exercises have been performed one time per shift. Patient is able to move easily in spite of monitoring cables and leads

SPECIAL NOTE

Treatment

Due to the intangible nature of ICU syndrome, recognition and resolution depend heavily on nursing. Pharmacological intervention has proven to be *ineffective* except to sedate the patient. Removal of the stressors is regarded as the treatment of choice. Symptoms then generally show improvement within a 24-hour period. Total resolution of the syndrome however may not occur for several days.

The Family

The symptoms exhibited by a patient with ICU syndrome are especially stressful for the family members. Special attention and support must be shown to the family during this emotionally taxing period in the patient's hospitalization.

Patient Awareness

The nurse must remember that patients may *not* be amnesic for events during this period. Support and compassion for the patient are essential caring skills that will decrease the patient's embarrassment and guilt following the confused period.

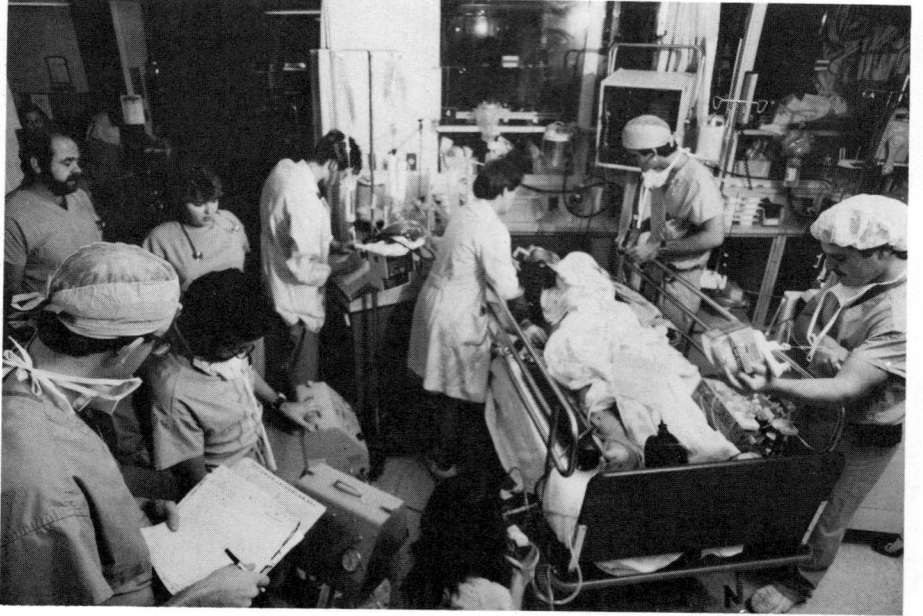

Figure 8–2. The ICU environment may seriously stress the patient psychologically, contributing to an alteration in perception of reality.

Care of the Patient's Family

NURSING DIAGNOSES	RATIONALE	DEFINING CHARACTERISTICS	EXPECTED OUTCOME
Coping, family: potential for growth Coping, ineffective family, compromised Coping, ineffective family, disabling Family process, alteration in	Since family members are interdependent, when one becomes ill, all experience stress. Often the event occurs suddenly, without time for the family to prepare psychologically. A loved one is abruptly separated from the family and is being cared for by an unfamiliar professional staff. The ICU environment is foreign; filled with bizarre machines, obtrusive odors, and alarming sounds. Often the patient's prognosis is guarded, at best, uncertain. Always present is the knowledge of a potentially overwhelming financial burden. The ICU nurse can often feel these pressures when the family members call or visit the unit. By developing the skill of caring for the family members, as an extension of the patient, the nurse can enhance the patient's recovery (Fig. 8–3).	Each family member, like each family unit, has a unique pattern of adaptive processes. Following are examples of behavior the ICU nurse may encounter: • Family members attempt to describe growth impact of crisis on their own values, priorities, goals, or relationships Family member is moving in the direction of health • Patient expresses or confirms concerns about significant members' responses to the patient's health problem Significant member describes an inadequate understanding or knowledge base that interferes with effective assistance or supportive behaviors • Family member(s) show neglectful care of the patient in regard to basic human needs and illness treatment Significant member displays agitation, depression, aggression, or hostility toward the patient or displaces these feelings toward the staff Member exhibits distortion of reality regarding the patient's health problem, including extreme denial about either its existence or severity • Family system is unable to meet physical, emotional, or spiritual needs of its members The family decision-making process is ineffective Family members are unable to send and receive clear messages	Stressors on the family associated with the ICU experience will be minimized or avoided

NURSING INTERVENTIONS

1. Support the family's hope by keeping them informed of each major improvement in the patient's condition
2. Provide daily honest and understandable explanations regarding the patient's progress
3. Assess the family's perception of the patient's current health status. Help them to sort out and direct their questions and feelings
4. Encourage the family to verbalize their emotions and seek additional support as necessary from the chaplain or liaison personnel
5. Reassure the family that the patient will receive close attention and that they will be notified at home about changes in status

6. Remain near the bedside during visiting hours to be supportive but provide a comfortable and private visiting period
7. Be sensitive to the patient's concerns, address him or her by name, and touch the patient in a reassuring manner

OUTCOME CRITERIA

1. The family's faith and hope in the patient's recovery will be realistic and supported
2. The family will receive adequate and honest information regarding the patient's condition
3. Anxiety of the family members will be minimized
4. Family members will be encouraged to share and express their feelings
5. The family will be assured that the staff is conscientious and concerned
6. The family will know that the staff is always present and will be near the patient during the ICU stay
7. The family will know that the individuality of the patient will be respected

DOCUMENTATION

Many ICUs have developed care plans that include pertinent information regarding the patient's living situation and significant family members. This information is valuable throughout the patient's stay in the unit, but essential during periods of unexpected crisis. Following are some suggested areas where documentation is helpful.

- Patient's customary living situation (alone or with others)
- Previous admissions to ICUs
- Accurate telephone numbers of patient's significant family members and friends (for notification during emergencies)
- Religious and clergy preference of patient
- Who will be visiting (relationship to patient)
- Date of patient care conferences with family members and physicians, nurses, and other professional services

SPECIAL NOTE

Enhancing Communication

Family members often have a sixth sense when it comes to anticipating a change in the patient's condition. Develop the art of sensitive listening in order to hear what the family's sixth sense is telling them.
Provide information to the family before they have to request it, and they will develop a sense of trust in the staff's ability to care.
Although the ICU nurse usually has daily contact with the family members, the physician can also allay family fears and concerns.
Be present when the physician discusses the patient with the family to be aware of what the family has been told.
Encourage the family to keep a list of questions and concerns to be discussed when they speak with the physician.
Encourage the physician to speak with the family, even if no new information can be given to them; this will help to keep the family members' anxiety manageable.

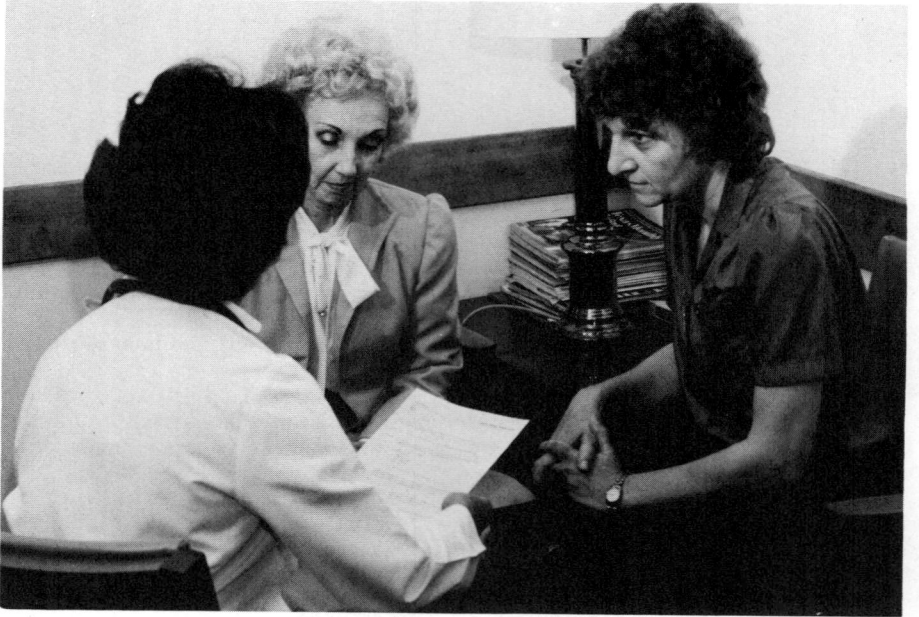

Figure 8–3. It is important for the ICU nurse to assess the family's perception of the patient's current health status, in order to help them sort out and direct their questions and feelings.

Care of the Patient and Family Experiencing Loss

NURSING DIAGNOSES	RATIONALE	DEFINING CHARACTERISTICS	EXPECTED OUTCOME
Grieving, anticipatory Grieving, dysfunctional	The skill of recognizing the stages and supporting the individual experiencing the grieving process is one of the highest levels of understanding a professional can achieve (Fig. 8–4). Bear in mind that this process is fluid and dynamic. Individuals within the family unit may manifest diverse responses as they move through their grief. One of the most difficult challenges ICU nurses must face is to refrain from imposing personal values and coping mechanisms on the patient and family unit experiencing loss.	Elizabeth Kübler-Ross pioneered the concept of psychological stages in the dying process. It is now generally accepted that these stages apply to loss in any form. Emotional reactions to loss are generally grouped in the following manner. Each response may last for varying periods of time or may exist simultaneously with another. • Denial and isolation: The patient and family member may ask repetitive questions of the staff related to prognosis or expected outcome, hoping each time that the answer will be encouraging. Another common occurrence is shopping for a doctor to obtain the positive response they so want to hear. The individual may appear detached from the situation. Vague somatic complaints may be evident. Signs of social withdrawal are common, and automatic or rote behavior is frequently displayed • Anger: The individual protests against the event and frequently directs hostility toward the physician and members of the staff. A person in this stage is constantly searching for explanations or reasons for these events and assigns blame whenever possible • Bargaining: In this stage, the individual seeks to postpone the inevitable by arranging situations to buy additional time. Most of these bargains are private promises with clergy and directed toward God—a vow to be a better person, lead a better life if only . . . • Depression: The individual is in despair and appears disorganized and restless. He or she may verbalize numerous vague somatic complaints or appear to be in a state of emotional shock • Acceptance: The individual displays some degree of reorganization and shows signs of being resigned to the inevitable. The patient's needs are usually fewer at this time. However, the family members may need more help, understanding, and support	The patient and family will experience the grieving process with assistance and support from the ICU staff members

NURSING INTERVENTIONS

1. Provide for the patient the information needed or requested. Answer specific questions and provide information that the patient is ready to hear
2. Determine what the physician has told the patient and family about the illness, treatment, and prognosis. Communicate with the physician if misperceptions or misconceptions are apparent
3. Encourage the patient and family to verbalize their thoughts and feelings, lending assistance in identifying areas of need. This can be done by asking open-ended questions
4. Decrease feelings of powerlessness and helplessness by providing the family with helpful and pertinent information regarding aspects of care
5. Evaluate the patient's and family's level of understanding regarding the illness, treatment, and prognosis
6. Provide the patient and family privacy and visiting time to share their feelings. Provide tools for communication if the patient is intubated. Encourage touching
7. Keep the patient comfortable and alleviate pain. Notify the physician when analgesia is ineffective
8. Maintain a nonjudgmental approach to any grieving reactions. The patient and all family members are unique individuals who will respond to the situation in accordance with their previous experiences with terminal illness and death

OUTCOME CRITERIA

1. The patient will be provided time to adjust to the diagnosis and prognosis
2. The patient's misconceptions will be corrected. Fears will be manageable
3. The patient will be provided with opportunities to share his or her thoughts and feelings
4. The family will achieve and maintain a sense of control regarding this event in their lives. They will be able to understand those factors they cannot control, such as visiting hours and phone calls to the patient
5. Information given to the family will be appropriate to their level of understanding
6. The patient's and family's need for privacy will be accommodated
7. The patient's physical needs will be met, and the patient's and family's comfort level will be maintained or improved
8. Individual responses will be accepted with compassion, nonjudgmental support and assistance

DOCUMENTATION

Documentation of the following types of situations will provide valuable information related to patient and family progress during the grieving process.

- Patient is requesting information regarding severity of the illness and expected prognosis
- Patient is verbalizing misconceptions or misperceptions about the illness
- Patient has (has not) verbalized regarding thoughts and feelings when opportunities have been provided
- The family has been informed of the most recent plan of care for the patient
- Both patient and family have received information regarding the expected outcome of the hospitalization and appear (do not appear) to understand the situation
- Patient visited privately with family members
- Analgesia appears to be (not to be) effective. Patient states that he or she is (is not) comfortable
- The patient and family have been reassured, and supportive measures have been provided

SPECIAL NOTE

Peer Support

Providing care for terminally ill patients may evoke strong emotions in the ICU nurse. These emotions may be manifest as anger, frustration, or avoidance of the patient and family. Team conferences and peer support help the nurse recognize these signs promptly and be cognizant of feelings underlying this especially stressful event.

Organ Donation

With death as the ultimate loss, many relatives are finally comforted by the fact that some good may result from their tragedy. Organ donation can make death appear less wasteful, and when approached with sensitivity, some families are assisted through the bereavement process by knowing that such a contribution has been possible.

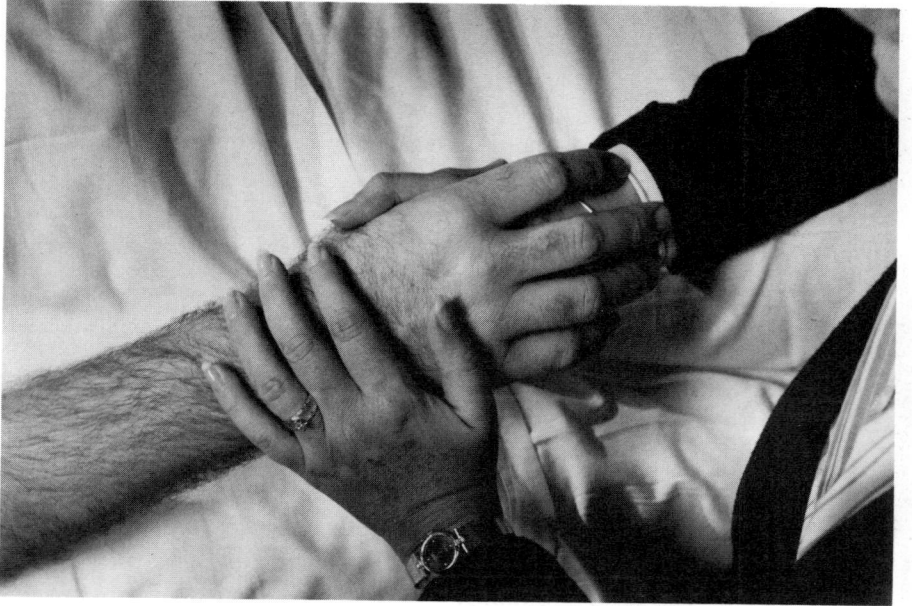

Figure 8–4. Provide the patient and family privacy and visiting time to share their feelings.

Care of the Patient and Family Experiencing Anxiety and Fear

NURSING DIAGNOSES	RATIONALE	DEFINING CHARACTERISTICS	EXPECTED OUTCOME

Anxiety
Fear
	Anticipation or threat of danger to a person's physical or psychological well-being elicits a pervasive uneasy feeling of apprehension. When the source or its consequences are vague, unknown, or unrecognized, anxiety results. When the source and its consequences become more specific, fear may emerge (Fig. 8–5).
	
	    Fear is generally traceable to an object, whereas anxiety is related to a threat to value. Both of these endanger the integrity of the personality, particularly feelings of self-worth and self-esteem. Fear and anxiety can range in intensity from mild to moderate, to severe, to terror and panic.
		The responses to fear and anxiety are indistinguishable. If the perceived threat remains unresolved or intensifies, the responses move from adaptive to maladaptive, with increased intensity and corresponding rise in level
		• Physiological responses are mediated by the autonomic nervous system. Responses, such as increased heart rate, increased blood pressure, rapid breathing, cold sweat, and dry mouth, as well as such indicators as restlessness, tenseness, increased startle response, and sleep disturbance, may be difficult to differentiate from symptoms associated with the patient's illness or the effects of medication
		• Psychological responses are commensurate with the level of anxiety being experienced
		    Mild anxiety: Increased alertness, energy, and responsiveness, such as that experienced in day-to-day tensions. Mild anxiety serves to motivate action and is generally considered adaptive in nature. As anxiety increases, psychological defense mechanisms that serve to deny or distort that part of reality that is in conflict with some value may be activated to protect the value and consequently alleviate the anxiety associated with the conflict
		    Moderate anxiety: Individual's focus of life and its surrounding events is turned to immediate needs and concerns, blocking out other areas. The patient becomes irritable, easily agitated, and angry. Anger serves to give a sense of power, which counters the feelings of isolation and helplessness accompanying this state
		    Severe anxiety: Focus continues to narrow and tends to fix on a specific detail, which takes on disproportionate significance. For example, a patient who complains of cold feet and
			Anxiety will be reduced and maintained at a level with which the patient or family member can adequately cope. Anxiety and fear levels will not be counterproductive to medical treatment, recovery, or family dynamics

wants his socks on may direct an all consuming effort to this task. Nothing else matters or will until this is accomplished. The longer it takes, the more agitated, intense, and excited the patient becomes. Responses may escalate to a state of panic

Panic: Loss of control, perceptual distortion, personality disorganization, and increased behavioral and motor response intensity are the hallmarks of this level

A mild level of anxiety does not usually lead to maladaptive coping mechanisms. Moderate and higher levels of sustained anxiety in a patient or family member with inadequate or exhausted coping mechanisms may be converted into psychological disorders in an effort to relieve the unpleasant and painful effects manifested by this otherwise unexpressed conflict. Severe neurotic disorders, such as phobias, obsessive and compulsive behaviors, conversion reactions (e.g., hysterical blindness, paralysis), psychomatic illness, and others, are characteristic of anxiety-based maladaptive coping mechanisms. Psychotic reactions can occur at the panic level as the personality structure starts to disintegrate

NURSING INTERVENTIONS

1. Familiarize the patient and the family with the ICU environment, expected procedures, personnel, and routine
2. Prepare the patient and family for even the most routine events, since these may provoke anxiety in the unknowing. Provide information for all interventions as to their purpose, procedure, and expected outcome
3. The patient and family should be advised of the function of all persons who enter and leave the room or approach the bedside
4. Provide the family with frequent reports of even routine procedures before they ask
5. Recognize that anxiety is contagious; mild to moderate anxiety may escalate in the patient or family as a result of exposure to other anxious people
6. A patient or family member who does not exhibit or minimally exhibits signs of anxiety may be using one of the psychological defense mechanisms that help to deny or keep him or her unaware of the significance of the illness. Do not confront this defense, as it serves to protect the person from the immediate threat perceived
7. The nurse should help the patient or family member exhibiting moderate anxiety who indicates a need and willingness to talk to identify his or her feelings. Simple identification of a feeling, with the acknowledgment that it is real to the person, understandable to the nurse, and acceptable to have it, tends to relieve a major portion of tension
8. People experiencing severe anxiety require interactions that are firm, clear, and delivered in a calm, caring, and organized fashion. Control is tenuous in these persons, and any fear or anxiety expressed by staff may intensify the reaction

(continued)

9. Patients in a panic state have lost control. Increased motor activity may result in lines and tubes being pulled out. The goals of intervention are to safely immobilize the patient to prevent self-injury and to help him or her regain control

OUTCOME CRITERIA

1. Preoperative patient teaching and information regarding the physical environment of the unit will be provided whenever possible
2. Information regarding the activities and procedures planned for the patient will be provided to the patient each morning and as often thereafter as necessary
3. All staff members will introduce themselves by name and title and state their reason for being in the patient's room or at the bedside
4. Current information regarding plan of care will be provided routinely to the patient and family
5. Patient care conferences will be held at regular intervals to allow the staff to identify and share their feelings regarding caring for the individual with increased levels of anxiety or fear
6. The individual's use of psychological defense mechanisms, such as denial and rationalization, will be identified and will not be confronted
7. Provide an atmosphere of caring in which the patient will be comfortable sharing his or her feelings and anxieties
8. Care will be provided in a calm, controlled manner for the patient or family member experiencing severe anxiety
9. The patient experiencing panic will be supported and safely immobilized to prevent self-injury

DOCUMENTATION

- Any patient and family education and teaching
- Explanations regarding unexpected procedures and routines to the patient and family members
- Orientation of the patient to the personnel of the unit
- Record when the family has been informed of plan of care and procedures
- Document any patient care unit conferences
- Document on the unit staff development programs and resources that help to identify various defense mechanisms so that these responses can be recognized by the staff and dealt with in an appropriate and supportive manner
- Document any statement that the patient makes regarding anxieties or fears. This will enable other staff workers to recognize and deal therapeutically with the patient's actions
- Notify the physician when the individual's anxiety or fear level appears to be increasing. All documentation that you can provide for the next shift will be extremely valuable in preventing the patient's anxiety level from reaching the severe stage
- Document if protective restraints are necessary, the time they were applied, and the patient's response to them. Also record when and how restraints are removed

SPECIAL NOTE

Panic

Patients or family members experiencing moderate, severe, or panic levels of anxiety may require a longer period of therapeutic intervention extending beyond the ICU experience. Psychiatric referral may be an option in this situation.

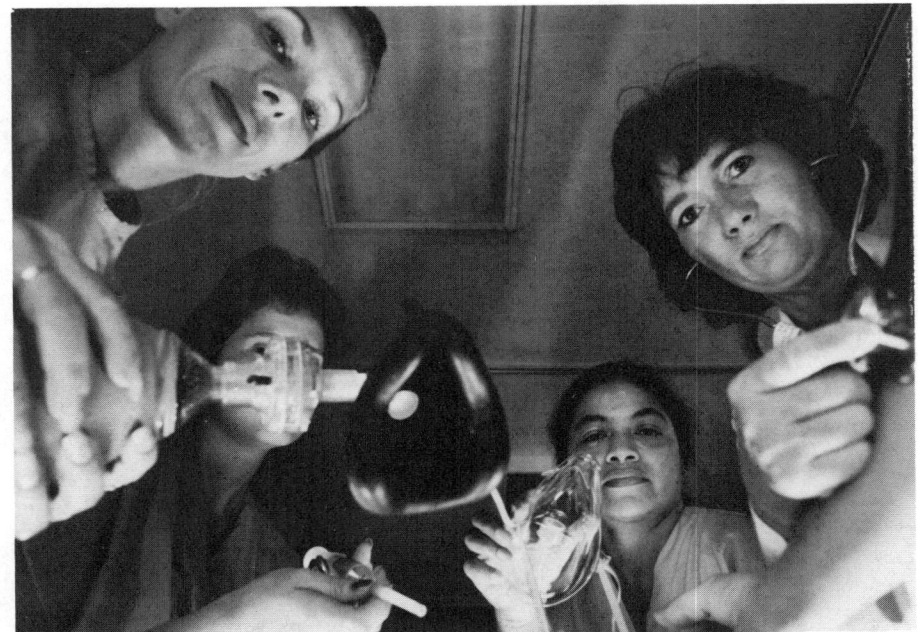

Figure 8–5. Prepare the patient and family for even the most routine events, since these may provoke anxiety in the unfamiliar.

Care of the Patient with a Disturbance in Self-concept

NURSING DIAGNOSES	RATIONALE	DEFINING CHARACTERISTICS	EXPECTED OUTCOME
	Self-concept is the sum of all the perceptions a person has about himself or herself, specifically, body image, self-esteem, role performance, and personal identity. Alteration in self-concept is a common finding in the individual whose illness, trauma, or surgery brings them to the ICU (Fig. 8–6)		A positive, reality-based self-concept will be regained and maintained
1. Self-concept, disturbance in: body image	1. Body image: Self-perception of physical body with biophysical, cognitive perceptual, psychosocial, and cultural or spiritual viewpoints.	1. Alteration in body image is indicated explicitly or implicitly by • Altered or removed body part, such that the functional capabilities of the person are changed; these changes may be actual or perceived, temporary or permanent • Significance of change in body image is dependent upon the importance of the altered or removed body part relative to age, sex, sociocultural roles, lifestyle, personal identity, and self-esteem	
2. Self-concept, disturbance in: self-esteem	2. Self-esteem: Value judgment that a person makes about his or her own worth based on how well he or she meets personally set standards or ideals; a self-appraisal of competence to handle reality and to function as a human being.	2. Disturbance of self-esteem is manifested by • Feelings of unworthiness and inferiority indicated by lack of eye contact or shying away from those offering help • Feelings of hopelessness and defeatism suggested by neglect of self-care or loss of desire for self-help; becoming self-indulgent • Feelings of inadequacy and incompetence, reflected by "setting one's self up" for failure, self-destructive behavior, and increasing dependency on others	
3. Self-concept, disturbance in: role performance	3. Role performance: Personally or socially expected level of performance of a set of behaviors either ascribed by virtue of an existing state of being, such as age and sex, or assumed with some degree of choice and control, such as occupation and lifestyle.	3. Disturbance in role performance is manifested by increased levels of anxiety and threatened self-esteem resulting from • Uncertainty regarding what behaviors are expected of a person with *patient* status • Incompatibility of role of *patient* with desire to resume customary roles • Fear of not being capable of performing important roles and fulfilling responsibilities after hospitalization	

4. Self-concept, disturbance in: personal identity	**4.** Personal identity: Awareness and acceptance of a cohesive set of characteristics as belonging to and reflective of one's self-definition: A statement of self-reliance and uniqueness.	**4.** Disturbance in personal identity resulting from or exacerbated by depersonalizing hospital procedures and attitudes may be manifested by • Activation of the identification process wherein the patient identifies with a known quantity, e.g., "I'm Dr. Smith's patient" or "I'm the triple bypass patient" • Engages in behavior that will result in some label (identity) being assigned, positive or negative • Lowered self-esteem, especially dignity, with associated behaviors, e.g., anxiety, self-depreciation, self-indulgence • Confusion, indicated by contradictory feelings about issues related to identity, which may result in escalating anxiety	

NURSING INTERVENTIONS

1. Self-acceptance is crucial and should be encouraged by showing acceptance, unconditionally and nonjudgmentally. Appearing disturbed at a diseased or disfigured body can be misinterpreted by the patient with low self-esteem as rejection of him or her as a person
2. The reality of the limitations imposed by the illness, trauma, or surgery are not to be hidden or understated, but the nurse should place emphasis on the capabilities of compensating strengths
3. Patients are often overwhelmed by the perceived complexity of their problems. Define the component parts of the problem at a level of simplicity that allows the patient to recognize what can be resolved within the constraints of their current condition and what will need to be set aside
4. Help the patient to clarify and organize achievable short-term goals to reduce feelings of helplessness, powerlessness, and incompetence

OUTCOME CRITERIA

1. The patient will be treated in a nonjudgmental, professional manner
2. The patient's strengths will be emphasized and limitations dealt with in a realistic manner
3. The patient will acknowledge the benefits and limitations of his or her condition and will capitalize on that focus in a more positive way
4. The patient will identify and solve short-term problems related to his or her condition and hospitalization

DOCUMENTATION

• Statements the patient makes regarding his or her body image
• Even the most minute self-care accomplishments. This will enable the following shifts to recognize progress the patient makes and provide a source of continued encouragement
• Seemingly small problems or areas of concern the patient may verbalize. This will provide continuity in the patient's care and more comprehensive understanding of his or her immediate concerns
• Problem-solving accomplishments of patient, family members, and health care providers

(continued)

SPECIAL NOTE

Identification

Each nurse must strive to recognize and cope positively with personal feelings and anxieties related to such conditions as amputation, stroke, burns, mastectomy, and colostomy, to be therapeutically effective with a patient experiencing a disturbance in self-concept

Projection

Attitudes of anger and resentment may be displaced onto the nurse when a patient or family is suddenly faced with the crisis of trauma, surgical procedures, or an unexpected, life-threatening diagnosis. Dealing with these attacks may be extremely stressful for the nurse. It requires a great deal of empathy, understanding, and sensitivity to handle them in a caring and nonretaliatory manner

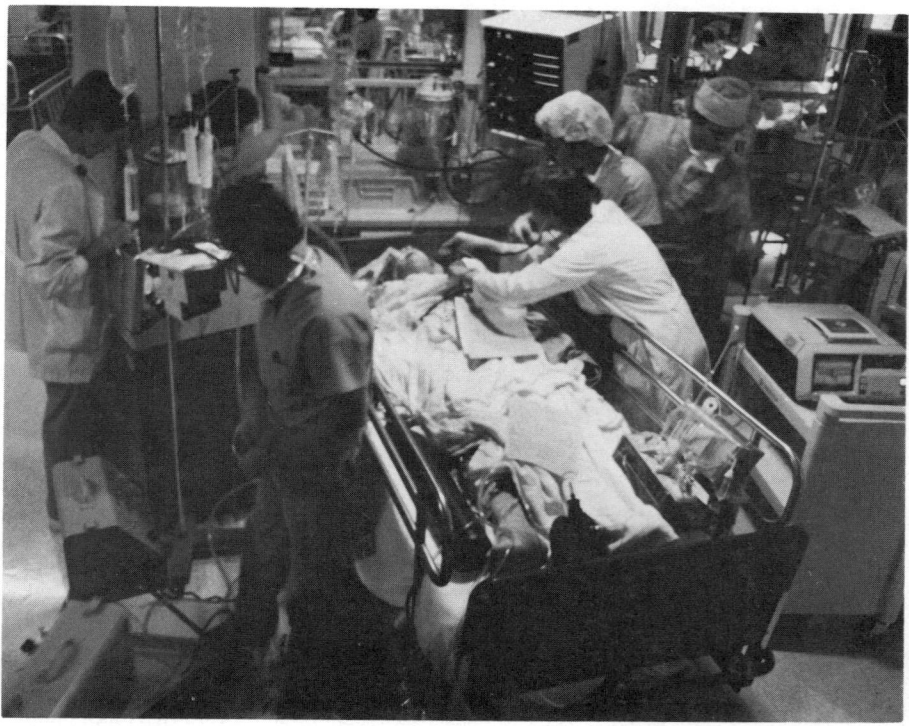

Figure 8–6. Alteration in self-concept is a common finding in the individual whose illness, trauma, or surgery brings them to the ICU.

Care of the Patient Exhibiting Self-destructive Behavior

NURSING DIAGNOSIS	RATIONALE	DEFINING CHARACTERISTICS	EXPECTED OUTCOME
Violence, potential for: self-directed or directed at others	Stressors experienced by an individual may be physiological, psychological, or sociocultural in nature. The individual's ability to tolerate stress is dependent upon coping ability: The use of internal as well as external resources. When the timing of stressor occurrence or the number of stressors occurring exhausts both internal and external resources, feelings of hopelessness and, more seriously, helplessness may emerge. This perceived loss of control and lack of options may result in the use of self-destructive or active, aggressive suicide acts (Fig. 8–7)	Indirect self-destructive behavior: Any activity that is detrimental to the physical well-being of the individual and potentially has the outcome of death. The individual may be unaware of the potential lethality of the behavior or of death as a goal. Examples the ICU nurse may encounter are • Abuse of alcohol and drugs • Eating disorders (anorexia nervosa, bulemia, obesity) • Self-mutilation Noncompliance with medical treatment Direct self-destructive behavior: Includes any form of suicidal activity: The intent of this behavior is death, and the individual is aware of this as the possible outcome	Self-destructive behavior will be identified, and measures will be taken to protect the individual from inflicting further harm

NURSING INTERVENTIONS

1. Develop an awareness of personal response to the individual exhibiting self-destructive behavior
2. Recognize that a therapeutic approach is empathetic and nonjudgmental
3. Physically protect the individual from inflicting further harm on himself or herself. Obtain a physician's order for restraints if necessary
4. If the patient presents with self-destructive behavior, verbally reassure the individual that you and the other members of the health care team will do their best to protect him or her from any further injury
5. Nonverbally reassure the individual by removing all potentially harmful objects from the immediate environment if possible
6. Obtain orders to administer medications in elixir or IV form to prevent the patient from sequestering oral medications for later ingestion
7. Provide one-to-one observation and an atmosphere that communicates caring by kindness and understanding
8. Previously agitated patients who may have come to a decision to commit suicide may be at highest risk when appearing more calm and conversant
9. Treat the patient with kindness. Self-esteem may be even more severely compromised following unsuccessful suicide
10. Elicit liaison support to educate family members regarding behavioral clues to suicide and community resources available to assist with crises

OUTCOME CRITERIA

1. Care will be delivered in a nonjudgmental manner
2. The patient will perceive the staff as nonjudgmental and concerned
3. The patient will express a feeling of safety while in the ICU environment
4. Self-destructive feelings will be verbalized rather than acted upon

5. Potentially harmful objects will be removed from the immediate environment
6. The patient will be observed closely during administration of medications
7. One-to-one observation will be provided to emphasize an atmosphere of caring and to assure patient safety
8. The patient will continue to be observed closely, especially when he or she appears to be coping better
9. The patient's self-esteem will be enhanced by the kindness and empathy demonstrated by the staff
10. The family members will be provided with helpful information enabling them to deal more effectively with this behavior

DOCUMENTATION

- Patient care conferences should be documented related to this specific patient
- Unit conferences should be documented to enhance the staff's therapeutic approach to patient behavior
- Time and type of restraints applied should be documented. The individual's response to protective restraints should also be noted
- Document that verbal reassurance is given to the patient
- Record when harmful objects are found and removed from the environment. Label personal belongings, such as glasses, and give to the family
- Record that the patient was observed to take the prescribed medication
- Documentation is done q30min by the person providing one-to-one observation
- Document verbal statements the patient makes regarding his or her state of mind, e.g.
  "You really don't have to stay with me any more; I'm feeling much better about everything"
  "Don't worry about me any more, I've worked everything out in my mind"
- Note the positive points and strengths of the individual so that his or her self-esteem can be enhanced
- Document family conferences and support services provided

SPECIAL NOTE

Noncompliance

Many people choose not to comply with prescribed health care programs or medications. They are usually cognizant of the fact that they have chosen not to follow medical recommendations but do not view this as indirect self-destructive behavior. They develop many rationalizations for noncompliance to which nurses should be attuned.
  "I feel fine, there's no need to take that medication"
  "I just don't have the money for the treatment right now"
  "I'm too busy right now, I'll do it later"
  "I really don't understand what I'm supposed to do"
  "I didn't know it was that important" (denial)

Conflicting Values

Self-destructive behavior is seen often in patients with life-threatening or chronic, painful illnesses. To these people, *quality* of life may be of more importance than *longevity*. This is a most difficult situation for the ICU nurse to face, as her own ethical and moral beliefs may be in direct opposition to this concept.

Exacerbation

Self-destructive individuals are not necessarily suicidal. Suicidal behavior can be an escalation of self-destructive behavior where death is perceived as "the only available option".

Risk Assessment

All self-destructive behavior is serious, and risk of suicide is evaluated by lethality, intentionality, and possibility of rescue.

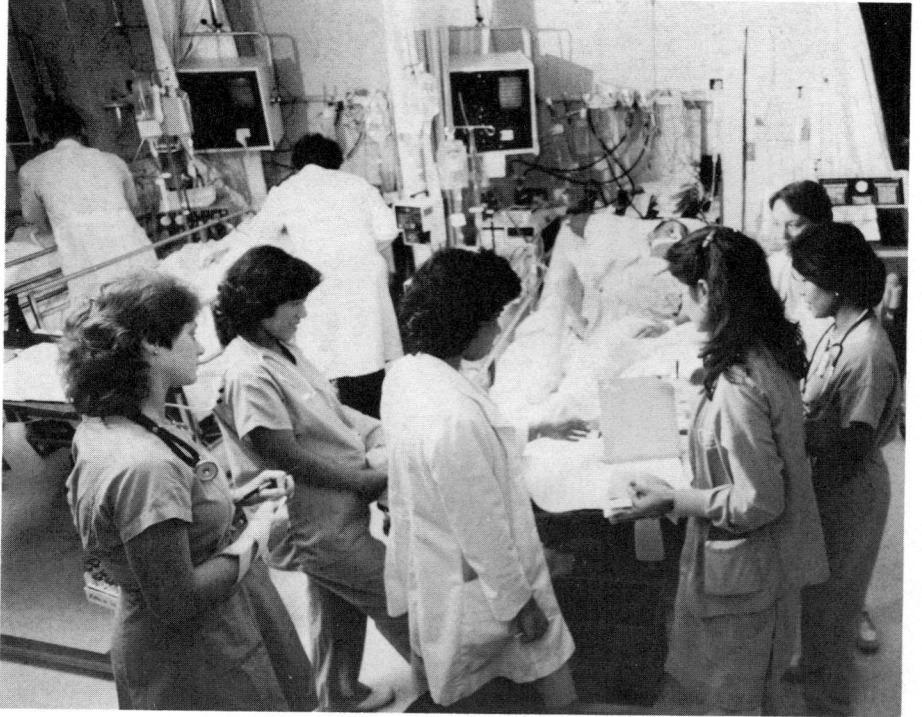

Figure 8–7. Unit conferences should be documented to enchance the staff's therapeutic approach to patient behavior.

Care of the Human Spirit

NURSING DIAGNOSIS	RATIONALE	DEFINING CHARACTERISTICS	EXPECTED OUTCOME
Spiritual distress	Distress of the human spirit is a disruption in the life principle that pervades a person's entire being and that integrates and transcends one's biological and psychosocial nature. Separation from strong religious and cultural ties threatens the integrity of an individual's belief and value system (Fig. 8–8)	The following responses are examples of the many ways the ICU patient may exhibit distress of the human spirit 　Expresses concern with meaning of life and death and belief systems 　Anger toward God (as defined by the individual) 　Questions meaning of suffering 　Verbalizes inner conflict about beliefs 　Unable to choose or chooses not to participate in usual religious practices 　Seeks spiritual assistance 　Questions moral and ethical implications of therapeutic regimen	The beliefs and value system of the patient will be strengthened and respected

NURSING INTERVENTIONS　Although it is unrealistic for the ICU nurse to be familiar with the attitudes and requirements of all the various religious groups, there are resources available that can assist staff to meet the spiritual needs of specific cultures. A brief overview of these religious tenets is provided in the Appendix to this chapter.

OUTCOME CRITERIA　Specific attitudes and spiritual needs of the patient will be identified and accommodated insofar as possible by the professional staff.

DOCUMENTATION　Documentation of spiritual needs being met should be made in narrative form in the patient's chart.

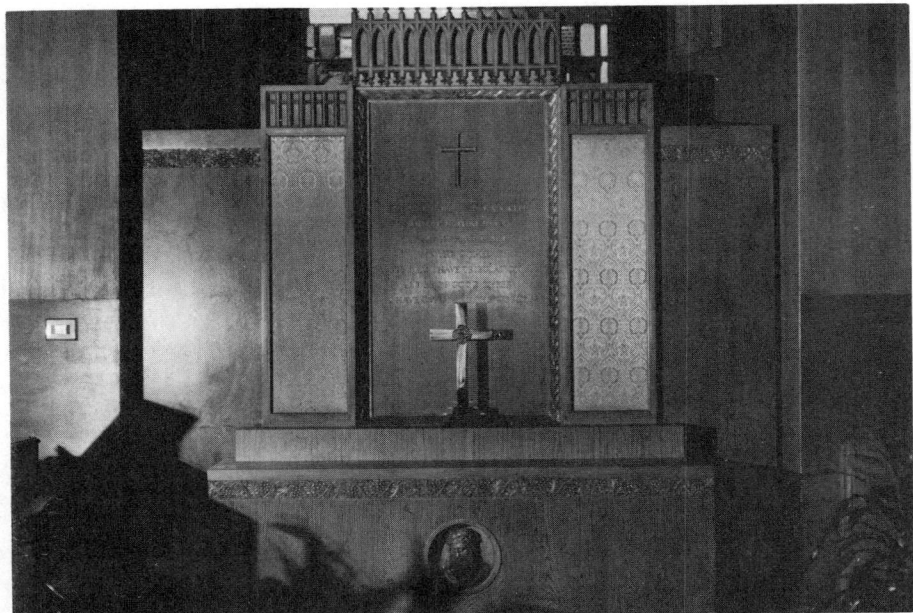

Figure 8–8. It is unrealistic for the ICU nurse to be familiar with the requirements of all religious denominations, however, specific spiritual needs of the patient should be accommodated in so far as possible.

Glossary

Affect: Feeling, mood.

Aggression: Mental drive to action that encompasses both constructive and destructive activities.

Alcohol-withdrawal delirium: A medical diagnosis for a serious alcohol withdrawal syndrome that is characterized by agitation, disorientation, anorexia, paranoia, insomnia, and visual hallucinations. Associated physiological findings include elevated temperature, tachycardia, tachypnea, hyperpnea, vomiting, diarrhea, and diaphoresis; may result in death if supportive intervention is not implemented.

Anger: An expression of the anxiety that is aroused by a real or perceived threat to one's rights, possessions, values, or significant others.

Anorexia nervosa: An eating disorder in which the person experiences hunger but refuses to eat, based on a distorted body image leading to a self-perception of fatness. Starvation ensues.

Anxiety: A diffuse vague apprehension associated with feelings of uncertainty and helplessness. It is an emotion without a specific object, is subjectively experienced by the individual, and is communicated interpersonally. It occurs as a result of a threat to the person's being, self-esteem, or identity.

Assertiveness: Behavior that is directed toward claiming one's rights without denying the rights of others.

Body image: Sum of the conscious and unconscious attitudes the individual has toward his or her body. It includes present and past perceptions, as well as feelings about size, function, appearance, and potential.

Cognition: Process of logical thought.

Compensation: Process by which a person makes up for a deficiency in his image of himself by strongly emphasizing some other feature that he regards as an asset.

Compulsion: A recurring irresistible impulse to perform some act.

Conflict: Clashing of two opposing interests. The person experiences two competing drives and must choose between them.

Confusion: A nonspecific term to describe a constellation of behaviors related to cognitive impairment, usually including disorientation, memory loss, loss of social skills, disruptive behavior, and difficulties with self-care.

Coping mechanisms: Any effort directed at stress management. They can be task oriented and involve direct problem-solving efforts to cope with the threat itself or be intrapsychic or ego defense-oriented, with the goal of regulating one's emotional distress.

Crisis: An internal disturbance that results from a stressful event or a perceived threat to self. Crises are self-limiting, and an adaptive or maladaptive resolu-tion usually occurs within 6 weeks. Crises are a time of increased vulnerability and can produce increased personal growth.

Crisis relativism: The idea that health and normality emerge within a social context and that the content and form of mental health and mental illness will vary greatly from one culture to another. Differences are due to variations in stressors, symbolical interpretation, acceptance of expression and repression, and cohesion of social groups and their tolerance of deviation.

Defense mechanisms: Coping mechanisms of the ego that attempt to protect the person from feelings of inadequacy and worthlessness and prevent awareness of anxiety. They are primarily unconscious in nature and involve a degree of self-deception and reality distortion.

Delirium: An organic mental disorder characterized by a cluster of cognitive impairments with an acute onset and the identification of a specific precipitating stressor.

Delusion: A false belief that may be persecutory, grandiose, or somatic in nature.

Dementia: An organic mental disorder characterized by a cluster of cognitive impairments that are generally of gradual onset and irreversible. The predisposing and precipitating stressors may or may not be identifiable.

Denial: Avoidance of disagreeable realities by ignoring or refusing to recognize them.

Depression: An abnormal extension or elaboration of sadness and grief. The term "depression" can be used to denote a variety of phenomena—a sign, symptom, syndrome, emotional state, reaction, disease, or clinical entity.

Disorientation: Inability to correctly identify the self in relation to time, place, or person.

Functional disorder: A mental or emotional impairment that is believed to be psychosocial in origin.

Grief: An individual's subjective response to the loss of a person, object, or concept that is highly valued. Uncomplicated grief is a healthy, adaptive, reparative response.

Hallucination: A sensory experience that is not the result of an external stimulus; may be visual, auditory, tactile, olfactory, or gustatory.

Illusion: Misinterpretation of a sensory input.

Noncompliance: The failure of the individual to carry out the self-care activities prescribed.

Obsession: A recurring thought that is unwanted but cannot be voluntarily excluded from consciousness.

Organic disorder: A mental or emotional impairment that is believed to be physiological in origin.

Orientation: The ability to correctly relate the self to time, place, and person.

Paranoid delusion: The false belief that one is being persecuted.

From Stuart, G. W., & Sundeen, S. J. Principles and practices of psychiatric nursing (2nd ed.). St. Louis, Mo.: Mosby, 1983, with permission.

Passive–aggressive: Term describing indirect expression, verbal or nonverbal, of angry feelings.

Perception: Sensory interpretation of a stimulus.

Psychosomatic reactions: Disorders in which the emotional tension is not discharged outwardly but is instead unconsciously channeled through the visceral organs.

Self-concept: All the notions, beliefs, and convictions that constitute an individual's knowledge of himself and influence his relationships with others.

Self-destructive behavior: Any behavior, direct or indirect, that if uninterrupted, will ultimately lead to the death of the individual.

Self-esteem: The individual's personal judgment of his own worth obtained by analyzing how well his behavior conforms to his self-ideal.

Stressors: Stimuli that the individual perceives as challenging, threatening, or harmful. They require the use of excess energy and produce a state of tension and stress within the individual.

Bibliography

Benzer, H., Mutz N., & Pauser, G. Psychosocial sequelae of intensive care. *International Anesthesiology Clinics*, 1983, *21*, 169–180.

Carlson, C. E., & Blackwall, B. *Behavioral concepts and nursing interventions*. Philadelphia: Lippincott, 1978.

Collins, M. *Communication in health care*. St. Louis, Mo.: Mosby, 1983.

Daley, L. The perceived immediate needs of families with relatives in the intensive care setting. *Heart and Lung*, 1983, *12*(3), 258–261.

Fisher, M. E., & Moxham, P. A. ICU syndrome. *Critical Care Nurse*, 1984, *4*(3), 39–45.

Geltman, R. L., & Paige, R. L. Symptom management in hospice care. *American Journal of Nursing*, 1983, *83*, 78–83.

Hodovanic, B. H., Reardon, D., Reese, W., & Hedges, B. Family crisis intervention program in the medical intensive care unit. *Heart and Lung*, 1984, *13*(3), 243–249.

Hoff, L. A., & Resing, M. Was this suicide preventable? *American Journal of Nursing*, 1982, *82*, 1106–1111.

Joyce, C. A time for grieving. *Psychology Today*, 1984, *18*, 42–43, 46.

Kinney, M. R., Dear, C. B., Packa, D. R., & Voorman, D. *AACN's clinical reference for critical-care nursing*. New York: McGraw-Hill, 1981.

Knowles, R. D. Building rapport through neuro-linguistic programming. *American Journal of Nursing*, 1983, *83*, 1011–1014.

Kübler-Ross, E. *On death and dying*. New York: Macmillan, 1969.

MacKinnon-Kesler, S. Maximizing your ICU patient's sensory and perceptual environment. *The Canadian Nurse*, 1983, *79*(5), 41–45.

Ostchega, Y., & Jacob, J. G. Providing safe conduct, helping your patient cope with cancer. 1984, *Nursing 84*, *14*, 42–47.

Saxton, D. F., & Haring, P. W. *Care of patients with emotional problems*. St. Louis, Mo.: Mosby, 1979.

Shragg, T. A., & Albertson, T. E. Moral, ethical, and legal dilemmas in the intensive care unit. *Critical Care Medicine*, 1984, *12*(1), 62–68.

Stillwell, S. B. Importance of visiting needs as perceived by family members of patients in the intensive care unit. *Heart and Lung*, 1984, *13*(3), 238–242.

Stuart, G. W., & Sundeen, S. J. *Principles and practices of psychiatric nursing*. St. Louis, Mo.: Mosby, 1983.

Attitudes and Requirements of Various Religious Groups

ADVENTIST (Seventh Day Adventist, Church of God, Advent Christian Church)

Birth. Opposed to infant baptism. Adults baptized by immersion.

Death. The dead are asleep until the return of Jesus Christ, at which time final rewards and punishments will be given.

Health Crisis. They believe in man's choice and God's sovereignty. Taking of communion or undergoing baptism may be desired. Some believe in divine healing and practice anointing with oil and the use of prayer.

Diet. No alcohol, coffee, or tea. Taking any narcotic or stimulant is prohibited because the body is the temple of the Holy Spirit and should be protected. Many groups prohibit the eating of meat.

Organ Transplants. The individual and the family have the right to receive or to donate those organs that will restore any of the senses or will prolong the life profitably.

Religious Sacraments. The serving of the bread and wine, called the "Lord's Supper" or "Communion," is taken to any patient upon request.

AMERICAN INDIAN

The approximately 300 different Indian tribal groups and geographically classified bands of Indians, each with its own culture, make it impossible to generalize about specific responses to specific situations. Religion, magic, folklore, disease treatment, and herbal medicine differ from tribe to tribe. Medicine men, shamans, and conjurers in various tribes perform, by use of many different symbolic actions, against illnesses, social taboos, powers of nature, and "enemy-oriented" diseases. Protection against disease is sought by the help of superhuman powers. These practices have two distinct forms according to the fundamental concept of the disease. Disease is conceptualized as taking two principal forms: one is the presence of a material object in the patient's body; the other is an effect of the absence of the soul from the body. Today, many Indians follow modern Christian religions, whereas some continue with traditional Indian beliefs.

The information in this appendix was compiled by Reverend J. W. (Bill) Turner, Chaplain, The Methodist Hospital, Houston, Texas.

ARMENIAN

Birth. Traditionally, baptism involves immersion 8 days after birth. Confirmation is immediately after baptism. On the fortieth day after birth, the parents bring the child to church.

Death. Last rites are practiced by the administration of Holy Communion.

Health Crisis. They advocate taking communion and the laying on of hands.

Diet. Fasting during Lent and for 6 hours before communion.

Beliefs. No conflict between modern medicine and religion.

BAHA'I

Birth. No baptism.

Death. No last rites.

Health Crisis. They advise prayer and, if medically permissible, fasting.

Diet. Alcohol and drugs permitted only on doctor's prescription.

Beliefs. No conflict between modern medicine and religion. The sick are specifically instructed in Baha'i scriptures to seek the advice of competent doctors. Spiritual health is felt to be conducive to physical health: Prayer adjunctive to healing by physical and chemical means is considered legitimate or even indispensable.

BAPTIST

Birth. Opposed to infant baptism. Only believers should be baptized, and it must be done by immersion.

Death. Clergy seeks to minister by counsel and prayer with patient and family.

Health Crisis. Some Baptists believe and practice healing by the laying on of hands.

Diet. Some groups condemn coffee and tea. Most condemn alcohol.

Organ Transplants. Organ transplants are generally approved when they do not seriously endanger the donor and when they offer real medical hope for the recipient. A transplant as an end in itself is not approved. It must offer the possibility of physical improvement and the extension of human life.

Religious Sacraments. Baptists do not attribute any physically healing powers to baptism or communion. These rites are understood by Baptists as "ordinances" rather than "sacraments" because the latter term suggests that the elements of these rites are "means of grace," and that they somehow transfer "power" from God to the recipient. Sacramentalism, therefore, is all too easily misunderstood as a potentially physically efficacious process, an idea that Baptists would not accept. The ordinances are to commemorate the baptism, death, and resurrection of Christ and as such are visible symbols of inner, spiritual transformation, a process that may occur independently of one's physical condition.

BLACK MUSLIM

Birth. No baptism.

Death. Carefully prescribed procedure for washing and shrouding the dead and performing funeral rites.

Health Crisis. Faith healing is not acceptable.

Diet. Prohibit alcoholic beverages, pork, and some foods traditional among American blacks, including cornbread and collard greens.

Beliefs. General adherence to Muslim tenets is overlaid in many instances by antagonism to Caucasians, especially Christians and Jews. They do not indulge in activities (such as sleeping) more than is necessary to health and always maintain personal habits of cleanliness.

BUDDHIST CHURCHES OF AMERICA

Birth. Rites, such as infant presentation, affirmation, confirmation, or ordination, are performed after the child has become mature enough.

Death. Last rite chanting is often practiced at bedside soon after death. Contact the deceased's Buddhist priest or have the family make the contact.

Health Crisis. A Buddhist priest should be notified for counseling. It should, however, be at the patient's or his or her family's request.

Diet. No restrictions on diet for most members, although some sects are strictly vegetarian. Most members practice moderation: they discourage the use of alcohol, tobacco, and drugs.

Beliefs. They are in harmony with modern science. There is no divine punishment; every occurrence depends on the law of causality, so illness is a trial to aid the development of the soul. This is a religion of supreme optimism as it teaches a way to overcome fears, anxieties, and apprehension. Special holy days are January 1 and

16, February 15, March 21, April 8, May 21, July 15, September 1 and 23, and December 8 and 31. Patients should be questioned about how they feel about medical and surgical treatment on these days.

CHURCH OF CHRIST

Birth. No baptism until a minimum of 8 years, then baptism by immersion.

Death. No last rites.

Health Crisis. Communion offered only to members of this church. Belief in the anointing with oil and the laying on of hands by the ministry for healing of sick. Ministers (elders) will visit any who desire.

Diet. No requirements or restrictions; most members refrain from using alcoholic beverages.

Organ Transplants. Organ transplants should not be a religious problem.

Religious Sacraments. Religious sacraments per se are not practiced by the church. Baptism and communion, however, are standard and encouraged. Members hospitalized need the assurance of God and the fellowship of fellow saints.

CHURCH OF CHRIST, SCIENTIST (Christian Scientist)

Birth. No baptism.

Death. No last rites; no autopsy, except in cases of sudden death. Individual decision regarding burial or cremation.

Health Crisis. They deny the existence of health crises; sickness and sin are errors of the human mind and can be eliminated by altering thoughts, not by drugs or medicines. They do not allow hypnotism or any form of psychotherapy that alters the "Divine Mind." A Christian Science practitioner can be called to administer spiritual support. The *Christian Science Journal* contains a directory of Christian Science nurses available to help bandage wounds, set bones, and perform other similar tasks.

Diet. Alcohol, coffee, and tobacco are seen as drugs, so are not used.

Beliefs. Disease is a human mental concept that can be dispelled by "spiritual truth." Many Christian Scientists adhere to this belief to the extent that they refuse all medical treatment, but each individual may decide whether he or she wishes to rely completely on Christian Science. Many adherents desire the services of a practitioner or reader. The church operates several nursing homes that rely solely on such "spiritual" means of health maintenance. They do not use drugs or accept blood transfusions, accept vaccines only when required by law, and do not seek biopsies or physical examinations.

CHURCH OF GOD

Birth. No baptism at birth; babies may be dedicated to the Lord upon request of the parents.

Death. No last rites; homegoing service for the deceased. Do not believe in cremation.

Health Crisis. Adherents believe in divine healing through prayer, though more liberal members do not prohibit medical therapy at the same time.

Diet. No requirements or restrictions; individual fasting may be practiced. Members refrain from all alcoholic beverages and tobacco.

Beliefs. "Speaking in tongues" is a mystical experience.

CHURCH OF JESUS CHRIST OF LATTER DAY SAINTS (Mormon)

Birth. Baptism by immersion at 8 years or older.

Death. They believe it proper to bury in the ground; cremation is discouraged. Baptism of the dead is held essential, although a living person may serve as proxy. Preaching the Gospel to the dead is also practiced.

Health Crisis. Devout adherents believe in divine healing through the laying on of hands, although many do not prohibit medical therapy. The church maintains an extensive and well-funded welfare system, including financial support for the sick.

Diet. They prohibit alcoholic beverages, tobacco, hot drinks (tea, coffee), or any other substance that may be injurious to the body. Sparing use of meats but no outright prohibition.

Organ Transplants. The question of whether one should will his or her bodily organs to be used as transplants or for research after death must be answered from deep within the conscience of the individual involved. Those who seek counsel from the Church on this subject are encouraged to review the advantages and disadvantages of doing so, to implore the Lord for inspiration and guidance, and then to take the course of action that would give them a feeling of peace and comfort.

Religious Sacraments. Within the beliefs of the Church, the term "sacrament" refers only to the celebration of the Lord's Supper wherein bread and water are blessed and partaken of in symbolic remembrance of the flesh and blood of the Savior and by the way of recovenant by the partaker to adhere to the Savior's teachings. The Church ordinance specifically related to the sick or dying is the laying on of hands by the elders for the healing of the sick.

EASTERN ORTHODOX CHURCHES (Turkey, Egypt, Syria, Rumania, Bulgaria, Cyprus, Albania, Poland, and Czechoslovakia)

Birth. Generally, these denominations believe in infant baptism by immersion, followed immediately by confirmation.

Death. Last rites obligatory if death is impending; cremation discouraged.

Health Crisis. Anointing of the sick is a form of healing by prayer.

Diet. Restrictions depend on particular sect.

Beliefs. No conflict with medical science.

EPISCOPALIAN

Birth. Infant baptism is mandatory and especially urgent if prognosis is poor, although aborted fetuses and stillborns are not baptized.

Death. Last rites (Rite for the Anointing of the Sick) are not mandatory for all members.

Health Crisis. Some believe in spiritual healing.

Diet. Some abstain from meat on Fridays, and some fast before receiving Holy Communion, which may be daily.

Organ Transplants. The Episcopal Church finds nothing offensive in organ transplants, provided the moral integrity of the donor is not violated.

Religious Sacraments. Holy unction, long regarded by Roman Catholics as a sacrament reserved for the dying, is commonly used in the Episcopal Church for the sick. This is a brief and simple ceremony that involves prayer and the laying on of hands or the anointing with oil of the patient by the priest. On Sundays, or before a serious operation, a patient is likely to request Holy Communion. This involves the patient in consuming a very small piece of bread and a sip of pure grape wine. In cases where there are strong medical reasons for the patient's not consuming such, the priest and patient should be so informed and an alternative form of "spiritual communion" can be substituted. When the death of a patient is imminent, the church has a very ancient rite for this occasion. If the family and their pastor are gathered, it is usually considered highly desirable to have the Litany at the Time of Death read. The sacraments are never regarded as magic. They are the Church's way of participating with the sick person in his or her sickness, of blessing and confirming the healing work of the physician and hospital personnel, and of integrating all these experiences for the patient and offering them up to Almighty God.

FRIENDS (Quakers)

Birth. Do not baptize; at birth, an infant's name is recorded in official books.

Death. They do not believe in life after this life.

Health Crisis. They have no restrictions and allow individual members to make decisions.

Diet. Up to the individual; most practice moderation, avoiding alcohol and drugs.

Beliefs. They are pacifists and conscientious objectors in wartime. They believe in plain speech and dress and refusal of tithes and oaths. God is in every person and can be approached directly.

GRACE BRETHREN

Birth. Do not practice infant baptism; baptism by immersion of those old enough to profess their faith.

Death. No last rites; individual decision regarding burial or cremation.

Health Crisis. Anointment with oil is practiced for physical healing and spiritual uplift.

Diet. No dietary restrictions; most abstain from alcohol, tobacco, and illicit drugs.

Beliefs. No conflict with modern science. Generally request noncombatant military service.

GREEK ORTHODOX

Birth. Baptism is recognized. Prefer to baptize the child at least 40 days after birth. If not possible to baptize by sprinkling or immersion, the church allows the child to be baptized "in the air" by moving the child in the sign of the cross as appropriate words are said.

Death. Last rites are the administration of the Sacrament of Holy Communion.

Health Crisis. In most cases each health crisis must be handled by an ordained priest, though a deacon of the church may also serve in some cases. Usually a priest administers Holy Communion in the hospital room in a procedure that takes only a few minutes. Some patients may also want the Sacrament of Holy Unction, which the priest can conduct in the hospital room in a brief time in an abbreviated service.

Diet. The church usually prescribes a fast period, which means avoidance of meat and, in many cases, dairy products. The usual fasting days are Wednesday, Friday, and during Lent. However, if these rules conflict with medical treatments, they need not be enforced. Some Orthodox patients will insist upon fasting even when in the hospital. If decision and desire to fast in the hospital do not interfere with medical procedures, there would be no reason for this to be refused. However, if this would adversely influence the medical condition of the patient, a priest should be called to convince the patient to forego fasting until his health is restored.

Organ Transplants. Organ transplants, such as skin grafting and blood transfusions from one human to another, always have been acceptable. This is extended to include kidney transplants, heart transplants, and so on. The life of the donor, however, is of equal importance.

Religious Sacraments. Sacraments in Orthodox Theology are essential to man's communion with God, and all patients should be afforded the opportunity of sacramental participation during treatment and before any surgical procedures that may involve a temporary loss of faculties.

HINDU

Death. Certain prescribed rites are followed after death: The priest may tie a thread around the neck or wrist to signify blessing; the thread should not be removed. Immediately after death, the priest will pour water into the mouth of the corpse; the family will wash the body. They are particular about who touches their dead, and the bodies are cremated.

Health Crisis. Some conditions, such as loss of a limb, represent "sins" committed in a previous life.

Diet. There are many dietary restrictions that conform to individual sect doctrine. The patient should be questioned when admitted.

Beliefs. Accept most modern medical practices: do not believe in artificial insemination because sterility reflects divine will.

ISLAMIC (Muslim, Moslem)

Birth. If abortion occurs before 130 days, the fetus is treated as any other discarded tissue; after 130 days, an aborted fetus must be treated as a fully developed human being.

Death. The patient must confess sins and beg forgiveness before death, and the family should be present. The family washes and prepares the body, then turns it to face Mecca. Only relatives or friends may touch the body, and unless required by law, there should be no portmortem; no body part should be removed.

Health Crisis. In pathological conditions, faith healing is not acceptable unless the psychological condition of the patient is deteriorating. Then it is done for the patient's morale.

Diet. All pork products are proscribed. In the ninth month of the Muhammadan year (Ramadan), daylight fasting is practiced.

Beliefs. Older and more conservative Muslims often have a fatalistic view that can militate against ready compliance with therapy.

JEHOVAH'S WITNESSES

Birth. No infant baptism.

Death. No last rites.

Health Crisis. Adherents are generally absolutely opposed to blood transfusion, although individuals can sometimes be persuaded in emergencies. When parents refuse consent for a child's transfusion, a court order may be sought to appoint some key hospital official temporary guardian of the child. The official may then legally consent to the transfusion.

Diet. They do not eat anything to which blood has been added; can eat animal flesh that has been drained.

Organ Transplants. No definite statement.

Religious Sacraments. The sacraments of baptism and communion are not recognized as such. Jesus gave only two things of symbolic nature to his followers, baptism and the Lord's evening meal.

JUDAISM

Birth. Ritual circumcision is mandatory among Orthodox and Conservative adherents on the eighth day after birth. Reform Jews favor ritual circumcision, but not as a religious imperative. A fetus is to be buried, not discarded.

Death. Human remains are ritually washed following death by members of the Ritual Burial Society, and the burial should take place as soon as possible. Cremation is not in keeping with Jewish law. All Orthodox Jews and some Conservatives are opposed to autopsy.

Health Crisis. They demand that an ill person seek medical care. Donation or transplantation of organs requires rabbinical consultation.

Diet. Orthodox and Conservative Jews observe strict kosher dietary laws, which mainly prohibit pork, shellfish, and the eating of meat and milk products at the same meal. There are complex proscriptions and prescriptions regarding food preparation. Reform Jews do not usually observe kosher dietary laws.

Organ Transplants. The sanctity of the human body covers each of its members and organs. So where any part of the body is separated from the corpus it, too, requires burial. However, where an organ is to be transplanted to save the life of a patient or improve his or her health, it is permitted.

Religious Sacraments. Wherever and whenever possible, the family and rabbi should be present when a patient seems ready to expire. There is a special formula known as "Vidui" (confession) that is recited at that time.

LUTHERAN

Birth. Baptize only living babies at 6 to 8 weeks after birth by pouring or sprinkling water or by immersion.

Death. Last rites are optional.

Health Crisis. If the prognosis is poor, the patient may request anointment and blessing.

Diet. No requirements or restrictions.

Organ Transplants. The ability to transplant organs from a deceased to a living person is considered a genuine medical advance.

Religious Sacraments. The Lutheran Church recognizes two: Baptism and the Lord's Supper. Congregations stand ready and willing to administer the sacraments privately for the ill and dying in the sick room. Pastors will respond to the request of the patient, his or her family, or his or her physician.

MENNONITE

Birth. Baptism during early and middle teens.

Death. No formal prescribed action. Personal assistance and prayer as appropriate while the patient is still conscious.

Health Crisis. No taking of communion or laying on of hands.

Diet. No official restrictions; many congregations require abstention from alcohol.

Beliefs. Not a sacramental church. There is a deep concern for the individual's dignity and self-determination which would conflict with shock therapy or medicine or treatment affecting the individual's personality and will.

METHODIST, UNITED

Birth. Baptism for children or adults.

Death. Believe in divine judgment after death. Good will be rewarded and evil punished.

Health Crisis. Communion may be requested prior to surgery or similar crisis.

Diet. No requirements or restrictions.

Organ Transplants. The Church encourages "men of ethical concern in various relevant fields together to engage in the study and direction of these developments," recognizing that they offer great potentialities for enhancing health while at the same time raising serious issues for traditional views of human nature and values.

Religious Sacraments. Two sacraments are recognized, Baptism and Holy Communion. Administration of these, especially of Holy Communion to the sick and other believers by an ordained clergyman, upon request and according to clergy and medical judgment, is regularly practiced. It is a means of conveying the love of God as expressed in the community. The sacraments partly aim, along with other resources, such as scriptures, prayer, and the pastoral relationship, to assist the patient in meeting his crisis with confidence in God as the power of new life, whether through physical recovery, renewal of faith and attitude, or life beyond death.

MORAVIAN

Birth. Infant baptism is usual, though they do not deny choice of adult baptism.

Death. No last rites. When illness is diagnosed as terminal, they do not believe that life should be extended at all costs; patient should be kept comfortable.

Health Crisis. Communion is received in both forms, public and private. Laying on of hands for consecration of ordained persons, both male and female. No restrictions on blood transfusions or organ transplants.

Diet. No requirements or restrictions.

Beliefs. Disease is not a form of divine punishment, although they feel that breaking God's laws of "good stewardship" can often lead to physical problems.

NAZARENE

Birth. Baptism is parent's option, not considered a saving sacrament. No need to baptize a baby or an adult who is dying.

Death. No last rites. Cremation is permitted; stillborns are buried.

Health Crisis. Local pastor will administer communion and laying on of hands, which are means of grace. Adherents believe in divine healing, but not exclusive of medical treatment.

Diet. Use of alcohol and tobacco prohibited.

Beliefs. No conflicts with modern science.

PENTECOSTAL (Assembly of God, Foursquare Church)

Birth. Water baptism by immersion after age of accountability.

Death. No last rites.

Health Crisis. No inhibitions against blood transfusions or medical care. Believe in possibility of divine healing through prayer. Anointing with oil may be practiced with laying on of hands.

Diet. Abstain from alcohol, tobacco, and eating strangled animals or anything to which blood has been added. Individuals may refuse pork products.

Beliefs. Some insist illness is divine punishment, but most consider illness an intrusion of Satan. Deliverance from sin and sickness are provided for in atonement. Pray for divine intervention in health matters and seek to reach God in prayer for themselves and others when ill.

ORTHODOX PRESBYTERIAN

Birth. Sprinkling most common in infant baptism.

Death. Last rites not a sacrament procedure; they read Scripture and pray.

Health Crisis. Communion administered when appropriate and convenient. Blood transfusion acceptable when advisable. No formal laying-on-of-hands ceremony. Prayer appropriate; local pastor or elder should be called.

Diet. No requirements or restrictions.

Beliefs. True science can be used for relief of suffering and recognized as a gift of the Creator. Full forgiveness through genuine repentance for any illness connected with a sin. Heaven and hell thought of in material terms.

ROMAN CATHOLIC

Birth. Infant baptism is mandatory, especially urgent if prognosis is poor. Baptism is demanded if an aborted fetus may not be clinically dead.

Death. The Rite for the Anointing of the Sick is recommended. If the prognosis is poor, the patient or his or her family may request it.

Health Crisis. The patient or his or her family may desire that a major amputated limb be buried in consecrated ground. There is no blanket mandate for this, but it may be required within a given diocese.

Diet. Most hospital patients are exempt from fasting or abstaining from meat on Ash Wednesday and Good Friday. Some older Catholics may still adhere to the former rule of abstaining from meat on Fridays.

Organ Transplants. The transplantation of organs from living donors is normally permissible when the anticipated benefit to the recipient is proportionate to the harm done to the donor, provided that the loss of such organ(s) does not deprive the donor of life itself nor of the functional integrity of his or her body. Organs necessary to sustain life may not be removed until death has taken place, according to commonly accepted scientific criteria. In accordance with current medical practice, to prevent any conflict of interest, the dying patient's doctor or doctors should ordinarily be distinct from the transplant team.

Religious Sacraments. Baptism: Except in cases of emergency (danger of death), all requests for baptism made by adults for themselves or for infants should be referred to the chaplain of the health facility. If a priest is not available, anyone having the use of reason and the proper intention can baptize. The ordinary method is to pour water on the head of the person to be baptized in such a way that it will flow on the skin, and while pouring the water, audibly to pronounce these words: "I baptize you in the name of the Father and of the Son and of the Holy Spirit." The same person who pours the water must pronounce the words. When the emergency baptism has been performed, the priest should be notified. The Catholic Church believes that the sick should have the widest possible liberty to receive the sacrament of the Eucharist (Holy Communion) often and the sacrament of Reconciliation (confession or penance) as the sick person may need or desire. In wards and semiprivate rooms, every effort should be made to provide sufficient privacy for confession. Catholics in danger of death are expected to receive Holy Communion, which in this case is called "Viaticum," while still in full possession of their faculties. Special care should be shown that those who are seriously or dangerously ill, due to sickness or old age, receive the Sacrament of the Sick (Anointing). A prudent or probable judgment about the seriousness of the illness is sufficient. A sick person should be anointed before surgery if in danger, and old people may be anointed if they are in a weak condition, even though no dangerous illness is present. The sacrament may be repeated if the sick person recovers after anointing or if the danger becomes more serious during the same illness. Normally, this sacrament is celebrated when the patient is fully conscious. It may also be conferred upon the sick or injured who have lost consciousness or the use of reason, if as Christian believers they would have asked for it were they in control of their faculties. In Catholic hospitals and institutions, those in charge will, with the consent of patients, promptly advise ministers of other faiths about the presence of patients of that faith and afford these ministers ample facility for visiting the sick and for giving them spiritual and sacramental ministrations.

RUSSIAN ORTHODOX

Birth. Baptism by priest only. Immersion three times and only on certain days.

Death. They do not believe in autopsies, embalming, or cremation. Traditionally, after death, arms are crossed, fingers set in a cross. Clothing at death must be of natural fiber so the body will change to ashes sooner.

Health Crisis. Cross necklace is important and should be replaced immediately when patient returns from surgery.

Diet. On Wednesdays, Fridays, and during Lent, they do not eat meat or dairy products.

Beliefs. Important not to shave male patients except in preparation for surgery.

UNITARIAN, UNIVERSALIST

Birth. Some practice infant baptism; most consider it unnecessary.

Death. Attitudes toward immortality vary widely. Cremation preferred to burial.

Health Crisis. No official sacraments. Reason and practicality are most important.

Diet. No requirements or restrictions.

Beliefs. They emphasize use of reason and knowledge and believe each person has the right to approach values individually: "God helps those who help themselves." At times, some may prefer not to have clergy visit them in hospital, since they assume responsibility themselves.